OT
Student Primer

A Guide to College Success

OT
Student Primer

A Guide to College Success

Edited by

Karen Sladyk, MS, OTR/L
Bay Path College
Longmeadow, Massachusetts

SLACK Incorporated, 6900 Grove Road, Thorofare, NJ 08086-9447

Publisher: John H. Bond
Editorial Director: Amy E. Drummond
Associate Editor: Jennifer J. Cahill
Creative Director: Linda Baker

Printed in the United States of America

Published by: SLACK Incorporated
              6900 Grove Road
              Thorofare, NJ 08086-9447 USA
              Telephone: 609-848-1000
              Fax: 609-853-5991

OT student primer: a guide to college success/edited by Karen Sladyk.
        p. cm.
    Includes bibliographic references and index.
    ISBN 1-55642-318-7
    1. Occupational therapy—Study and teaching. I. Sladyk, Karen.
    [DNLM: 1. Occupational Therapy. WB 555 087 1997]
RM735.42.08 1997
615.8'515—dc21
DNLM/DLC
for Library of Congress   97-7852

DEDICATION

This book is dedicated to our past, present, and future students. May you take the science, art, and ethics your teachers give you and touch the mind, heart, and soul of those you treat.

CONTENTS

ACKNOWLEDGMENTS

Writing a book is a challenge in itself. I am thankful to my peers for their outstanding contributions. You will find some of the chapters written by OTRs and some chapters written by other professionals. The people invited to write chapters for this primer are some of the best educators of today. Their names might not be famous but they teach with a love in their heart and a fire in their soul. I am proud to know each of them.

As is true of most book writing, there are many people to thank. A very special thank you to Amy Drummond, Debra Christy, and Jennifer Cahill at SLACK Incorporated for always stopping what they were doing to answer my questions and reassure me.

Five senior OT students were very helpful with their feedback on the manuscript: thank you to Christine Carbine, Kelly Carew, Deanna Ceniglio, Victoria Frechette, and Kari Ann Gilland. I have worked with these students on fieldwork and I know they will be fine OTRs.

We acknowledge the help of Maria Stephens, whose résumé and cover letter were adapted as examples for our chapter.

All the writers could not have been successful without the support of their families and friends, especially Jeanine English and Louise Matson. These two moms of OT professors volunteered to proofread their daughters' chapters.

CONTRIBUTING AUTHORS

Karen Sladyk, MS, OTR/L, has a bachelor's degree in occupational therapy from Eastern Michigan University and a master's degree in community health from Southern Connecticut State University. She is currently a doctoral candidate in adult and vocational education at the University of Connecticut. Karen recently accepted a new position as program director at Bay Path College in Longmeadow, Massachusetts. As program director, she has developed a student-centered curriculum. As an occupational therapy teacher, Karen's interests include clinical reasoning and fieldwork. *OT Student Primer: A Guide to College Success* is Karen's second book written for students. *OTR Exam Review Manual* was written with peers to guide students through the NBCOT exam. Karen's focus is on meeting students' needs through her informative books. She resides in Vernon, Connecticut, in a very old house with two cats. When she is not busy with academic challenges, she enjoys quilt making.

Mary Alicia Barnes, OTR/L, is the Level I fieldwork coordinator at Tufts University—Boston School of Occupational Therapy. Her clinical and academic interests include fieldwork education, occupational therapy with children and adolescents with mental illness, and school-based practice. She has published in the areas of community-based practice, occupational therapy in child psychiatry, vocational programming with adolescents with emotional disturbances, and fieldwork education. She enjoys walking, bike riding, camping with her husband, and following fashion trends.

Debra Francoeur Bowler, MS, OTR/L, received a bachelor's degree in psychology from the University of Hartford in 1981 and a master's degree in occupational therapy from New York University in 1985. She specialized in neurorehabilitation with an emphasis on program development for clients with brain injuries. Debra began a new life in academia while raising her family. She and her husband, Leo, recently built a home in Northford, Connecticut, where they live with their two children, Zachary and Chelsea. When not at work, you will find her painting, planting, and playing outdoors.

Marilyn B. Cole, MS, OTR/L, has a bachelor's degree in English from the University of Connecticut and a master's degree in clinical psychology from the University of Bridgeport. Marli has a certificate in occupational therapy from the University of Pennsylvania and has practiced mental health occupational therapy for more than 24 years. She is currently a tenured associate professor of occupational therapy and an occupational therapy consultant. Her clinical interests include group process, sensory integration, geriatrics, and research. Marli has two grown children, Charlot and Bradley. She and her husband, Marty, enjoy downhill skiing and scuba diving.

Rosellen S. East, CPRW, has a bachelor's degree in Spanish from Southern Connecticut State University and is certified as a professional résumé writer by the Professional Association of Résumé Writers. She began her career with the Connecticut Department of Labor in 1971 and currently is an internal consultant, providing training and performance management services. Rosellen volunteers with Connecticut Special Olympics and was involved in the World Games in 1995. She is beginning to explore the world through travel with upcoming trips to Bermuda and Alaska.

Mary E. Evenson, MPH, OTR/L, is the academic fieldwork coordinator at Tufts University—Boston School of Occupational Therapy and teaches in the areas of fieldwork education and clinical reasoning. Her professional interests include the application of clinical reasoning in the fieldwork process, particularly in the supervisor-student relationship. Clinically, her experience is in physical disabilities and chronic disease management. Mary received her bachelor's degree at the University of Puget Sound and her master's degree in public health from the University of California at Los Angeles. She enjoys traveling, photography, collecting arts and crafts, and outdoor fitness activities, such as biking, hiking, and cross-country skiing.

Tara J. Glennon, MS, OTR/L, is the director of Pediatric Occupational Therapy Services, Inc. in Fairfield, Connecticut, the director of The Connecticut Center for Pediatric Therapy, LLC in Wallingford, Connecticut, and an assistant professor of occupational therapy. Tara is hooked on audiotapes of suspense novels, and enjoys home decorating and gardening. She never misses a morning walk with her roommate, Johanna, and their two dogs, Abbey and Shelby (a golden retriever and Jack Russell terrier).

Kimberly D. Hartmann, MHS, OTR/L, FAOTA, is chair of occupational therapy at Quinnipiac College. She is currently a doctoral candidate at the University of Connecticut studying learning disabilities. Kim believes that teaching is a primary way to change the future and practices that belief through her teaching at the college level, consulting to public schools on assistive technology, and remaining active in local school endeavors. She lives in the country near the sea in Guilford, Connecticut, with her husband, Shawn, and daughters, Calla, Jennifer, and Katie, and their four cats. As a family, they live for adventures at Disney World, family parties, tennis, art shows, cello concerts, the theater, and equestrian events. In her "free time," Kim collects art, Disney memorabilia, and enjoys creating topiaries and crafts with her children.

Sandra L. Hastings, PhD, has a bachelor's degree in sociology from Arizona State University, and a master's degree and doctorate in adult and vocational education from the University of Connecticut. While in her current position as the director of staff development at the Connecticut Department of Labor, Sandra designed the Strategic Quality Training model which won the United States Department of Labor's 1995 National Capacity Building Award. Sandra and her husband, Marty, share the joys and challenges associated with the parenting of their three terrific teenage sons, Jeremy, Jonathan, and Brian.

Marijke Kehrhahn, PhD, has a bachelor's degree in fine arts and a master's degree in special education. She completed her doctorate in adult and vocational education at the University of Connecticut in 1995. Marijke has devoted 12 years of her working life to developing systems that support people with disabilities to live full lives in their community through collaboration with people with disabilities, professionals, paraprofessionals, policy makers, and private and public agencies. For the last 3 years, Marijke has worked with college students to develop effective ways to manage time, tasks, and goals in pursuit of advanced degrees. Marijke lives in Middletown, Connecticut, with her husband, Ray, and their 6-year-old daughter, Jasmine.

Signian McGeary, MS, OTR/L, has a master's degree in adult education from Southern Connecticut State University. Her current clinical interests include outcome studies using the A-One for ADL evaluations. She studies Mandarin Chinese to enhance her work in China with the World Health Organization. She is finalizing plans to take occupational therapy students to China in the summer of 1997. Signian and her husband, Ken, both college faculty, share an interest in promoting international field studies for students.

Catherine Meriano, MHS, OTR/L, has a bachelor's degree in occupational therapy and a master's degree in education from Quinnipiac College. She teaches occupational therapy full-time and is currently vice president of the Connecticut Occupational Therapy Association. In addition, she works part-time treating residents in a sub-acute rehabilitation setting. When not working, Catherine enjoys spending time with her husband, John, and her two young children, Kathleen and Jay. Catherine lives by the shore in Branford, Connecticut, and thoroughly enjoys the beach with her children.

Beth O'Sullivan, OTR/L, is the academic fieldwork coordinator for Quinnipiac College. She is currently completing her thesis for a master's degree in public health at the University of Connecticut. Besides being responsible for the 200 students she places on fieldwork, she is currently expecting her first "real" child. She and her husband, Tim, enjoy watching drag racing and in their free time can be found restoring old cars.

Andrea Passannante, OTR/L, has a bachelor's degree in occupational therapy from Quinnipiac

College. She is presently working in the Brain Injury and Coma Recovery Unit at Southside Hospital on Long Island, New York. In addition, she carries a home care caseload. Being a fairly new therapist, she has been focusing on continuing her education on the treatment of brain injury, specifically cognitive and visual impairments. At home, she and her husband try to spend as much time together rollerblading, cooking for friends, and relaxing with family.

Henriette Pranger, MA, has a bachelor's degree in philosophy from Trinity College and her master's degree in adult and vocational education from the University of Connecticut. She is currently a doctoral candidate studying teaching strategies designed to improve problem solving in adults. Her teaching interests lie in portfolio assessment and college survival skills. She enjoys entertaining, gardening, and is preparing for the arrival of her first child prodigy soon.

Ellen Berger Rainville, MS, OTR/L, FAOTA, is an assistant professor for the occupational therapy program at Springfield College in Springfield, Massachusetts. She is responsible for teaching research, pediatrics, and preclinical courses. Ellen has a master's degree in management from Lesley College and is currently a doctoral student in therapeutic studies at Boston University. Ellen has had extensive experience in management, supervision, team development, and consultation. She lives in Conway, Massachusetts, with her husband, Mike, and their three children, Nicole, David, and Kellie. As a family, they enjoy country fairs and peaceful walks.

S. Maggie Reitz, MS, OTR/L, has both her bachelor's and master's degrees in occupational therapy from Towson State University in Maryland. After 10 years of clinical practice, she returned to Towson State to teach. She is currently completing her dissertation on coronary heart disease for a doctorate in health education. She resides with her husband, Fred, and their daughter, Jessica. The family was recently enlarged by the addition of an unusual cat by the name of Splotch.

Lori G. Sladyk, MS, CSE, has a bachelor's degree in social work from Southern Connecticut State University, a teaching certificate in special education, and a master's degree in language arts from Central Connecticut State University. She is currently pursuing an advanced graduate degree in learning disabilities at the University of Connecticut. When not busy with work and school, she is active in community activities with her three sons, Brent, Seth, and Blake. Lori also holds a teaching position, lives in an old house in Vernon, Connecticut, and enjoys quilt making, but is much different from her sister, Karen, in that she only has one cat.

Roseanna Tufano, MFT, OTR/L, has her master's degree in marriage and family therapy from Southern Connecticut State University. She has worked in a variety of mental health settings since 1980 as a staff OTR and consultant. Her expertise in mental health has led to teaching in both occupational therapy and physical therapy programs. Her teaching interests include psychopathology, group dynamics, and clinical media. In addition, Roseanna coordinates Level I fieldwork. She resides with her husband, Lou, and their two children, Carissa and Brett. The family recently welcomed a new addition to their home, a black and white puppy named Jake.

Linda Waak, RPT, has a bachelor's degree in physical therapy from The University of Michigan at Flint. She is currently working to complete a master's degree in orthopedic physical therapy. Linda is employed by Sundance Rehabilitation Corporation as a regional physical therapy clinical director where she oversees physical therapy operations in a variety of sub-acute and long-term facilities in southern Connecticut. She enjoys skiing, sports, and playing the flute.

PREFACE

Looking at the selection of outstanding textbooks available in OT makes me proud of my profession and my colleagues. OT has provided me with the best career I could have hoped for. It is from those outstanding textbooks that I learned my art.

There were many times when learning OT was difficult for me. Even now, I occasionally have a difficult time understanding a new concept, theory, or technique. Even as an OT professor, it is difficult to stay abreast of the newest information in so many areas. Our profession is seeing exciting growth in public awareness, need, and research. Being an OT student in today's world is very exciting but more difficult than ever.

The authors of this book set out to help you through the process of becoming a COTA or OTR. This book is designed to give you all the advice we would give you if you were sitting in our office with a problem. The reason we called the book a primer is because it contains basic information you can use to build your knowledge of OT. We never intended this book to be the OT textbook for a particular class. Instead, the primer is designed to be your companion, like an older sister or brother. The book is designed to relieve anxiety about test taking, to provide you with reviews of basic OT concepts, and to give you advice to avoid problems and advice on handling problems if you find yourself in one. We paid particular attention to the problem-avoiding and problem-solving aspects. Whether you are an "academically challenged" student or an A+ student, we hope you find what you need in this primer. This was written for you.

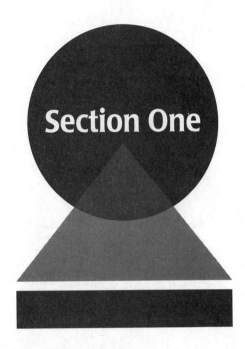

Section One

General Information

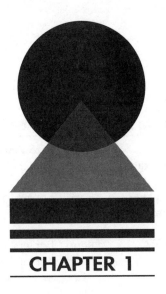

CHAPTER 1

INTRODUCTION

Karen Sladyk, MS, OTR/L

HOW TO USE THIS BOOK

This book is designed to be your companion as you begin to master new OT skills. It is written to give you advice and assistance to some basic OT concepts. Some students will find they do not need much of this book, but most students should find something helpful. The primer is not designed to substitute for your teacher's advice, but is designed to get you started in the right direction. While developing the book, we authors asked ourselves the following questions:

- What basic OT concepts are essential to set a student on the path to success?
- What advice do we routinely give students about succeeding in their studies?
- What common problems come up during academic studies, and how can we prevent them?
- How can we help students develop their best professional image?
- How can we ensure students have a good understanding of how they fit in to the future of OT?
- What skills do students need to succeed on fieldwork and on their first job?

This book is part academic advisor, part tutor, part companion. It contains **figures, tables**, **worksheets** to fill out for better self-understanding, and **exercises** (with **answers**) to check what you have learned. All of the primer is written to help students succeed in their OT program.

GETTING STARTED

This primer is designed to be read in parts. You do not need to start at the beginning of the book to understand the end. Where you start depends on what your needs are at the moment. Some chapters may be assigned in one class, while other chapters may be assigned

Table 1-1
Where to Start Problem-Based List

Problem	Chapters to Read
OT classes are about to start and I am not sure what will happen.	Read Chapters 2, 3, 6, and 7.
OT classes have been going for a few weeks and I am beginning to get overwhelmed.	Read Chapters 6, 7, 10, and 12.
I do not see why I should join AOTA.	Read Chapters 2, 3, and 4.
I am out of money for school.	Read Chapter 5 and the book buying section of Chapter 7.
I am not getting the grades I want.	Read Chapters 6, 7, 8, 9, and 10.
I need help on OT papers, projects, and presentations.	Read Chapter 8 and the time management section of Chapter 10.
I am not passing a class.	Start with Chapter 9, then review Chapters 6, 7, and 10.
I think (or know) I have a disability.	Start with Chapter 11, then review Chapter 9.
My professional image is tarnished.	Start with Chapter 10, then read Chapters 6 and 8.
I am stressed.	Read Chapter 10, then review Chapters 6 and 9.
I am not balancing school with non-school activities.	Read Chapter 12.
I do not see why uniform terminology is so important.	Read Chapter 13.
I do not understand frames of reference.	Read Chapter 14.
I need help on medical terminology, ROM, or documentation.	Read Chapters 16, 17, and 18.
I need help in communicating with my peers or my patients.	Read Chapters 15 and 19, and the group project section of Chapter 8.
I have an ethical problem.	Read Chapter 21.
I need to review some clinical skills.	Read Chapters 20 and 22.
I do not understand what fieldwork is all about.	Read Chapters 2 and 23.
I am getting ready to find my first job.	Read Chapters 24 and 25.
What about graduate school?	Read Chapter 26.

in a different class. You may have bought the book for yourself without it being required reading or you may have kept the book after a class was completed. You will find the Table of Contents to be a good starting place or you can use Table 1-1 for some direction.

A FEW WORDS ON SUCCESS

There are many books on the market about success. Many have been bestsellers for long periods of time. So what makes success books so successful? Most people want to succeed in life and like advice from others who have been successful. Often people have invested a lot of time and money, such as tuition, into becoming successful. As an OT student, you may have bought this book to make the most out of your student career. Here is some general advice to help you become successful in both your OT career and your personal life.

John Anderson wrote an article for *Reader's Digest* (1996) where he outlined several steps to being successful. Anderson suggested that you start by following your dream. When things get tough, visualize your dream. Set time aside to work on your goals. Managing your time is an important skill. Take one step at a time and remember that nothing of significance comes easily. This is very true of a college degree. If earning a college degree was easy, everyone would have one. It takes hard work, one step at a time.

Manage your weak points by working hard to overcome them. Many people fail at their goals because they stick with the things they are good at while avoiding improving their weak areas. Once you are managing the weak areas, you will find everything is manageable. When things are going well, stop and look back on your accomplishments. Take a break and reflect on how far you have come. Enjoy your success along the way.

SETTING YOUR PERSONAL GOALS

Only you can decide what your goals will be while you are in OT school. Most likely, you will have a variety of goals both personal and professional. Remember that you are only in OT school once and you will likely want to get the most education for the dollar. Set goals that are challenging yet within your reach. Seek input from your family, friends, and professors but use your best judgment for setting your own goals. You may find guidance in this primer. OT is a rewarding career; make the profession proud of you and be proud of your profession.

SUMMARY

This brief chapter is designed to get you familiar with this primer. The primer is designed to help students succeed in OT school. The book can be read from start to finish or the appropriate chapters can be read out of order. The focus of the primer is on advice and tutorials to make your journey through OT school more successful for the reader. This chapter specifically looks at common problems and gives suggestions on where to start.

BIBLIOGRAPHY

Anderson, J. E. (1996, May). If you really want to succeed. *Reader's Digest*.
Bolles, R. (1991). *What color is your parachute?* Berkeley, CA: Ten Speed Press.
Ellis, D. (1985). *Becoming a master student.* Rapid City, SD: College Survival, Inc.
Smith, L., & Walter, T. (1995). *The adult learner's guide to college success.* Boston: Wadsworth Publishing Co.

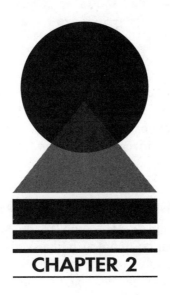

CHAPTER 2

UNDERSTANDING OT

Karen Sladyk, MS, OTR/L

INTRODUCTION

People who work in OT will tell you it is a wonderful career, but a career that is not well known to the public. You may have found out about OT from family or friends who benefited from OT services. You may have found out about OT from a career class or from college recruiters. This chapter will help you understand some basic ideas about OT. OT personnel and where they work will be discussed. Developing your own personal definition of OT will be covered. In addition, you will have a place to track your progress in your OT career.

THE ROLE OF COTAS AND OTRS

Currently, OT has two levels of personnel: the Certified Occupational Therapy Assistant (COTA) and the Occupational Therapist, Registered (OTR). Although you may hear the OTR called "a registered occupational therapist," the initials are always OTR, not ROT. Generally, a COTA has an associate degree from an approved OT assistant program, and an OTR has a bachelor's degree, post-bachelor certificate, or entry-level master's degree from an approved OT program.

The AOTA, or the American Occupational Therapy Association, in Bethesda, Maryland, has developed essential requirements for all approved OT programs. When a school has met the requirements, it is awarded accreditation from AOTA and the students from the school become eligible to sit for either the OTR or COTA exam. As a student in your OT program, it is important that you be aware of your program's accreditation status.

The employment outlook for both COTAs and OTRs is good. Even with the health care system changing rapidly, there continues to be a need for OT personnel. A great variety of employment opportunities are available in OT. COTAs and OTRs work in a variety of settings from hospitals to home care. In addition, OT services are used by people of all ages, from newborns to senior citizens. A career in OT can provide you with a wealth of experiences across the age span.

BECOMING A COTA

The COTA must first complete an accredited or approved program for the OTA. Generally, these programs can be found at junior, vocational, technical, or community colleges. There is no "on the job" training such as the OT aide that might be found in some hospitals. The COTA is an educated and trained technician different from an OT aide. The COTA works with an OTR to meet the needs of their patient or client. After a student finishes the academic aspect of his or her program, fieldwork is begun. Fieldwork is arranged creatively to provide the student with experience in OT. Although fieldwork is different in each program, the COTA student generally can expect to do 16 full-time weeks, usually 8 weeks in one site and 8 weeks in a different site. After the academic and fieldwork components are completed, the student can sit for the exam to become certified (COTA). A person cannot call him- or herself a COTA until he or she has passed the exam. State laws, accreditation agencies, and workplace requirements make it impossible for a person to work as an OTA without passing the certification exam.

BECOMING AN OTR

The OTR must first complete an accredited or approved program for the OT. Generally, these programs can be found at colleges or universities. The OTR is an educated and trained professional different from the COTA. The OTR is responsible for evaluating the patient or client and developing a treatment plan. The OTR and COTA work together to meet the needs of their patient or client. After a student finishes the academic aspect of their program, fieldwork is begun. Fieldwork is arranged creatively to provide the student with experience in OT. Although fieldwork is different in each program, the OTR student generally can expect to do a minimum of 24 full-time weeks, usually 12 weeks in one site and 12 weeks in a different site. Some schools require a third fieldwork, while other schools suggest it. After the academic program and fieldwork is completed, the student can sit for the exam to become certified (OTR). A person cannot call him- or herself an OTR until he or she has passed the exam. State laws, accreditation agencies, and workplace requirements make it impossible for a person to work as an OT without passing the certification exam.

TRACKING YOUR PROGRESS IN OT SCHOOL

Whether you are in school to become a COTA or an OTR, you will likely follow a similar plan of study. Understanding what is in front of you will help you plan for the future and avoid surprises. Worksheet 2-1 is provided to help organize your long-term plan of study and help you plan for your financial needs. Remember that the outline is a "typical plan." If you are a part-time student or a student who requires special accommodations for a disability, your plan might be different. Fill in your plan and update your progress when appropriate.

Worksheet 2-1

Plan of Study

Task to be Completed	Projected Date	Completed Date
Accepted into COTA or OTR School		
Complete Liberal Arts and Sciences: COTA 2 Semesters, OTR 4 Semesters, Graduate Degree Finish Prerequisites		
1st Semester		
2nd Semester		
3rd Semester		
4th Semester		
Complete OT Classes: COTA 2 Semesters, OTR 4 Semesters		
1st Semester		
2nd Semester		
3rd Semester		
4th Semester		
Fieldwork One: 8 to 12 Weeks		
Fieldwork Two: 8 to 12 Weeks		
Fieldwork Three: 8 to 12 Weeks		
Complete All Paperwork to Sit for the Exam		
Take the Exam		
Look for First Job		
First Day of Work		

WHERE COTAS AND OTRS WORK

Understanding how you fit in to the profession of OT comes after you begin to examine the profession. More than likely you visited OT clinics and observed OT services before you started your OT career. Many OT programs have students visit OT clinics as part of the introduction classes. As mentioned earlier, OTs and COTAs enjoy working in a variety of setting including:

- General hospitals
- Psychiatric hospitals
- Nursing homes
- Public schools
- Home health agencies
- Rehabilitation hospitals
- Pediatric hospitals
- Community programs
- Private practice

OT personnel work with a variety of health problems, both physical and mental. A COTA or OTR might assist a person with a stroke, developmental delays, depression, head injury, hip fracture, schizophrenia, attention deficit disorder, or cerebral palsy. Some COTAs or OTRs might specialize in adaptive equipment, technology, hand treatment, work hardening, or even education. It is very likely that most of your faculty are OTs. In this chapter, some of the workplaces will be further explored. Because of the great variety of places OT personnel can work, it would be impossible to address each area in this primer. If you have a particular interest in learning more about an OT specialty, see your academic fieldwork coordinator to discuss your ideas.

OT in Mental Health

OT has strong roots in the area of mental health. At one time, half of all OT personnel worked with people with schizophrenia, depression, bipolar disorder, and other psychiatric diseases. Today, COTAs and OTRs work in both hospitals and community-based programs to help people with mental illness improve their lives. Children, adolescents, adults, and the elderly vary in their mental health needs, but OT can use purposeful activities to improve functioning with people across the age span. Besides the diagnostic categories mentioned above, OT works with people with:
- Borderline personality
- Chemical dependencies
- Autism
- Eating disorders
- Adjustment disorders
- Anxiety and stress disorders

Examples of treatment may include:
- Job coaching for a person with depression returning to his or her job
- Coping skills for a group of survivors from a natural disaster
- Parenting skills for teens with new babies
- Sensory motor activities for people with schizophrenia
- Community living skills, such as taking the bus, for people with chronic mental illness

OT in Physical Rehabilitation

A large number of OT personnel work in physical management. With better medicine and technology, people are living longer and surviving accidents or injuries. Today, COTAs and OTRs are seeing a huge growth in the area of physical rehabilitation. You may find COTAs and OTRs in acute care hospitals, rehabilitation hospitals, nursing homes, outpatient clinics, and home care. Children, adolescents, adults, and the elderly vary in their physical management needs, but OT can be effective in physical rehabilitation, as in mental health. OT is common with persons with stroke, head injury, heart attack, and work injuries. In addition, you will find OT working with the following diagnostic categories:
- Multiple sclerosis
- Hand injuries
- Arthritis

- Hip fractures
- Burns
- Amputation

Examples of treatment may include:
- Safety training for the homemaker with a stroke
- Driver education for a young man after a head injury
- Energy conservation for the mother with arthritis
- Personal hygiene for the teen with burns
- Adaptive equipment for the pianist with a hand injury

OT in Pediatrics

OT has grown in the area of pediatrics. COTAs and OTRs may work in public schools, pediatric hospitals, pediatric outpatient clinics, and home care. Just like in any other area, pediatric OT finds meaningful activities to aid children in developing the skills they need to succeed in school and home life. OTRs treat premature babies, teaching them impoved sucking, and both COTAs and OTRs work with adolescents to assist them in the adjustment to adult roles. In general, pediatric OTs work on encouraging normal development from birth to adulthood. In addition to the diagnostic categories mentioned above, you will find OT working with:
- Muscular dystrophy
- Developmental disabilities
- Sensory integration dysfunction
- Learning disabilities
- Juvenile rheumatoid arthritis
- Delayed motor development
- Congenital anomalies

Examples of treatment may include:
- Wheelchair positioning for the second grader with spina bifida
- Building an obstacle course for fourth graders with delayed motor development
- Playing with blocks with a 4-year-old who just got prosthetic arms
- Developing a behavioral contract with a preteen who acts out in class
- Practicing handwriting with a child with visual problems

OT With the Elderly

As our population begins to age, OT with the older adult has seen a huge growth. Many elderly are actively participating in wellness programs and living longer than ever. OT uses goal-oriented activity to treat people impaired by normal aging, accident, or illness. Function and independence become the focus when working with the older adult. Just like any other specialty area in OT, you will find COTAs and OTRs working in hospitals, nursing homes, outpatient programs, and community programs. In addition, you will find OT in adult day care programs, retirement programs, hospices, and senior centers. The diagnostic categories for the elderly are the same as mentioned in the mental health and physical rehabilitation sections of this chapter. Treatment specific to the older adult might include:

- Adaptive golf club for the retired person with a hand injury
- Organizing a room at home to improve memory
- ROM exercises to music popular with the older adult
- Adapted daily living activities for poor vision or hearing
- Maintaining independent living skills and meaningful activities for a person with terminal illness

EXPLAINING OT

Now that we have talked about where COTAs and OTRs work, the next logical step is figuring out how to explain it to others. More than likely someone has asked you about school and the conversation has gone something like this:

Friend/relative: "How's school going?"

You: "Great! I really love my classes."

Friend/relative: "Good. What are you studying again?"

You: "Occupational therapy."

Friend/relative: Long pause. "What exactly is that?"

You: Silently, you think, "Boy, if I only had a dollar for every time I answered that!"

There is some advantage to everyone not knowing what OT is. If they did, everyone would want to go to OT school and it would be impossible to get into your OT program. But seriously, you are likely to explain what OT is 100 times before you finish your first year of working. Whether you are a future COTA or OTR, you will have to explain OT to many different people. How you explain OT will depend on who you are talking to. As an OT student, you should prepare several different answers.

The first step in developing your own definition of OT is to look at what OT is all about. If you were to reread the section of this chapter that addressed where COTAs and OTRs work, you will see some key phases that are unique to OT. These include *meaningful* or *purposeful activity*, *function*, and *independent living skills*.

People will likely ask you if you find jobs for people and you will have to explain that the word occupation means "all roles for all people." For example, each person has several roles besides his or her job. A secretary with a hand injury from keyboarding may also be:

- A mother of three teenage boys
- A daughter and caregiver to an aging mother
- A volunteer at the soup kitchen
- A student of ceramics
- A tennis player

The word *occupation* means all roles in work, activities of daily living, and play and leisure.

Later in this book, you will review Uniform Terminology. Uniform Terminology provides the framework for our profession. If you are unfamiliar with the document from AOTA, review Chapter 13 in this primer before proceeding with this chapter. Uniform Terminology will help you define OT to other people. When it comes time to tell people about OT, you may want to start with something that sounds like this:

OT uses purposeful activities to improve function in clients.

The second step to developing your own definition of OT involves evaluating who you are talking to. You will want to take different approaches with friends, family, doctors, other professionals, and patients. Be sure to give a definition that the person can relate to. Fancy professional terminology will only confuse people.

You may want to add the differences between OT and PT. Discuss how PT works on strength, endurance, balance, and gait. Include examples of how PT and OT work together in many rehabilitation facilities. For example, explain how a PT might work on balance and endurance with a person with a head injury and the OT would focus on balance while completing ADLs using adaptive equipment.

The last step in developing your definition is evaluating how much time you have to convey your thoughts. You should have two sets of definitions. The first is the "elevator" definition. This definition should be short and simple enough to tell on an elevator trip. The second is a longer (but still short) definition that you can use face-to-face when you may have 2 to 3 minutes to explain OT. Write out your an elevator definition and a face-to-face definition of OT in Worksheet 2-2.

Worksheet 2-2

How I Would Define OT

Elevator (15 Seconds)	Face-to-Face (2 to 3 Minutes)
Family:	
College Friend:	
Medical Doctor:	
Patient:	

SUMMARY

This chapter has reviewed how to become a COTA or OTR. In addition, some typical OT services are reviewed. The importance of developing a working definition of OT is addressed. Worksheets to track your progress in your academic career and on developing your own working definition of OT are provided.

BIBLIOGRAPHY

Christiansen, C., & Baum, C. (Eds.). (1991). *Occupational therapy: Overcoming human performance deficits*. Thorofare, NJ: SLACK Inc.

Hettinger, J. (1996). Who are we? *OT Week*, March 28.

Punwar, A. J. (1988). *OT principles and practice*. Baltimore: Williams & Wilkins.

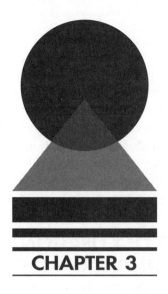

CHAPTER 3

THE AMERICAN OCCUPATIONAL THERAPY ASSOCIATION

Tara J. Glennon, MS, OTR/L

INTRODUCTION

What is AOTA? The basic answer would be AOTA is the American Occupational Therapy Association. This chapter will attempt to fill you in about AOTA and adjunct organizations that are affiliated with AOTA.

AMERICAN OCCUPATIONAL THERAPY ASSOCIATION (AOTA)

The AOTA, located at 4720 Montgomery Lane, PO Box 31220, Bethesda, MD 20824-1220, is a national association or society for OT professionals founded in 1917. This professional community, including OTRs, COTAs, and OT students, offers many benefits to help you in many aspects of your professional life. Some affect you directly at your current level of professional development, while some benefits are broader in scope and relate to the growth of the profession. Benefits that come with membership will be further discussed later in this chapter.

As a professional organization, AOTA becomes the voice of our profession in the public, legal, and professional communities. AOTA must provide quality assurance for OT services right down to whether the school you are enrolled is accredited. This accreditation is necessary for you to obtain your certification or state license. AOTA also sets forth standards of practice for our profession and supports state regulation of practice through licensure and other regulatory laws. Quality management is one of the major areas on which AOTA focuses attention. Within this domain, promoting professional development through continuing education, publications, practice information, and other services enable therapists to continue to monitor and improve quality of care. As a student, your membership and participation in AOTA is extremely important.

AMERICAN OCCUPATIONAL THERAPY FOUNDATION (AOTF)

Although physically located in the same building as AOTA, the AOTF is a completely separate entity. AOTF is a "charitable, nonprofit organization dedicated to refining and expanding the body of knowledge of OT and promoting understanding of the value of occupation in the interest of the public" (AOTF, 1996). Funding sources for AOTF include private contributions from individuals, corporations, and other charitable organizations. The Foundation's mission, to support development of the OT knowledge base and increase public understanding, guides the projects and services. The Foundation strongly supports research and education by offering scholarships, research grants, doctoral fellowships, and faculty development opportunities. Obviously, the most important foundation service to the OT student is the scholarship opportunities. The 1996-1997 scholarship program offered more than 100 scholarships to students deserving support. Eligibility requirements are outlined in the brochure available through the Foundation (301-652-2682). The applications are generally mailed out from September 1st through December 15th. Complete applications must be postmarked by January 15th and applicants are notified in April (AOTF, 1995). Remember, AOTA membership is a requirement to qualify for all scholarships.

AMERICAN STUDENT COMMITTEE OF THE OCCUPATIONAL THERAPY ASSOCIATION (ASCOTA)

ASCOTA is made up of student members of AOTA and is considered to be a vibrant, integral component of AOTA. ASCOTA "provides a mechanism for the expression of student concerns and offers a means whereby students can have effective input into the affairs of the AOTA" (AOTA, 1995a). Student delegates from all accredited educational programs are elected to represent their fellow students at yearly national meetings. This meeting occurs at the national conference to coincide with the meeting of AOTA's Representative Assembly (RA). ASCOTA's immediate past president serves as the RA Student Representative and represents the student voice. The ASCOTA representative has a vote in the RA. ASCOTA also has input to the Executive Board of AOTA through its past president and the Steering Committee Officers (Figure 3-1). The student association is currently considering a name change to better serve student needs.

PI THETA EPSILON

The Greek interpretation of Pi Theta Epsilon is Advancement, Therapeutic, and Occupation. In other words, advancement in OT. This organization is the national OT

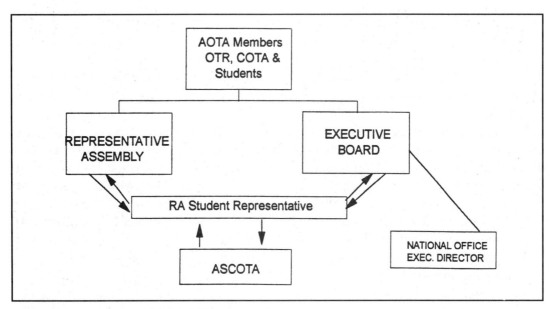

Figure 3-1. Diagram of ASCOTA relationships.

honor society which recognizes and encourages superior scholarship and service among OT students enrolled in an entry-level program. This honor society originated at the University of New Hampshire in 1958. For approximately 30 years, various chapters were formed and ran fairly independently. In the 1980s, at the annual meeting of ASCOTA, an ad hoc committee was formed to investigate the possibility of nationally organizing the society. After a few years, the committee approached AOTF for assistance. AOTF's desire to foster scholarship and research endeavors led to their agreement in sponsoring this endeavor. Advisory and working committees were formed which resulted in policies and procedures being formulated, the production of a constitution, and a promotional campaign. In 1991, AOTA adopted a resolution to recognize Pi Theta Epsilon as the national OT honor society.

Via a letter to the honor society's national office dated March 28, 1996, Pi Theta Epsilon was welcomed into the Association of College Honor Societies. The constitution and an informational pamphlet on how to start a chapter at your school is available from the Pi Theta Epsilon national office, located in the AOTA building in Bethesda, Maryland.

AOTA BENEFITS AND SERVICES

Publications

As a member of AOTA, you would receive the *American Journal of Occupational Therapy (AJOT)*, the official publication. In this journal, you will find articles related to theory, techniques, differing approaches, research, and educational activities. *AJOT* is distributed monthly, except for bimonthly distribution in July/August and November/December. In November 1995, *OT Practice* began appearing in the same mailing as *AJOT*. This magazine was designed to address more specific practice needs. In essence, the AOTA wanted to hear what the practitioner was doing out in the field. Participation and dialog are strongly encouraged through *OT Practice*. The publications of *OT Practice* that have come out since its inception have been quite creative and exciting. If a student wishes to receive this practitioner periodical, a small fee would be incurred.

Another free resource for student members of AOTA would be semiannual issues of the *Journal of Occupational Therapy Students (JOTS)*. *JOTS* provides the student with an opportunity to publish as a student. Consider submitting a paper from class with the help of a professor.

Newsletters are also part of your membership benefits. You would receive *OT Week*, a newspaper that is circulated to approximately 60,000 OT personnel. Although this newsletter is promoted as the profession's leading employment bulletin, it has some great articles as well. These articles are also listed in a yearly index. So, if you are looking for information on a topic, just check the yearly indices for the topic area.

The second newsletter that you would be entitled to receive as part of your membership is the quarterly special interest newsletter. A special interest section is an area of interest for which AOTA publishes a quarterly newsletter. The current areas are:
- Administration and Management
- Developmental Disabilities
- Education
- Gerontology
- Home and Community Health
- Mental Health
- Physical Disabilities
- School System
- Sensory Integration
- Technology
- Work Programs

When you join AOTA, you are entitled to choose one area of special interest to receive the quarterly newsletter. If you choose more than one interest area, you simply pay an additional $15 fee for each additional area of interest. For students, there is an additional student newsletter called *The OT Line* that you would also be entitled to receive.

Products

AOTA has a product catalog that would be beneficial for OT professionals to obtain. They have balloons, buttons, self-sticking notes, paper clips, pencil grippers, rulers, calendars, brochures, posters, mugs, lunch bags, bumper stickers, key chains, and T-shirts, all with an OT logo or catchy phrases. These are good for promoting the profession during OT Month (April).

AOTA offers books and videos on various topics, everything from arthritis to wellness. Everything in between includes ethics, information on specific diagnoses, fieldwork resources, management, documentation, development, assessments, splinting, public information, and even the history of OT.

Besides these books and videos, AOTA offers self-study series on specific topic areas. A self-study series is designed for therapists in need of specific information in a practice area and who wish to gain continuing education information. As an OT student, you do not have to worry about continuing education until after you graduate. Currently, the self-study series topics include neuroscience, school-based practice, cognitive rehabilitation, assessing function, and the practice of the future.

Additional Benefits

Other benefits of joining AOTA as a student would be the weekly job placement bulletin, reduced rate for AOTA-sponsored conferences, information and consultation resources, and reduced prices on publications and products. The last benefit which should be mentioned, which might be of significant importance, would be the availability of a credit card program. Also, AOTA is continually expanding the methods through which members can access information. In addition to *The Reliable Source*, a state-of-the-art computerized information system, AOTA has recently instituted a benefit called AOTA's Fax-On-Request. A member can simply call a special toll-free number and supply the code number for the information needed. The information is then promptly faxed back to you, free of charge. AOTA is continually striving to improve member services and the ability to gain information.

WHY SHOULD YOU BECOME A MEMBER OF AOTA?

With all of the information and resources available to you through AOTA, the question really becomes, "What would make me not join AOTA?" Your response might be "the money." The current student cost is $42.50. This membership goes for 1 year. The savings on textbooks alone will likely cover your membership fee. Even if you pass your registration exam and are now a full-fledged COTA or OTR, your membership will not increase until your anniversary date of membership. To join, you can call AOTA to get a membership application.

When you do join AOTA, you should get used to saying "AOTA, AOTA, AOTA," because it will soon become a good part of your life. Even the membership telephone number is 1-800-SAY-AOTA. Remember, this is only the telephone number if you have a membership, otherwise, you will not get past the operator. Also, always have your member identification number when you call AOTA.

SUMMARY

This chapter reviewed the importance of becoming a student member of the AOTA. The voice of our profession in the public and legal arenas, the AOTA also promotes growth and development of our profession. This is accomplished through the many membership benefits, such as journals, newsletters, continuing education, and products. Students have a voice in the AOTA through the ASCOTA. Also, as a member of AOTA, students can access the financial resources of the AOTF. Participating in AOTA as a student can start your career off on the right foot.

BIBLIOGRAPHY

American Occupational Therapy Association. (1994a). *About AOTA.* Bethesda, MD: Author.
American Occupational Therapy Association. (1994b). *How does ASCOTA relate to AOTA.* Bethesda, MD: Author.
American Occupational Therapy Association. (1995a). *ASCOTA mission statement.* Bethesda, MD: Author.
American Occupational Therapy Association. (1995b). *ASCOTA 1995-1996 Strategic plan and operational objectives.* Bethesda, MD: Author.
American Occupational Therapy Association. (1995c). *OT Practice.* Bethesda, MD: Author.
American Occupational Therapy Association. (1996a). *OT Week.* Bethesda, MD: Author.

American Occupational Therapy Association. (1996b). *The AOTA 1996 winter catalog.* Bethesda, MD: Author.

American Occupational Therapy Foundation. (1995). *Informational brochure.* Bethesda, MD: Author.

American Occupational Therapy Foundation. (1996). *AOTF connection.* Bethesda, MD: Author.

Association of College Honor Societies. (1996). East Lansing, MI: Author.

Pi Theta Epsilon National Office. (1996). *Pi Theta Epsilon: The national occupational therapy honor society.* Bethesda, MD: Author.

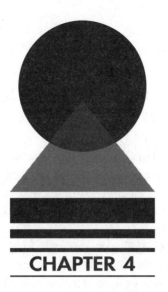

CHAPTER 4

OT AND POLITICAL ACTION

Debra Francoeur Bowler, MS, OTR/L

INTRODUCTION

During your career as a COTA or OTR, you may come to examine your profession from many different perspectives. When you apply to an OT program, your focus is on the best points. While in your last year, you may wonder if you will ever make it to the clinic. While on your first affiliation, you will be amazed at all the knowledge you have retained and all the learning taking place that does not come from books. Your last hurdles involve finishing school, passing the exam, and, finally, looking for the right job that challenges both mind and spirit.

Students often complain that being in an OT program makes it hard for them to have any kind of life that is "connected to the real world." And yet it is important for you to do just that. Your chosen profession is part of a greater health care system that changes almost daily as lawmakers, insurance companies, and service providers look for cost-effective ways to deliver quality care. These changes will directly impact your future in OT. The workforce you witnessed as a freshman may evolve into something very different by the time you finish your OT program.

As the trend toward government involvement grows in the area of health care, so does the need for individual involvement. Thomas Jefferson said that the basis of our political system is the right of its people to make and alter their constitutions of government. This chapter will help you understand how AOTA participates in legislative action. It also outlines ways that you can become involved in the political process to ensure that the OT career you are working so hard to achieve will remain part of the health care field.

HISTORY OF POLITICAL
ACTION COMMITTEES (PACS)

During the late 1960s and early 1970s there were many campaign contribution abuses reported at the federal level. This prompted Congress to pass the Federal Election Commission Act of 1971, which provided a legal framework for campaign contributions to federal candidates. This law and its amendments helped pave the way for corporations, labor unions, and professional organizations to have a vital and legitimate interest in the operation of the government.

Political Action Committees (PACs) permit individuals or groups of individuals who share concerns to participate in the political process and help elect candidates with similar concerns. A PAC is a legally sanctioned vehicle through which organizations can engage in otherwise prohibited political action and work to influence the outcome of federal elections. It is the only legal and ethical way a profession can unite behind the candidate of its choice (AOTA, 1995).

Federal law limits the amount of money groups can contribute. For example, it prohibits large corporations from using treasury funds for campaign contributions. Organizations can establish PACs and solicit voluntary donations from certain eligible groups specified by law. Individual state laws vary with regard to limits and some impose restrictions only. Both the contributing group and the candidate must file periodic reports of expenditures and receipts with the Federal Election Commission (FEC). The FEC is a regulatory body charged with enforcing federal election law. This makes the election process better documented and open to the public, which has access to FEC records.

TYPES OF PACS

There are two types of PACs. The first, Party and Candidate Committees, raise funds to support local and state political parties as well as individual candidates. The second, Nonparty Committees, has two categories, Connected and Nonconnected PACs.

Connected PACs are formed by sponsoring groups such as professional organizations. The laws permit the sponsoring group to pay for the administrative soliciting costs of fundraising so that every dollar made can contribute directly to the candidate of their choice. Connected PACs can solicit money only from members and their families.

Nonconnected PACs operate as independent entities without sponsoring organizations and may represent all ranges of the political spectrum. They may solicit funds from any American citizen. A percentage of the money raised is used to offset soliciting costs.

PACs provide a dual service to our political system. First, they help federal, state, and local candidates to raise money. Second, they provide an effective way for people of all political persuasions to have an impact on politics, both at state and federal levels. This strengthens representative government by getting more people involved in the political process (AOTA, 1995).

AOTA'S POLITICAL ACTION COMMITTEE (AOTPAC)

AOTPAC is AOTA's federal Political Action Committee. It is a voluntary, nonprofit, unincorporated committee of AOTA members who are exercising their rights as American citizens. In 1976, the Representative Assembly authorized AOTPAC and it has been in operation since 1978. Its mission is to further the legislative aims of the AOTA by influencing or attempting to influence the selection, nomination, election, or appointment of any individual to a federal public office. In addition, AOTPAC supports any OTR, COTA, or OT student member of AOTA seeking election to any state or local office (AOTA, 1995). AOTPAC supports candidates who share issues and concerns that affect our profession and ensure that our government represents all sectors of society.

For almost 20 years now, AOTPAC has made political contributions to candidates in almost every state. This political involvement in the election process for both House Representatives and Senators has enabled AOTA to broaden its contacts in legislative and executive branches of government. Through AOTPAC, OT practitioners have a collective voice which will be heard in the debates over the ever-expanding number of health care issues that come before Congress (AOTA, 1995).

The money raised by AOTPAC is called "hard dollars" and must be placed in seperate funds for direct campaign contributions. The operating costs used to raise this money (e.g., office space and telephone service) are called "soft dollars." This money is made available by AOTA which generates the funds through membership applications, mail solicitation, and AOTPAC night at the Annual Conference.

CANDIDATE SUPPORT—
WHO GETS AOTPAC FUNDED?

There are many factors that go into making decisions regarding candidate support from AOTPAC:

- Recomendations of AOTA members and officers.
- Leadership of State Associations.
- Advice of the Legislative and Political Relations Department (LAPD). The staff analyzes and interprets Congressional voting records. LAPD is able to distinguish who are important players in the health care legislative process and will support the profession of OT.
- Activity of those politicians who have supported specific proposals and policies advanced by the profession.
- Those who may chair or are members of important committees or subcommittees who may be sympathetic to OT goals.

LOBBYING—THE ART OF INFLUENCE

One of the ways AOTA stays active in the political process is through lobbying. Lobbying efforts involve activities aimed at influencing public officials toward a desired legislative action. AOTA lobbyists work to further professional agendas in two ways: first, through the legislative process of how a bill becomes a law, and second, through the regulation-making process which is how those laws get implemented.

THE LEGISLATIVE PROCESS

Before lobbying efforts can begin, lobbyists must be familiar with how the legislative process works and all the steps of how a bill becomes a law. Try to think back to your high school civics classes while we review the process. Our focus here will be on how a lobbyist gets involved at each stage to ensure passage of a desired bill.

When a group wants changes in a law brought about they will seek out a legislator who will be sympathetic to their cause. This individual will then sponsor a bill and introduce it to the legislature. Educating both the public and the legislators is a crucial activity at this stage in order to enlist support for the bill. Choosing as many individuals as possible who are respected in that area of concern will also increase the chances for successful passage.

The bill is now assigned to a committee or subcommittee to review the proposals. Lobbying can occur here, too, as bills are often assigned according to jurisdiction. For example, bills related to health care will go to the health committee. Doing your homework and finding out legislators' voting records is an important step in preparing your lobbying strategy.

Public hearings by the legislators are required to allow groups and individuals to gather information and voice concerns. Writing, calling, and visiting your representatives prior to the hearing will keep them informed of relevant issues regarding this proposal.

Next, the language of the bill may be modified to reflect any changes made. This is an excellent opportunity to continue making requests. Subcommittees formed must now report back to full committees and legal intentions regarding the bill are reviewed. How lawyers and judges will interpret this bill in the future is a concern and lobbyists now must focus on inclusion of explanations so that no misinterpretations about the law can be made later.

Now it is time for the House and Senate floors to vote. If there are differences, members from each floor form a Conference Committee to reach a compromise. Lobbying efforts are aimed at reaching a version that satisfies the original intent (Scott & Acquaviva, 1985). Once a compromised version is created, it gets passed on for approval by both the House and Senate floors. The last step is onto the President for signature. During this whole process, lobbyists are monitoring the administrative processes, identifying resources, and providing legal services. Local staff at representatives' offices are very helpful in providing information needed.

REGULATION-MAKING PROCESS

Vocational rehabilitation and workers' compensation are just two examples of agencies that will take these new laws and translate them into policies and procedures that may directly affect programs that deliver OT services. An agency will formulate the rules for implementing the law and this information is published daily in *The Federal Register.* Some states may vary on how this is published; some may publish rules in local newspapers only. An invitation for a public hearing will follow. Now is the time for members of organizations affected by these proposed rules to attend and voice their concerns.

The agency proposing the rules will send the rules to related agencies for comments. It is important for OTs to have contacts with all agencies relating to their interests. These proposals are sent to the government for review where they are either accepted or rejected and sent back for revisions. This is a good time to contact your government office with your concerns and requests.

Legislative review or intervention may occur if the legislator thinks an agency has misinterpreted the law's intent. If an organization is aware of this, they may enlist the support of legislators sympathetic to their cause to facilitate a review (Scott & Acquaviva, 1985).

The COTA or OTR in the clinic and in the community can be very influential in helping shape policy by demonstrating that OT services represent a cost-effective alternative to dependence (Christiansen & Baum, 1991).

AOTACTION NETWORK

The AOTAction Network is a group of OT representatives from key states, organized to coordinate the grassroots lobbying efforts for health care reform. The states targeted are those that have U.S. Senators or Representatives seated on key committees of Congress that will be directly involved in preparing health care reform legislation for full Congressional review.

The goal of the network is to educate the specific U.S. Senators or Representatives on the importance of OT and other related issues in health care reform. This is being done in several ways. Arranging for Senators or Representatives to visit a facility and see OT in action, meeting with Senators or Representatives in their state/district offices, and communicating by phone or letter are all productive strategies.

TAKE ACTION

This section of the primer presents information about action taken by AOTA. However, there are many things which you can do now as a student to prepare you for life as a "political practitioner." The following are some ideas to jumpstart your involvement.

- **Become a member of AOTA.** Student rates are less expensive than full fees and you get the same great benefits. Membership also entitles you to access such great resources as the Government Relations Department and AOTPAC. AOTA publications such as *OT Week* and *OT Practice* are full of up-to-date happenings in the political arena.
- **Become a member of your state OT association.** There are legislative committees always at work on some issue related to health care reform. It is also a great way to meet other students in your state as well as practitioners who may someday be working side-by-side with you. State associations sponsor conferences throughout the year and you may use this opportunity to learn about health care reform issues.
- **Become involved with AOTAction Network.** The network is always looking for people to assist with their efforts. Call and ask AOTA to send you an updated listing of network contacts in your area.
- **Communicate.** One of the most important roles you can play as a responsible citizen is to communicate effectively with your elected representatives. Seek them out, and offer assistance to keep them informed on key issues concerning OT. Do your homework first. Find out who they are and learn all you can about them. Your state OT association and AOTA's LAPD staff can help you. Organizations such as the state or local Chamber of Commerce also publish directories and manuals which list elected officials, legislative committees, and other pertinent information. The local public library is an excellent source of political information. Stay abreast of your politician's position on issues through public statements made, votes taken on issues, and media coverage (AOTA, 1995).
- **Write letters.** Letter writing is an effective way to communicate with legislators who spend a lot of time in Washington. The guidelines in Table 4-1 are designed to assist

---

Table 4-1
Legislator Letter Writing Guidelines

- Address the letter correctly referring to the elected official as "The Honorable (name)".
- State the reason for writing.
- Provide brief background information about yourself.
- Keep comments short and to the point, covering only one issue per letter.
- Identify the subject clearly. Use the House or Senate bill number if available when writing about a bill.
- Explain how this issue would impact you, your community, and your state.
- Be reasonable, courteous, and respectful.
- Be constructive in your proposals.
- Avoid form letters or stereotyped phrases and sentences.
- Write when the lawmaker does something that deserves approval. A word of appreciation will create a more favorable light for the next communication.

---

you in this process (AOTA, 1995).

- **Maintain a constituent relationship.** Keep up on voting records and let lawmakers know how you feel. Get to know the administrative assistants who work with your legislators. They can provide you with a wealth of information and may be more accessible than politicians at times. Attend political functions and fundraisers. They are a great way to get involved in political campaigns.
- **Educate the public.** As a student, you have a college-wide audience. Set up a table during lunchtime to display AOTA publications, adaptive equipment, and other tools of the trade. Answer questions and provide resources. Visit your old high school during career day to promote your profession. Contact AOTA for materials that can be distributed or create your own "fact sheet." You are going to need the practice, because many people still do not know what we do. Survey your work environment for those who could benefit from knowing more about OT. April is OT month—Get out into the community wearing buttons purchased from AOTA and answer questions posed.
- **Review your insurance policy.** Check your health insurance policy for coverage of OT services. If you are not satisfied, write, call, or make an appointment to meet with your agent. Better yet, gather signatures of others you know with this coverage who are also dissatisfied to present a more powerful proposal.
- **Lobby.** Review the lobbying process presented in this chapter. Make phone calls, write letters, gather support among other students, and attend public hearings. These are all activities that are designed to get you involved.
- **Power in numbers.** Any of the activities outlined in this chapter can be done on your own. They can also be done with others as a great way to divide up the work, cover more ground, and show increased support.

These are just a few ideas to get you headed in the right direction. If an idea pops up, perhaps the guidelines in Table 4-2 will help you determine if your action project will be one you can be proud of.

Table 4-2
Developing New Political Action Ideas

- What is the purpose or goal of this project?
- Who is the target goup or individual for this project and why did you chose this group or individual?
- What resources were used to create this project (i.e., literature, materials)?
- How might this project be carried with you during various stages of your professional career?
- How will this project affect public policy regarding health care delivery for OT services? Rights for individuals with disabilities?

SUMMARY

This chapter reviewed how your national organization represents you in the political process. Your role in political action will help further the profession of OT. You have many options available to you. Match them up to your interests, your learning style, resources available to you, and your schedule, and then go out and make a difference!

BIBLIOGRAPHY

American Occupational Therapy Association. (1995). *AOTPAC national legislative conference handbook*. Bethesda, MD: Author.

American Occupational Therapy Association Government Relations Department. (1995). *AOTPAC information packet*. Bethesda, MD: Author.

Christiansen, C., & Baum, C. (Eds.). (1991). *Occupational therapy: Overcoming human performance deficits*. Thorofare, NJ: SLACK Inc.

Scott, S. J., & Acquaviva, J. D. (1985). *Lobbying for health care*. Bethesda, MD: American Occupational Therapy Association.

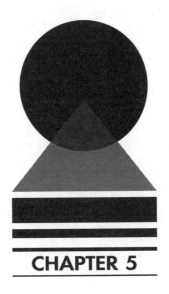

CHAPTER 5

OT FINANCIAL AID AND SCHOLARSHIPS

Karen Sladyk, MS, OTR/L

FINANCING YOUR EDUCATION

Finding the money to pay for your education is a challenge in today's economy. Most students find they need to work, but working can affect the time they have to focus on studying. Since scholarships are based on academic achievement and/or financial need, working can reduce your chances of winning a scholarship. This can be frustrating. This chapter will address scholarships and loanships that are available to OT students.

TRADITIONAL FINANCIAL AID

Any student who has applied for financial aid is familiar with the lengthy process. The best approach to federal aid is to apply as early as possible and keep detailed and accurate financial records. There are three forms of federal aid. First are grants such as the Pell Grant. This type of financial aid does not have to be paid back. Second are loans such as Stafford Loans for students and Plus Loans for parents. Loans must be paid back, usually at a lower interest rate than commercially available. Lastly, federal aid can include work-study programs. Work-study provides you with a job on campus. The job types vary greatly and can include anything from newspaper photographer to secretarial help. Since the government subsidizes the school, you are paid for your services under financial aid packages. Undergraduate students may receive all three types of federal aid, but graduate students can only receive loans and work-study.

The first step in applying for federal financial aid is to complete the *Free Application for Federal Student Aid* (FAFSA). You can get the application at any college or university. Apply as soon after January 1st of the academic year before you need the aid. Aim for no later than March 1st as many schools give priority to early applications. You will need to provide information from your and/or your parents' federal income tax report. It is important that you and your parents complete your respective tax returns as soon as possible after January 1st. If you have any questions about the application process, call 1-800-4-FED-AID (1-800-433-3243).

Your school will likely require you to complete an additional college application. This application will vary greatly from school to school. When applying to OT programs, visit the financial aid office and get an application for each college. If you are already enrolled in your college, visit your financial aid office as soon as possible; however, avoid the office the first week of classes as there are likely to be long lines.

The key to receiving the maximum financial aid package from federal or school programs is planning ahead and being persistent. Be careful about agencies that say they will find financial aid for you for a fee. Many experts believe these agencies do not provide any more information than is easily available to you on your own. Check your local library or bookstore for several guides on college financial aid.

Do not assume you are ineligible for financial aid; research your options carefully because many programs have special criteria that you may qualify for. Look for scholarships awarded by local organizations. Even if you graduated from high school several years ago, check with the high school guidance office to see what community scholarships might be available. If you have access to the Internet, visit the Washington, D.C.-based National Association of Student Financial Aid Administrators (http://www.finaid.org). This site provides free searches of more than 200,000 private scholarships (Weinstein, 1997). The federal government also has a website home page (http://www.ed.gov). At the federal government site you will find timely news and will be able to click on the 40-page student financial aid guide. If you want to go directly to the student financial aid guide, type http://www.ed.gov.prog_info/SFA/StudentGuide/.

In addition to the programs already mentioned, check with your OT program director to see if special financial aid is available to OT students at your school. The following sections will tell you about special financial aid programs for OT students.

AOTF SCHOLARSHIPS

The AOTF has as its goal the development of scholarship and research in OT. To meet the goal, AOTF has established many creative programs such as honor programs, student research grants, and scholarships. AOTF awards more than 100 OT scholarships per year. The AOTF scholarship panel reviews more than 200 applications each year. The funding is generally in the range of $500 to $1,000. Scholarships are available to associate, bachelor's, and master's degree students who apply and meet the funding requirements.

About half of the scholarships administered by AOTF are provided through state OT associations. Table 5-1 lists the states that have AOTF manage their scholarships. Residents of these states may want to investigate whether they meet the state qualifications. In addition, AOTF manages memorial scholarships created through donations in memory of prominent OT practitioners.

Students interested in applying for an AOTF scholarship should contact the Foundation through AOTA. Student members of AOTA can call 1-800-SAY-AOTA. Students who are not members can call 1-301-652-2682. Students should be aware that some scholarships require membership in AOTA or have other special requirements.

Table 5-1		
States With AOTF-Managed Scholarships		
• Arizona	• Michigan	• Oregon
• Arkansas	• Nebraska	• Pennsylvania
• Illinois	• New Hampshire	• South Carolina
• Kentucky	• New York	• Tennessee
• Louisiana	• North Carolina	• Texas
• Maryland	• Ohio	• West Virginia
• Massachusetts	• Oklahoma	• Wisconsin

LOANSHIPS

During the early 1990s, a new type of recruitment tool was developed by health care agencies to recruit OTRs. With a shortage of OTRs, health care agencies, such as hospitals, would provide scholarships to junior and/or senior OTR students if they would agree to work for the facility upon graduation. Generally, 1 year of work is required for each year of funding awarded. The funding is generally between $5,000 and $10,000 for 2 years of work. The student who accepts the scholarship agrees to repay the gift as a loan if he or she decides not to accept a job at the facility. Salaries for students who accept loanships appear to be competitive with students who do not accept loanships. Contracts are usually developed and students should seek advice before accepting this type of scholarship. Students have reported that they are happy with this type of program because it relieves the financial strain of the last 2 years of school.

Loanship information can usually be found through either your academic fieldwork coordinator or your program director. Both faculty usually are on several mailing lists and may post or file loanships. Currently, loanships are available for both COTAs and OTRs. If you find that a loanship is not offered by a facility you are interested in, consider calling the personnel office to see if they offer one. If they do not, ask if they might be interested in developing one.

Some loanships are from large agencies such as the VA Hospital System. Upon graduation, students are offered a list of hospitals across the nation with openings. Students are able to pick one of the hospitals from the list and the VA hospital assists the new OTR in relocating.

There are, of course, some negative aspects of loanships. The new OTR must fulfill the contract fully. In addition, if the student accepts another position, the scholarship must be repaid with interest agreed upon at the contract signing. Whether or not a student accepts a loanship is a personal decision that should be considered along with the student's family.

LOAN PAYBACK

A program similar to the loanships mentioned above is loan payback. Some facilities recruit new therapists by agreeing to pay back student loans. For each month the new graduate continues to work for the facility, a loan payment is made. If the COTA or OTR decides to leave, the therapist then takes over the loan repayment. This arrangement is good for the graduate with high loans at graduation. Since most college loan payments are spread out for up to 10 years, the therapist would have to work in a loan payback facility for a long time if the graduate wanted all of the loan paid. Before looking for a loan payback program, the new graduate should compare and contrast salary with other benefits such as sign-on bonuses or tuition assistance for returning to college.

BIBLIOGRAPHY

Mohan, S. (1995). AOTF 1995 scholarship awards. *Occupational Therapy Week,* June 8, 14-15.

Tobias, A. (1996, March). How to borrow like an expert. *Parade Magazine.*

U.S. Department of Education. (1996). *The student guide to financial aid.* Washington, DC: Author.

Weinstein, B. (1997, Jan 26). Shopping for college money the painless way. *The Boston Sunday Globe,* J25, J27.

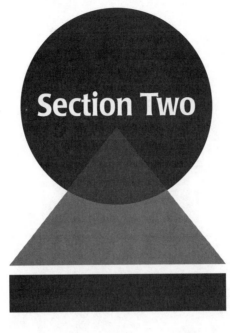

Student Skills

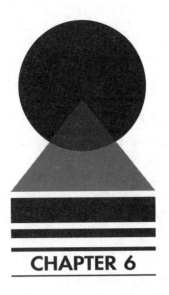

LEARNING AS A COLLEGE STUDENT

Henriette Pranger, MA

INTRODUCTION

One of the greatest problems college students face is managing their studies. Whether you are new to college or are returning for another semester, you know that developing an effective work style is critical to college success. This chapter contains ideas to help you improve your study skills. The chapter begins by advising you on how to deal with the "college crunch", a well-known phenomenon that happens to almost every student. Consider reading the chapter on self-management after you finish this chapter.

DEVELOPING A WORK STYLE THAT WORKS

The college crunch happens when you leave your schoolwork to the last minute. The situation worsens when you settle down to study and realize you underestimated how much work must be done. To deal with the college crunch, students usually adopt a survival work style that involves one of two actions. Students either cram seemingly unrelated bits of information into their heads, which is forgotten quickly after an exam, or they write a poorly organized term paper at the last minute. In both cases a passing grade may result, but what was learned? Not much. A work style characterized by procrastination and last minute bursts of energy may lead you to graduate, but this approach will not prepare you for success in the work world. The possible long-term outcomes of this work style are a low paying job and wasted college years.

What else can you do? Decide to develop an efficient work style that results in time to balance schoolwork and leisure activities. College offers the chance to learn how to han-

---

Table 6-1
Benefits of an Effective College Work Style

- More time to enjoy your life and less time spent studying.
- The ability to learn anything anywhere.
- A selective approach to reading rather than trying to read everything.
- Relative success no matter who teaches the course or what subject you take.
- Good grades, good memories, and a satisfying post-college job.

---

dle a heavy workload successfully. Even though many students do not believe so, instructors assign lots of work for a reason. The heavy workload simulates the pressures professionals experience on the job. Although you cannot change the amount of work required in college, you can decide to develop an efficient work style that enables you to avoid the college crunch and to earn good grades (Table 6-1). This chapter covers three strategies for developing an effective work style: understanding your learning style, making a positive impression on your instructors, and building general study skills that may help you organize and complete your schoolwork more effectively.

YOUR LEARNING STYLE

Developing an effective college work style begins by figuring out how you learn best. Every person does not learn in the same way. The way you learn affects what you need to learn. For example, some people need quiet in order to concentrate, while other people need background music to help them focus on a task. The person who needs quiet but decides to study in a noisy environment will take longer to complete his or her work. You can minimize the amount of time you spend studying and maximize the outcome of your study time by making choices that result in a study environment that meets your learning needs.

Psychologists have published numerous books to help students determine their learning styles and related learning needs. The college library, academic counseling center, or campus bookstore staff can help you locate written resources. A book on learning styles will describe the different ways that people learn so you can discover your learning style through reading. For example, reading a chapter or two may help you realize that you learn best through discussion. You might then choose to form a study group or to enroll in a class where the teacher relies heavily on collaborative learning groups. Or you may realize that you learn best with plenty of quiet because you need time to reflect on abstract concepts. In this case, you might choose to study in a private library room that has minimal distractions.

Completing a self-scoreable instrument is another way to obtain valuable clues to your learning style. Learning style instruments (Table 6-2) can be located with the help of your college librarian or academic counselor. Your college counselor may give you a written learning style assessment that you can complete and your answers can provide you with specific, detailed feedback about your learning needs.

An example of a learning style inventory that looks at your preferences for reading, writing, conversing, thinking, or doing is presented in Worksheet 6-1.

Table 6-2
Examples of Learning Style Inventories

- The Myers-Briggs Type Indicator
- Kolb's Learning Style Inventory
- Gardner's Multiple Intelligences
- 4MAT
- Gregoric Learning Styles Inventory

YOUR STRONGEST LEARNING PREFERENCE

Most learning style instruments help you think about ways that you take in, store, and retrieve information. Worksheet 6-1 will help you discover one of your strongest learning preferences. For example, this instrument can help you determine if you learn better by

---

Worksheet 6-1

Learning Style Characteristics Checklist

Check the following characteristics that apply to you.

1. [ ] When I have a problem, I usually tell someone right away.

2. [ ] I keep a journal.

3. [ ] I often take notes, although I do not always refer to them.

4. [ ] I take good notes and then rewrite them at a later time.

5. [ ] I read in my free time.

6. [ ] I have the TV on even if I am not watching it.

7. [ ] I have good intentions of writing to people but usually call instead.

8. [ ] I often shut my eyes to help me concentrate.

9. [ ] When studying or solving a problem, I pace back and forth.

10. [ ] I would rather hear a book on audiocassette than read it myself.

11. [ ] Forget the cassette, I would rather wait until it comes out on film.

12. [ ] I prefer reading the newspaper to watching the news on TV.

13. [ ] I prefer to study in a quiet setting.

14. [ ] To remember a spelling, I see the word in my mind.

15. [ ] I would prefer an oral exam to a written one.

16. [ ] I prefer a multiple choice format on a test.

17. [ ] I would rather do a project than write a paper.

18. [ ] I would rather give an oral report than a written one.

19. [ ] I remember better what I read rather than what I hear.

20. [ ] I keep a personal organizer.

21. [ ] I reread my notes several times.

22. [ ] I would rather take notes from the text than attend a lecture on the material.

23. [ ] I often "talk to myself."

24. [ ] I learn best when I study with a partner.	
25. [ ] I can locate a passage that I have read by "seeing it."	
26. [ ] I find it hard to sit still when I study.	
27. [ ] If I forget why I walked in the kitchen, I retrace my steps from the bedroom.	
28. [ ] Once in bed for the night, I shut my eyes and plan the next day.	
29. [ ] I cannot clean unless the music is on.	
30. [ ] I would rather read directions than have someone tell me about them.	
31. [ ] I can put something together as long as the directions are written.	

From Sladyk, K. (1996). OTR exam review manual. *Thorofare, NJ: SLACK Inc.*

listening to or by writing about a particular subject. Your learning style may be characterized by one preference or a combination of strategies may work best for you.

Scoring the Checklist

Compare your answers from your checklist to the following list. Circle the number/letter combinations that correspond to your answers.

1. S	6. L	11. V	16. V	21. R	26. D
2. W	7. S	12. R	17. D	22. W	27. D
3. DW	8. V	13. L	18. S	23. SL	28. V
4. W	9. D	14. V	19. R	24. SL	29. L
5. R	10. L	15. S	20. W	25. V	30. R
					31. R

Tally the number of S, W, D, R, L, and V responses and record the totals:

S	W	D	R	L	V

If you have three or more responses of one letter, you most likely have a preference for that learning style. Most people have at least one preference, but you may have more than one. The following descriptions provide more detail about your particular strength. As you read the descriptions, think about decisions you could make to improve your current approach to studying.

Speaking (S). Three or more checks in this area indicates a preference for learning information by saying it. Talking or conversing about the information you need to learn really helps you to learn it. Strategies that rely on speaking to learn include reading your notes and text aloud, or at least the chapter headings. You may also find it beneficial to have a study partner, or to speak into a tape recorder and play your tape back. You may ask someone to listen to you as you explain a principle. After reviewing information, play the part of a teacher by asking questions aloud. Repeat concepts aloud and ask questions of others. Any activity that involves speaking about the material will help you learn more quickly than the types of activities described below.

Writing (W). If your strength is writing, then any activity during or after class that involves writing will help you learn the material more quickly. Your study strategies should include lots of note taking from your readings. Other strategies might include rewriting your notes on paper or index cards that you can use to quiz yourself or your study partner with later. Consider making tests for yourself and take them. Make it a habit to write notes in the margins of your texts and notebooks. You may naturally do better in classes that involve lots of essay writing.

Doing (D). Often thought of as the kinesthetic modality, students who have this preference learn best by doing. If you have this type of preference, you know that you enjoy becoming involved with the material. Effective study strategies are active (e.g., making a model, map, or diagram of the information you need to learn). You may enjoy studying in an empty classroom and writing on the board. You might also find it helpful to carry index cards with the information you are trying to learn because you can pull out the cards while you are walking or exercising. Activity is the key action for this learning style and any study strategy that involves activity will help you learn the material more quickly and easily than strategies emphasizing the other preferences.

Reading (R). Learners with this preference pick up material easily through reading. Effective study strategies include borrowing other students' notes so you can read them and fill in any information you may have missed. Also consider highlighting text passages to easily locate information. Read additional articles or texts on the subject to be learned. Read and reread information because this is your preferred learning preference.

Listening (L). Learners with a preference for listening would benefit from participating in a study group or at least studying with a partner. Effective study strategies include having others read to you. Consider listening to tapes of course lectures or review sessions as often as possible. You may also find it helpful to call classmates and have them read their notes to you or quiz each other over the phone. These last two ideas may sound awkward, but if you team up with a partner who learns by speaking, you will both benefit.

Visualizing (V). If this is your learning strength, you learn best by picturing information in your head. You are apt to "see" a page of information. You benefit from closing your eyes and recalling information. You can take advantage of your gift for visualization by taking note of the way information is written, as well as the shape, color, and size of the paper. This will help you recall the information later. Effective study strategies would include using different color pens to take notes. Use these and other strategies to help your mind highlight when and where the information was learned and to facilitate recall.

Most theories emphasize that it is beneficial for you to study in more than one way. Studying that involves the use of different preferences reinforces the ideas or skills in your mind. The key is to begin studying the way you learn best and then to gradually incorporate other styles into your repertoire of study habits. The larger your repertoire, the easier you will be able to meet the demands of different types of classes and different learning challenges. Remember, your learning profile is unique, and just because your friend studies best when listening to music does not mean that listening to music will help you learn. Reading about learning styles or completing several different learning inventories will help you to be strategic about study habits. Take the time to inventory your strengths so you can develop a work style based on the way you learn best.

PROBLEM CLASSES

What happens if you take a class that requires you to learn in a way that doesn't come easily to you? Usually, you hate the class. One of the hardest times in college is when you have a teacher you don't like or you have a required class in a subject you find boring because the work doesn't come easily to you. You can be successful in these situations by developing a flexible work style. Use your knowledge of learning styles and interpersonal skills to appreciate a teacher who is very different from you. Reinterpret your dislike for the instructor as a possible mismatch between your learning needs and the teacher's instructional style. Some teachers may consider your learning style when they create assignments or teach the class. Other teachers may feel it is important to challenge you by assigning tasks that are difficult for you and that require you to use your less preferred learning styles. Learn all you can from every teacher and flex your style to adapt to the situation. To summarize, when you find yourself in a situation where your work style is very different from your teacher's style, flex. Students with effective work styles will flex their style according to the demands of the situation. This strategy, or ability to flex your work style, will bring you success in both collegiate and work environments.

Students can develop a strategy for dealing with a challenging class by paying attention to environmental clues. Keeping a brief journal the first 3 weeks of class may help. Consider jotting down observations about your teacher during the first few class meetings. Remember, how teachers learn may affect their work style or approach to teaching. Noticing a teacher's work style may prove useful to you as you figure out how to learn in class and to complete class assignments. For example, teachers who prefer to learn by listening and observation may devote the bulk of class time to lectures. Teachers who prefer to learn through discussion may devote most of class to lively dialog or collaborative work groups. If the teacher's style is opposite to your learning style, you may leave the class feeling tired or frustrated. You can decide to work smart by scheduling an activity that energizes you either before or after class. For example, you might schedule either a quiet jog or a lively lunch with friends depending on what energizes you.

Experiment and keep a learning journal in which you jot down activities you find helpful or situations that you find frustrating. Then do what works. Doing what works means making decisions that result in an effective work style. Making decisions to meet your learning needs will save you valuable time. If keeping a journal doesn't appeal to you, completing Worksheet 6-2 is another alternative.

CLASSROOM ENVIRONMENT EXERCISE

Complete Worksheet 6-2 to help determine what behaviors are part of your work style. Past behaviors provide clues on how to best deal with new classes. First, think of a course in which you did well. Read the first column and check the behaviors that best describe your memories of the course. Second, think of a course in which you did not do well. Check the items that describe your memories of the course.

When you have finished, answer these questions:

- Do you notice any patterns?
- What kinds of behaviors were helpful or not helpful?
- Based on your answers, what types of courses do you think will be easy for you and what courses will be difficult?
- What can you do to ensure success?

Developing an awareness of your learning styles and those learning requirements associated with different courses will pay off. You can use this information to make decisions about how you will tackle class assignments. For example, teachers who learn best when they focus on specific details and practical applications of theories may give high grades

Worksheet 6-2

Classroom Environment Exercise

Best Class: _____

Worst Class: _____

Behavior	Best Class ✓	Worst Class ✓
Arrived to class early.		
Asked questions before I went too far into an assignment or exercise.		
Developed a positive relationship with the teacher (e.g., stayed after class and talked).		
Enjoyed discussions that focused on the facts of the situation or theory.		
Enjoyed talking in small groups about class ideas.		
Enjoyed working with a study partner.		
Exercised choice and freedom in assignments.		
Experienced conflicts with other students.		
Experienced feelings of competitiveness.		
Felt distracted and bored.		
Felt the teacher didn't like me.		
Followed a regular study schedule.		
Followed logical, clear, detailed instructions and asked questions when the instructions were not clear.		
Found it helpful to watch films or videos on the topic.		
Gave my paper to someone else to comment on and to proofread.		
Made an outline before writing.		
Made to-do lists.		
Missed several class meetings.		
Participated actively in class exercises.		
Read the lessons before class.		
Set deadlines and met them.		
Studied alone in a quiet place.		
Studied in the library with a group.		
Studied with background music playing.		
Thought about practical applications of the theory.		
Thought for a while before I started talking or participating in a discussion.		
Understood things and mastered the task by doing it the right way.		

Behavior	Best Class ✓	Worst Class ✓
Used written assignments to think about how things could be and proposed a new way of doing things.		
Used written assignments to think about the implications or connections between ideas.		
Was creative and thought of a novel way that was a little different from the assigned task and that reflected my ingenuity.		
Worked on the easiest tasks first.		
Worked on the hardest tasks first.		
Wrote my paper the night before it was due.		
Wrote my paper without an outline.		

to practical, detail-focused essays and lower grades to more creative essays. With an awareness of work styles, you can recognize quickly different learning styles and then flex your style to match your teacher's preferences. Following this example, you might decide to devote extra time and energy to writing a practical essay and resist the temptation to write a more creative essay, despite the fact doing the latter comes more easily to you. Making assignments for problem classes a priority may also help ward off the college crunch. To avoid feeling frustrated, remind yourself that your adjustments are temporary.

IMAGE MANAGEMENT

Your decision to create a study environment that meets your learning needs will help you master course content, but college success is more than content mastery. A goal of a college education is to help you develop an *educated persona* that reflects inquisitiveness, energy, flexibility, and a passion for learning. Consequently, to earn a good grade from a teacher, you also need to manage your image. Teachers are human and the personal impression you make on teachers influences their opinion of you as much as your ability to master course content. Developing the ability to make a good impression is part of an effective work style. There are several ways you might persuade the instructor that you have become an educated person (Table 6-3).

The steps to making a good impression in college are simple: attend class, come prepared, participate, and convey a positive attitude. Teachers appreciate and admire conscientious, interested, and hard-working students. Often the teacher's course content reflects his or her life's passion. Showing respect for the teacher's ideas as well as a genuine interest in the subject will go a long way in making a good impression. In addition, try to convey an air of flexibility and adaptability.

Why are flexibility and adaptability important? Flexibility and adaptability in your interpersonal relationships with other students and teachers show that you are not narrowminded and inflexible. During your college years, you will meet people with ideas, values, and beliefs that are very different from your own. You will be asked to read, write, and participate in activities and conversations on topics and with people that you might never meet outside of college. You can develop the ability to suspend judgment tem-

---

Table 6-3
Ways to Convey an Educated Persona

- Arrive to class on time and attend all class meetings.
- Sit up front and look interested in the lecture or discussion.
- Ask pertinent questions that illustrate reflective thinking.
- Come to class prepared (e.g., read the assignments before class).
- Take notes diligently.
- Ask permission to submit written assignments to the instructor early and ask for preliminary feedback that you can address in the final work.

---

porarily by listening and considering new ideas or ideas with which you disagree. Conveying an air of flexibility and adaptability is critical to success in college as well as in the modern workplace. The modern workplace is characterized by constant change as our society adapts to the creation of new technologies. Success in a rapidly changing workplace requires the ability to be open to learning and thinking about new ideas and techniques, as well as working with teams of people quite different from yourself. Strong interpersonal skills that enable you to manage your image and to convey an air of flexibility are critical to success.

STUDY TIPS AND TRICKS

If something works, do it. Having trouble? Then try something different. The key is to learn from your experience. This applies to the topics already covered in this chapter: learning styles, classroom environments, and teacher relationships. Learning from your experience also relates to study skills. There are several ineffective study habits that have become myths on college campuses. People with ineffective collegiate work styles perpetuate these myths through their advice to other students. These myths include that you can be successful in college when you:

- Wait until the night before an exam and stay up all night cramming and drinking caffeine
- Either go to class or read the assigned books, but you do not need to do both
- Study in long, full-day marathon study sessions instead of following a study schedule that consists of short, 2-hour study sessions

These three pieces of advice are myths. Consider the advice in Table 6-4, which was generated by students with effective work styles. Which strategies you decide to use, if any, will depend on what you decide works well for you.

COLLEGE FUN

A successful work style integrates classroom learning and life experiences. A successful college student does not spend 24 hours a day, 7 days a week in the library. A successful student spends a great deal of quality time with friends because his or her effective work style enabled him or her to tackle college tasks in an organized, efficient way. He or she has time to spend enjoying leisure activities. Successful students learn, through trial and error during the college years, what personal combination of work and leisure activities gives their lives meaning. You can achieve a healthy balance between work and

Table 6-4
Effective Study Habits

Before Class

- Meet a half hour before class with a study group and discuss interesting course content.
- Find a study partner and quiz each other regularly.
- Buy a personal calendar and mark classes and assignment due dates; use a coding system to prioritize work and always do the hardest work first.
- Talk to former students who have taken the class (e.g., What was the teacher's style?).
- Ask for the syllabus before class starts. Buy the books and read before the first class.
- Complete all assigned reading before class. Reread after class.
- Read the syllabus closely and check it often.
- Tape the lecture, then listen to the tape after class. Stop the tape and ask yourself questions.
- Turn in all assignments on time. If you must miss a class meeting when an assignment is due, turn it in early.

During Class

- Arrive to class on time, consider arriving early, never arrive late.
- Sit in the first or second row of lecture classes.
- Take notes on what you do not know, not what you do know.
- Ask questions.
- If you are called on and do not know the answer, politely say so.
- Keep side conversations during class to a minimum.
- Ask yourself key questions to help relate new information to past experiences, beliefs, and ideas.
- Attend all classes. If you must miss a class, call the instructor beforehand and explain why you won't be there. Arrange, on your own, to have two or three other students take notes for you. It is your responsibility to figure out what you missed.

After Class

- Realize studying is more than reading. Shut the book, ask yourself questions, and recite the answers aloud. Then take notes on the questions you could not answer.
- Visit the teacher once or twice during office hours and ask an intelligent question.
- Start a phone/address list, index card file, or database table to record resources that you can use later in your professional life. For example, teachers provide addresses of health associations you can use in later classes.
- Consider converting your notes to flash cards (i.e., question on front, answer on back). This is a helpful technique for classes that require a great deal of memorization like medical terminology.
- Keep flash cards with you at all times and quiz yourself in your spare moments.
- Squeeze in study time, always carry a book, and learn new things in small chunks (e.g., one page at a time).
- Schedule regular times on your personal calendar to study for a class in 2-hour blocks.
- Study what you do not know, not what you do know.
- Ask someone else to proofread your written papers.
- Copy over your class notes using colored pens and highlight key ideas.
- When information is difficult to memorize (i.e., anatomy and physiology classes), make giant posters on newsprint and post them around your room. Look at them and think about the information while you are doing simple tasks such as dressing or cleaning.

school. Your effective approach to studying will leave you time to spend with friends and family. One way to balance activities is to integrate them. For example, you can take advantage of the cultural and intellectual activities offered at college because they deepen your knowledge of classroom topics. Consider the following list of ways to integrate collegiate and extra-collegiate activities:

- Read the school newspaper and submit articles or letters to the editor.
- Attend lectures on topics of personal interest or related to class assignments.
- Participate in cultural festivals, movies, plays, and concerts. Listen for opinions that support or challenge ideas covered in class.
- Spend time with family and friends discussing how ideas learned in college are supported, challenged, or changed when applied in the work world.
- Attend classes and do homework following a daily schedule that has leisure activities scheduled as part of the week.

Attempts to achieve balanced and integrated thinking will lead to college success. Use extra-collegiate activities not as opportunities to escape classwork, but as opportunities to think about and apply classroom learning on a deeper, more personal level. This is the last goal of a college education.

SUMMARY

To help you avoid the college crunch, this chapter presented some ideas on how to develop an effective work style. The chapter discussed the value of understanding how you learn best, creating a helpful study environment, and conveying an educated persona. The chapter ended with some advice from successful college students about how to develop good study habits. Although students may disagree about the definition of college success, graduates agree that the college experience provides an opportunity to develop an effective work style that will lead not only to success in college but in the work world. Hopefully, this chapter gave you a few ideas to help you strengthen your current approach to your studies.

BIBLIOGRAPHY

Ellis, D. G. (1985). *Becoming a master student*. Rapids City, SD: College Survival Inc.

Gordon, L. (1989). *People types and tiger stripes*. Gainesville, FL: Center for the Applications of Psychological Type.

Kolb, D. A. (1984). *Experiential learning: Experience as a source of learning and development*. Englewood Cliffs, NJ: Prentice Hall.

McCarthy, B. (1990). Using the 4MAT system to bring learning styles to schools. *Educational Leadership, 48*(2), 31-38.

Meisgeier, C., Murphy, E., & Meisgeier, C. (1989). *A teacher's guide to type: A new perspective to individual differences in the classroom*. Palo Alto, CA: Consulting Psychologists Press.

Sladyk, L. (1996). How to study for the exam. In K. Sladyk (Ed.), *OTR exam review manual*. Thorofare, NJ: SLACK Inc.

Smith, L. N., & Walter, T. L. (1995). *The adult learner's guide to college success*. Boston: Wadsworth Publishing Co.

Steltenpohl, E., Shipton, J., & Villines, S. (1996). *Orientation to college: A reader on becoming an educated person*. Boston: Wadsworth Publishing Co.

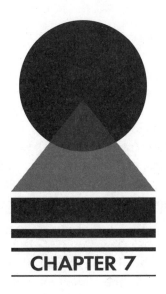

CHAPTER 7

LEARNING AS AN OT STUDENT

Karen Sladyk, MS, OTR/L

INTRODUCTION

The previous chapter of this primer discussed learning as a college student, but there is no doubt that being an OT student makes you different from other college learners. You have chosen a career that involves helping other human beings in a very personal way. It is your faculty's responsibility that you learn how to take care of this valuable resource. As an OT student, you are likely to be tested in many challenging ways. There will be information that must be memorized not only for a test but for the rest of your life. There will be many experimental and experiential projects for you to participate in. At the very least, you will have more fieldwork experiences than most students at the associate or bachelor's degree level.

As an OT student you will likely be attentive to your grades. Your program may require a minimum GPA to get into the program and a minimum GPA to stay in the program. Even if there is no minimum GPA, you may find that your classmates, as a whole, are high achievers and this may lead to a competitiveness. You may have as a goal to maintain a certain level of grades yourself. Perhaps you want to make dean's list or graduate with honors. You may want to work at a special facility that has many applicants, so you want your schooling to stand out. Whatever the motivation, doing well in OT school requires some careful planning.

GETTING ORGANIZED

This primer has several chapters that are designed to get you going in your studies. If you have not done so already, review Chapter 6 on learning in college. Later in this book you will find chapters on what to do if you are not passing and how to manage your time. This chapter will look at issues that develop because you are an OT student. Specifically, this chapter will discuss OT instructors, OT textbooks, note taking in class and from your textbook, and, finally, getting ready for OT exams. The section on studying for exams will review getting ready for practicals, multiple choice, and problem-based tests.

ANATOMY OF AN OT PROFESSOR

Before you even arrive in OT classes you are likely to have experienced many types of classes with many types of teachers. Once you have begun your OT classes it is time to "decode" your OT professors. So what is a typical OT professor like? The answer is "It depends." Just like OTs who work in the clinic, you will find great variety of OTs who work in education. Here are some unique qualities that OTRs who specialize in education share in common.

- Almost always, the OT educator took a substantial cut in pay when he or she moved from the clinic to education. There must have been some special reason why a person would do this. It is likely that the desire to teach new COTAs and OTRs was so strong that he or she was willing to reduce his or her income to be part of the experience.
- OT professors are generally available to their students, not only to advise them about class material, but to help in developing the professional person. You will find that OT professors are involved in many academic activities outside of the classroom and that they are willing to share their experiences with students.
- OT professors have similar characteristics to OT personnel in the clinic, but OT professors transform their love of meaningful activities into creative assignments. The goal is to develop a new COTA or OTR with flexible and adaptable thinking. As a student, you may not like every assignment, but your faculty has developed a long-range plan for your professional development.
- Although an OT professor may only be in the classroom 12 to 20 hours per week, you can guarantee that three times as many hours are spent preparing, writing lectures, developing tests, and correcting papers, projects, and presentations. In addition, your professors are likely to be doing clinical work, research, or going to graduate school all at the same time.

So what does all this mean? OT educators are a special breed of OTs. They are creative, bright, adaptive, and flexible. They appreciate students who are taking an active role in their education and OT professors enjoy helping students grow professionally. On the flip side, OT professors become upset when students whine about workloads, want to be spoonfed classroom material, or look for the easy way out of every assignment. These are traits that are not professional and show a resistance to growth. When a student gets a reputation of unprofessional behavior, it is difficult to change. The best attack for a reputation of professional behavior is to be professional from the start.

Now that we have looked at what makes OT professors tick, it is time to look at how to study OT. The next section of this chapter will address books, note taking, and test taking. Key to this idea is developing your own study environment. Your study environment will be a place where you can successfully sit down and attend to the serious task of studying OT. Consider reading the chapters in this book about learning in college, self-management skills, and OT papers, projects, and presentations.

HOW YOU LEARN BEST

Each person has a particular way that they learn information best. Even when you look at OT students who are all learning the same information, each student has a particular way they prefer to study. Return to Chapter 6 in this primer to examine your learning style. When setting up your study environment, consider your learning strengths and weaknesses. Reflect on how your learning style will affect your reading textbooks, taking notes, and preparing for exams. Consider all these issues as you read the following sections of this primer. By integrating your learning style with the advice that follows, you have custom designed your own learning environment.

OT TEXTBOOKS

The cost of your OT books will likely be twice as much as your friends' in other majors. This is not because OT books are so expensive, it is because you may have to buy more books than another major. As you write the check in the bookstore, you may ask yourself, "Why so many books?" The answer to that question lies in the fact that you will be treating human beings. There is no room or tolerance for not knowing what you are doing. A business or humanities major has time for great thinking; as a future COTA or OTR, you may not have the luxury of time. The best advice is to buy all the OT books you can and keep them for your professional library after graduation.

Now for reality. OT faculty know that students do not always buy every book and often sell books back at the end of the semester for cash. There are many reasons why students do not buy all the books required for an OT class and there are many reasons why students sell books back at the end of the year. Table 7-1 lists some of the reasons you should buy all the books.

Ask yourself this important question: Would you want a COTA or OTR to treat you or your parents if you knew he or she had only bought half of the textbooks in OT school?

Solutions to Book Buying Problems

There is no doubt that buying $700 worth of books your first semester is going to hurt. Table 7-2 lists some creative ways of saving some money.

Enough said about books. The bottom line is: It is your responsibility to be professionally prepared when you graduate. This means having the books you need to be prepared.

TAKING NOTES IN OT CLASS

By this time in your academic career, you have likely managed to develop a note taking pattern that is successful. Many OT students find that they become more successful by developing a more refined system of taking notes. Note taking is the process of taking auditory information and transforming it to visual information. This cognitive skill seems simple enough until you add a fast-talking teacher, information that is new to you, or information that you do not understand.

You can always ask a teacher to slow down, but this is often as difficult as asking a 5-year-old to wait for Santa. OT professors teach because they are excited about what they are talking about. Sometimes it is difficult for a professor to understand why the whole class is not as excited as they are. In addition, teachers know that they can only spend a

Table 7-1
Buying and Keeping OT Books

Reason Not to Buy	Reason to Buy	Reason to Keep
No money.	Having no money in college is no fun, but books should be a priority if you want the best value from your education.	Selling books back may give you quick cash but that will be gone quickly. You rarely get the book's real value.
Upperclassmen said you don't really need that book.	Ask yourself if this is a person who acts as professional as you want to be. Maybe this advice is from a person who missed the point.	
The book is on a topic that you are sure you will never practice in once you graduate.	You never know if you like something until you have tried it.	All topics are covered on the certification exam. Will you have the information you need to study for the exam?
The book is way over your head and you do not understand it.	What seems hard in the beginning of the semester seems so easy at the end. Give yourself a break, you'll get it soon.	As a professional, schoolwork will seem easy. Once you are working, you will want more advanced books to read. (Honest, this is true!)
Other students say that the reading is never on the tests.	That doesn't mean that you do not need to know the information. Your goal should be to be the best COTA or OTR possible, not to only learn what is on the tests.	A true professional wants to know more than what had to be memorized for the tests in school.

Table 7-2
Saving Money

Ways to Save	How Much It Will Help
Buy used books	You likely already know about saving with used books. Generally you will save 25% by buying used over new at your college bookstore. Before you buy your books, check the area bulletin boards. Sometimes you can buy from a former student at even greater discounts.
Cost spreading	Plan ahead and find out what books are needed next semester or next year. Buy them in the summer when you may have a little more cash. Since the bookstore generally pays half price for a book that will be used again, buy the book directly from a student at 60%. They get more and you save 40% off new.
Cost sharing	If you are unsure about a book, split the cost with room-mates or class peers. When the semester is done you can

	raffle off the book or if someone really wants it, they can buy it from their peers.
Join AOTA as a student member	OT books bought from AOTA are discounted for members. Usually the discount will cover the cost of membership plus you still get the journals, newspaper, and conference discounts.
Check discount book chains	Some books used in OT classes can be found in general public bookstores at discounted prices. If the book is something that might be read by the general public, check the discounted stores first.
Join a co-op bookstore	You maybe lucky enough to have a co-op bookstore on campus but most bookstores are for profit. A co-op bookstore gives you a refund check depending on how well the bookstore does and how much you spent. Most co-ops let outside members join and will order books for you.
Form your own mini co-op	Publishers are likely to give a discount if you buy from them in volume. Form a group of 10 people and see if you can buy directly from the publisher and save. Share the responsibility of organizing the task.

limited amount of time on a topic and they want to give you as much information as possible. The bottom line is that fast-talking teachers are not speed talking on purpose. They truly are trying to give you a wealth of information in a short time. Examine the ways of dealing with this problem:

- **Use "I" statements** to politely ask the teacher to slow down. Example: "I am having a difficult time keeping up with my notes. I would appreciate it if the lecture pace could be slowed a bit. Avoid "you" statements. Bad Example: "You must think we are speed writers. Can you slow down?"
- **Use shorthand or abbreviations.** Example: pt = patient, b/c = because, w = with, (I) = independent, ^ = increased. Do not worry about getting every word down unless you are writing a definition.
- **Use a tape recorder** and copy your notes down later. This allows you to listen to the original lecture and think about what is being said.
- Make an agreement with a peer or two to **share notes**. Have deadlines to provide each other with photocopies.
- **Sit in the front row.** Time and time again, the best students are the ones who sit up front.

When information is being presented that is new or confusing to you, it is easy to get overwhelmed and not be able to keep up with note writing. The first question that must be asked is "Is it just me or is the whole class confused?" Even if you are not the only one, the teacher may not slow down because he or she may believe you should understand what is being discussed. No one said college would be easy. Either way, here are some ways of dealing with this problem:

- **Read the assigned readings before and after class.** Before class, focus on the words that will be used in lecture. Develop an abbreviation list to start your notes out. Keep a list of abbreviations on the inside front cover of your notebook. After class, read the assignment for content and understanding.

- **Use a tape recorder** and copy your notes down later. This allows you to listen to the original lecture and think about what is being said.
- Make an agreement with a peer or two to **share notes.** Have deadlines to provide each other with photocopies.
- Go to the learning center on campus and **sign up for a tutor.** Tutors are usually former students who got As in the class. Ask them how they did it.
- **See the professor during open office hours.** Go into the office with a specific list of prepared questions. Have your notebook ready for inspection. No whining or complaining—remember, your professional image is being formed.
- **Recopy and organize your notes ASAP after the lecture.** This way you are likely to still remember details. Get the task done and out of the way as soon as possible.
- **Sit in the front row.** Time and time again, the best students are the ones who sit up front.

The best students do a lot of these coping skills as part of their everyday note taking. If you are a commuter student, you can take advantage of driving time while listening to a lecture. You can even listen to lectures while taking a walk or exercising. Sharing notes with peers allows you to pick up missed information in your notes, but can be a problem if one person takes advantage of the others. Recopying your notes allows you to organize the material in a way that is best for you. Many OT students use different colored pens and markers to visually organize their notes. Lastly, it is true that students who sit in the front row stay more alert and therefore take better notes.

TAKING NOTES FROM YOUR TEXTBOOKS

Sometimes you will be expected to cover more information in your OT readings than was covered in class. Taking good book notes becomes a key to mastering a large volume of information. There are many different ways to take notes from your books. The easiest way to note the important information is to use a highlighting marker to point out the important text. One problem with this approach is that students sometimes over highlight, resulting in paragraphs of pink or yellow smudge. Another way is to annotate the text. This means that the reader writes notes in the margins of the book. This method may be more effective than highlighting because it requires you to be more alert. The last way to take notes from a text is similar to taking notes in the classroom. On a separate paper, the student summarizes what has been read in the textbook. One benefit of this type of book note taking is that the student can add the book notes to the class notes for ease in studying.

The task of taking notes from your textbooks can seem overwhelming at times because the book is often full of details you might not understand yet. No matter what method of book note taking you use, there are some guidelines for making the task efficient. Use the following plan to map your way through a textbook and arrive at the destination of understanding more effectively.

- Do not start highlighting, annotating, or note taking until you have quickly read the entire assignment first.
- Read one section of the assignment at a time and then go back and note the important aspects.
- Continue reading sections and noting until the entire assignment is read.

- Note the generalizations, relationships, or main ideas.
- Consider using different color pens, such as pink for definitions, green for main ideas, etc.
- Use a paper or electronic dictionary to look up every word you do not know. Often, poor vocabulary is the main reason for not understanding a test question.
- Summarize each assignment with a key sentence.
- Do not overdo it. Too much highlighting or note taking makes studying more difficult.

STUDYING FOR TESTS—MEMORIZE AND APPLY

I am reminded of an OT professor explaining how some of her OT freshman memorize range of motion (ROM). She said some learn the directions and store the information in their brain. In the brain, it is available for the next step of learning manual muscle testing (MMT). Some students learn ROM directions and store the information in their bladder. As soon as the test is done they relieve themselves so that they can have room to memorize the new material. The professor called this the "Diuretic Effect" and it speaks to the importance of building skills on skills.

Students are often surprised to learn that they will be held accountable for information learned in earlier classes and will be responsible for integrating information in upper level classes. Integration means that you are expected to not only remember ROM from freshman intro class, but also muscles from anatomy and physiology and movements from kinesology, and apply that knowledge in MMT lab. This is different from your liberal arts and sciences classes. A history professor would never expect you to build on your literature class in Western civilization. So what does this mean to you the OT student? It means a different approach to memorizing information.

MEMORIZING

The goal of memorizing in OT school is adding the information to long-term memory so you can retrieve it later. Information stored in short-term memory is not likely to stay with you and will make learning more difficult later. The key to memorizing information in long-term memory is slow and gradual study. Last minute "all nighters" will only result in short-term memory. If you are lucky, the short-term memory will hold out for the test but even that might be too hopeful. A slow and steady approach works best.

Generally, any information that might be considered basic to another more complex concept is the kind of data that can be memorized. Medical terminology is a perfect example of information that must be memorized and retained for later. Medical terminology is basic for documentation. Muscle movement is basic to MMT. ROM is basic to activity analysis, which is basic to treatment planning, which is basic to quality assurance.

The first step in memorizing information is organizing the data. Keep in mind your learning style and make a plan on how the information can best be organized so that you learn it.

The second step is to develop different ways of presenting the information to yourself. Will you use visual posters as well as practice with a peer? Examine Table 7-3 for different modalities to memorize information.

The last step in memorizing data is applying the information. Can you take the directions for ROM and perform it on a peer? Do not attempt to apply the information until you have mastered enough of the data to understand what you are doing. If you try to apply too soon, you will only get confused and frustrated. You will know you have both memorization and application down when "lightbulbs start turning on." When you have reached the application phase, it is good to practice with a peer. Once you have mastered the skill you have been learning, try changing the problem a little. For example, let us say that you are learning ROM. You will have a practical exam in lab and will be expected to show you can do ROM on a peer. Practice until you are good and then ask your peer to cause a slight problem, such as being crabby or having a weak arm. Problem solve what you would do. This will reinforce the application aspect of memorizing the ROM directions.

TAKING OT TESTS

Tests are a natural part of going to OT school. Exams have a long history of measuring your progress in classes. Even if you have a teacher who says that he or she does not give tests, what the teacher likely means is no pen and paper tests. The key to succeeding on OT tests is keeping up with your studies all along. Never leave reading assignments or practice homework until the last minute. It is impossible to try to complete a month's assignments in 24 hours before a test. Make sure you understand what is expected of you well before your final studying. Ask appropriate questions of the instructor such as:

- What format will the test take?
- If there are essay questions, will I have a choice?
- Will I know the weight of each question?
- Is the test comprehensive or focused on a certain area?

Students often get in trouble by asking inappropriate questions that upset the professor such as:

- Do we have to know this for the final? The teacher may not know yet.
- Does spelling count? Yes, a college student should know how to spell.
- How fast will we know our grade? As fast as the teacher can get to them.

Just like the variety that comes with OT papers, projects, and presentations, OT tests come in a variety also. Tests are likely to be pen and paper tasks, but can include practical exams as well. One thing is for sure, after you have completed all your classes and your fieldwork, you will have to take the "big test," the National Board for Certification in Occupational Therapy (NBCOT) exam. The NBCOT exam certifies that you are a competent health care professional ready to treat patients. To get you ready for the NBCOT exam, your faculty will provide you with many different ways to show that you have mastered the OT material they have covered. The following sections will discuss different approaches to taking tests in OT school. If you need more help, consider visiting your school's learning resource center. They likely have many programs for problem test takers.

Practical Tests

A practical test usually involves the student demonstrating competence by showing the faculty they have mastered the assignment. Examples might include doing ROM on a peer or giving part of a standardized assessment. Most students get more nervous about a practical test than any other type of exam. This is probably because the teacher is watch-

Table 7-3
How to Memorize Information

Technique	How It Works Best
Study peer group	Form a group of peers to review the information. Make sure that each member understands his or her responsibility to the group. Avoid asking only friends so that socializing does not interfere with studying. Share study techniques and resources, and quiz each other.
Copy your notes over	Keep two notebooks for each class. One is for class and contains your original notes. The second notebook has your originals copied over. Use the second notebook to organize and highlight your notes. Keep notes on the readings in your second notebook.
Flash cards	Put the information you are studying on index cards. Take the cards with you and review when you have 10 minutes before class, between studying for other topics, or while you wait for an appointment or ride.
Wall posters	Use large sheets of newsprint (craft store) or freezer paper (grocery store near tinfoil) to make large study sheets. Hang the posters in places you spend time, such as the kitchen while you clean up or bathroom while you brush your teeth.
Cassette tapes	Say a question into a tape recorder, pause, and then say the information. While listening, try to say your answer before the tape gives you an answer. Share tapes with peers.
Recite	Walk around reciting what you are learning. The verbal feedback will reinforce what you are reading. This works well with your outlines or flash cards.
Develop acronyms	Remember in fourth grade music class you learned G clef—Every good boy deserves fudge.
Worksheets	Develop your own worksheets and share them with peers.
Game night	Invite your study peers over for game night. Model your game after a favorite TV game show. Ask each participant to come to game night with a category ready. Follow the rules of the game completely but substitute the information you are studying for the questions. Use snacks as prizes.

ing just you during the exam. Practical tests require that students not only memorize information but also apply the information in a correct way. Because this can be so nerve-racking, the key to success means early studying. Have the information you need to have memorized completed at least 3 days before the test. Start to practice the application with yourself. Pretend you are the patient and talk out loud to yourself. Once you are confident, begin practicing with a peer.

Always start a practical test by greeting your "patient." Explain what you are doing to the patient and ask him or her to give you feedback (i.e., "Let me know if this hurts, Mrs. Smith."). By greeting and explaining first, you show the teacher that you know what is to be done even if you make a mistake in the application. In addition, the explanation will help you get over the initial anxiety and make you more comfortable. If you are so nervous that you are forgetting everything, simply ask the instructor for 1 minute to gain your composure and then continue.

Sometimes there is too much information for the teacher to check with every student. For example, you may have learned six pediatric assessments in lab but the teacher will only test one. It is assumed that you were a responsible student and you learned all six. You may walk into the test and pull a card from a pile of the possible assessments. Never say to the teacher "Oh good, I studied that one" or "Oh, I was hoping I did not get that one." These types of statements are like saying, "I really did not have the time or interest in studying all the work you gave me, so I just did the minimum I thought I could get away with." It does not add to your professional image and it certainly will not put the teacher in a good mood.

Multiple Choice Tests

Multiple choice tests are often students' favorite because there is something reassuring in knowing that the right answer is there, you just have to find it. Generally, teachers do not like to give multiple choice tests because they may not accurately measure what the student knows. If the class is large, the material is appropriate, or if there are time limits to the test, than multiple choice tests are a logical choice.

The key to mastering a multiple choice test is reading the question clearly and knowing the answer before looking at the choices. Many students miss a correct answer because they do not read the question clearly or read too much into the question. It is important to pay attention to your learning style as you approach a multiple choice test. If you learn best by auditory input, read the question out loud to yourself. If your friends say you hyper-analyze everything, then keep the question simple. If you are easily distracted, bring white paper with you and use it as a bookmark to cover your answers. Learn about how you learn before you take the test.

Students are almost always nervous in a test. Occasionally, students feel that the teacher is trying to stump them on a test. Generally, teachers try to make multiple choice questions clear and concise. Usually, there are no trick questions; it's just the nervousness bubbling up. Before you label a question a trick question, read each word out loud to yourself. Sometimes what your eyes see and what your brain sees are different. Check Table 7-4 for other helpful multiple choice test hints.

Problem-Based or Essay Tests

When test questions require long answers, the teacher is usually looking for evidence that the student has mastered concepts or integrated different levels of information. Preparing for this type of test means understanding the important concepts covered in class and your textbook. The best way to approach this type of test is to practice writing answers to your own questions. If the questions are likely to cover some math, such as biokinematics, practice solving formula questions. If the questions are likely to involve comparing and contrasting, such as frames of reference, practice case studies. Make practice tests and share them with your peers. Set time limits to answer different questions. Use the plan in Table 7-5 to map your way through a problem-based or essay test.

Table 7-4
Helpful Multiple Choice Test Hints

- Look for qualifiers first. Are there any *all, none, never, often, except* options?
- Whenever possible, answer the question before looking at the available answers.
- The best answer will likely be grammatically correct with the question. After you have picked the best answer, read the question followed by your answer. Does it flow?
- When a question involves numbers, the answer is usually in the middle.
- Look for obviously wrong answers that are flippant or humorous.
- Always fill in every question. A blank answer is always wrong. You at least have a chance at a guess.
- Reason actively. Cross out any answers that you know are untrue and then make an educated guess at the remainder.
- Look for clues in other questions to help you understand a difficult question.
- If you are recording your answers on a separate bubble sheet, make sure the numbers always correspond.
- Do not get distracted by irrelevant information. Ask yourself, "What is the point of this question?"
- Make sure your name is on both the test and the bubble sheets. As simple as this sounds, many students forget to put their name on tests.

Table 7-5
Helpful Hints for Problem-Based or Essay Tests

- Never jump right into an essay test. Take a few minutes to read the test questions, establish a plan of action, make an outline, and decide how much time to give to each answer.
- Start with the questions you can easily answer but do not spent too much time with them. The hard questions will require more time.
- Answer "short answer" questions without outlining, but always outline an essay question before writing.
- If you run out of time, pass in your outline.
- If the answer will be longer than eight sentences, have an introduction and summary.
- Watch grammar and spelling.
- Always write neatly. If this is a problem for you, print all answers.
- Cross out errors with one line through it and rewrite the correct answer. Do not black out parts of an answer.
- If a question is too difficult, break it into small parts and answer each part individually.

SUMMARY

The key to succeeding in your OT program is making your goal to be the best COTA or OTR you can be. This chapter discussed issues special to OT students, including your professional library, studying like an OT, and succeeding on OT exams. Specific examples of studying techniques were offered, as well as managing your professional image during exams.

BIBLIOGRAPHY

Apps, J. W. (1982). *Study skills for adults returning to school*. New York: McGraw-Hill.

Armstrong, W. H. (1983). *Study tactics*. Woodbury, NY: Barron's Educational Inc.

Coman, M. J. (1990). *How to improve your study skills*. Lincolnwood, IL: VGM Career.

Davies, D. (1986). *Maximizing examination performance*. New York: Nichol Publishing.

Feder, B. (1979). *The complete guide to taking tests*. Englewood Cliffs, NJ: Prentice-Hall.

Frender, G. (1990). *Learning to learn*. Nashville, TN: Incentives Publications.

Semones, J. (1991). *Effective study skills*. Fort Worth, TX: Semones Publishing.

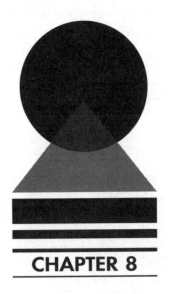

CHAPTER 8

OT PAPERS, PROJECTS, AND PRESENTATIONS

Karen Sladyk, MS, OTR/L

INTRODUCTION

OT faculty usually take their love for activity and transform it into student papers, projects, and presentations. In your career as an OT student, you may have close to 100 different tasks to do for evaluation and grades. Although you may prefer one type of assignment over another, a variety of challenges will add to the flexibility of your thinking. The key to all assignments is allowing yourself thinking and organization time.

OT PAPERS

No doubt you have written many papers before you even started your classes in OT. OT faculty will assume that you have the minimal writing skills of an upper level college student. If writing has been a problem for you, this is the place to get everything in order. Do the quick self-assessment (Worksheet 8-1) to evaluate your level of college writing. If you have several answers in the "no" column, you are a candidate for improved writing. Even minor changes in your approach to writing can improve your grades. Evaluate where you missed the writing skills you need and how you can correct the problem (Table 8-1).

You may ask yourself, "What's the big deal about doing only fair on my papers?" OT faculty will tell you that writing is one of the most important skills a COTA or OTR has. Writing is required for mastery of documentation, and documentation is essential in today's health care environment. A COTA or OTR must be able to communicate effectively if the profession of OT is to continue to grow like other health professions. Poor

Worksheet 8-1

Is Writing a Problem?

Question	Yes	No
Do you generally get a high grade on your paper?		
Are you happy with the grades your papers get?		
Do your papers come back with less than three spelling corrections?		
Do your papers come back with less than two grammar corrections?		
Do you think that the reader of your papers got the point?		
Have you ever used the writing lab, academic tutoring center, or learning center at your school for extra help?		
Do you think about possible topics or content for a paper at least 1 week ahead of the due date?		
Do you outline your idea in your head or on paper before you start?		
Do you include theories, opinions, and arguments to the main point?		
Do you include an introduction and summary in every paper?		
Do you have bridges between each paragraph or section, such as "In the next section,...will be discussed in detail."?		
Do you start with a first draft then revise and edit several times?		
Do you have a paper done 24 hours before the deadline?		
Do you ask at least one other person to read your paper for grammar and spelling?		
Do you ask someone to read the paper to see if the main point is clear?		
Do you take advantage of special learning programs in your school's learning center?		

writing skills give a poor image to both the professional and the profession. To be respected by others, it is important that you project your best personal and professional image.

No one likes to get negative feedback on their writing. When we get feedback, both negative and positive, we tend to take it personally and allow it to affect our self-image. If your writing is not your best work, make a commitment to improve your writing this semester. Students are more likely to succeed at improving their writing if they write out a plan of action. Write your goal and your plan in Worksheet 8-2.

EVALUATING YOUR OWN WRITING

You may not always be able to run to the learning center on your campus to get help on a paper. There will be times, especially late at night, when you will have to count on yourself for a thorough review of your paper. Use Worksheet 8-3 to evaluate each paper before you turn it in.

Table 8-1
Starting a Writing Improvement Plan

Did not do well in high school writing, English is a second language, never had a lot of writing to do before college.	Each school usually has an academic center where students can get extra help in college work. Consider speaking with someone in your school's learning center to find out what services are available to you.
Took English Composition 101 in your first year but did not do as well as you wanted.	Retake the class, reread the text and your class notes, or see if the learning center has a refresher workshop. Ask your peers to read your paper before you pass it in, make corrections, and mentally make a goal not to repeat the problem areas.
Your writing is good when you take the time, but usually you pull an "all nighter" to get your papers done.	Read the chapter on self-management skills in this primer.

Worksheet 8-2

Writing Improvement Plan for This Semester

Goal	Plan

APA FORMAT FOR OT PAPERS

Each OT faculty might ask you to follow a particular style when writing a paper for OT class. As a general rule, most professional OT papers published in journals follow the format detailed by the American Psychological Assocation (APA). You can purchase the *Publication Manual of the American Psychological Association* (4th ed.) (1995) at your local bookstore. The manual is generally in stock because it is used by so many people in health care, education, and research.

This primer includes the basics of APA format for OT papers. Before completing a paper for OT class, be sure you have asked the instructor what is expected in the style. If the instructor says to use APA format, be sure you understand to what degree the teacher

---

Worksheet 8-3

Paper Self-Evaluation

[ ] Introduction and summary paragraph. Every good paper has one of each.

[ ] Main point clear. Will the reader understand my point?

[ ] Support. Theories, opinions, and arguments support the main point.

[ ] Integration. Terms and information talked about in class are integrated into the paper.

[ ] Bridges. Paper has "The next section will discuss...For example,...Analysis shows..."

[ ] Flow. If the paper was read aloud, it would sound smooth not choppy.

[ ] Typed. Unless specifically told to hand write, all work should be typed for a professional look.

[ ] Spelling correct. Paper is free of spelling errors including words missed by the spellchecker.

[ ] Grammar correct. Basic rules of grammar are followed, the paper has a smooth flow.

[ ] No contractions. No *couldn't, shouldn't, wouldn't, I'll*. Write out both words.

[ ] No run-on sentences. Each sentence has no more than two thoughts and only one *and, but, or*.

[ ] No vague words. Leave out *a lot, a real lot, so many, very, a ton, hardly any*.

[ ] No blackened words. If you make an error, put one line through it and correct it neatly above.

[ ] Use correction liquid as appropriate. No teacher likes to read a paper that is painted with correction liquid.

[ ] All ideas not your original ideas are referenced. Plagiarism is a serious matter.

---

expects. If the instructor says complete APA, then buy the 368-page APA publication manual from the bookstore and follow it completely. Many times the instructor will accept the title page, citations, and reference list to follow APA, which are the three elements we will focus on here.

CITATIONS APA STYLE

The type of paper you are writing will dictate how many references you are using. If the paper is an opinion paper, you will have less references than if the paper is research based. Either way, any idea that is not your original idea must be referenced in two places. First, in the text of the paper, and second, in the reference list in the back of the paper. Citations in the text will be discussed first.

There are three different ways to cite a reference in the body of the text. All three include the author's last name (surname) and the year of publication. Choose one of the following.

Christiansen (1991) discussed the role of occupational performance assessment related to dysfunction.

In 1991, Christiansen discussed the role of occupational performance assessment related to dysfunction.

The role of occupational performance assessment was related to dysfunction (Christiansen, 1991).

If the information you are referencing is written by two authors, you must include both surnames. Notice how the word "and" or "&" is used.

Struther and Schell (1991) addressed the effect of public policy on performance.

In 1991, Struther and Schell discussed the effect of public policy on performance.

Public policy has had an effect on performance (Struther & Schell, 1991).

If the information you are referencing is written by three, four, or five authors, you must include all the names the first time you cite them. After the first citation, use only the surname of the first author followed by "et al." Notice that et al. has a period after al. In addition, pay attention to how commas are used. In APA format, a comma is always before the word "and" with three or more words, but not for only two words.

Allen, Earhart, and Blue (1992) used a cognitive approach to psychosocial illness. Allen et al. believes this approach is helpful to understanding mental illness and functioning.

In 1992, Allen, Earhart, and Blue used a cognitive approach to psychosocial illness. Allen et al. believes this approach is helpful to understanding mental illness and functioning.

A cognitive approach to psychosocial illness was used (Allen, Earhart, & Blue, 1992). Allen et al. believes this approach is helpful to understanding mental illness and functioning.

Other unique citations in the text of the paper include:
- Group as the author: (American Occupational Therapy Association, 1995)
- Unknown author: (Anonymous, 1994)
- Same last name: (P. Smith & R. Smith, 1993)

REFERENCE PAGE OF OT PAPER

After you have completed all the citations in the text, it is time to develop the reference list at the back of the paper. Some students wait until the paper is completely done before doing the reference page, others develop the reference page as they go along. Generally, the reference page will take longer than you think, so plan accordingly.

The reference page has some rules.

The typing format is as follows:
- Indent the first line
- Type the author's surname followed by a comma. Example: Smith,
- Type first initial period space then second initial period. Example: Smith, H. J.
- Use an "&" to separate two or more names Example: Smith, H. J., & Melling, B. S.
- Use a comma to separate several names. Example: See below
- Type the year in parentheses followed by a period. Example: (1996).
- Type the title in lowercase letters followed by a period. Example: Reliability of the BaFPE.
- If title is a book, underline. Example: <u>Elder care</u>.
- If title is a journal article, do not underline. Example: Reliability of the BaFPE.
- If title is a journal, type journal name underlined followed by a comma and the volume number and a period. Example: <u>American Journal of Occupational Therapy, 45</u>.
- Only books and journal names are underlined
- If title is a book, follow title with the city of publication comma the state colon pub-

lisher period. Example: Thorofare, NJ: SLACK Inc.
- Use only official two-letter post office approved state abbreviations. Both letters are capitalized and the are no spaces or periods in them.
- Finish the citation with page numbers if appropriate followed by a period. Example: 763.

Allen, C. K., Earhart, C. A., & Blue, T. (1992). <u>Occupational therapy treatment goals for the physically and cognitively disabled</u>. Bethesda, MD: American Occupational Therapy Association.

There are rules to arranging the actual reference list as well.
- Alphabetize the names, letter by letter.

Allen, C. K., Earhart, C. A., & Blue, T. (1992). <u>Occupational therapy treatment goals for the physically and cognitively disabled</u>. Bethesda, MD: American Occupational Therapy Association.
Burke, J. P., & DePoy, E. (1991). An emerging view of mastery, excellence, and leadership in occupational therapy practice. <u>American Journal of Occupational Therapy, 45,</u> 1027-1032.
Christiansen, C., & Baum, C. (Eds.). (1991). <u>Occupational therapy: Overcoming human performance deficits</u>. Thorofare, NJ: SLACK Inc.

- If several works are by the same person, arrange oldest first.

Fleming, M. (1989). The therapist with the three track mind. In <u>AOTA Practice Symposium</u>. Bethesda, MD: American Occupational Therapy Association.
Fleming, M. (1991). Clinical reasoning in medicine compared with clinical reasoning in occupational therapy. <u>American Journal of Occupational Therapy, 45</u>, 988-996.

- Use lowercase letters to separate same author same year works.

Fleming, M. (1991a). Clinical reasoning in medicine compared with clinical reasoning in occupational therapy. <u>American Journal of Occupational Therapy, 45</u>, 988-996.
Fleming, M. (1991b). The therapist with the three track mind. <u>American Journal of Occupational Therapy, 45,</u> 1007-1014.

- Put one-author works before multi-author works.

Crepeau, E. B. (1991). Achieving intersubjective understanding: Examples from an occupational therapy session. <u>American Journal of Occupational Therapy, 45,</u> 1016-1025.
Crepeau, E. B., & Leguard, T. (1991). <u>Self paced instruction for clinical education and supervision</u>. Bethesda, MD: American Occupational Therapy Association.

TITLE PAGE OF OT PAPER

Although the title page is the first page your OT teacher will see, students are likely to prepare the title page last. One good reason for doing the title page last is that you are likely to have several ideas for the title as you write the paper. After you have decided on the title, typing the title page is usually quick and painless (at least compared to the reference page). Center on the page, the title followed by the author, and the class or affiliation. Use a running head and page header if your teacher requires them. A running head and page header will keep your paper together in case the pages are accidentally separated.

Sample APA Pages in an OT Paper

There are a few other helpful tips for writing an OT paper using APA format. Generally, headings for each section are in upper- and lowercase letters centered across the line. In most cases, do not use abbreviations but write out the whole word. Try to remain gender bias free in your writing by using only the author's last name. Examine the samples of a title page (Figure 8-1), text with citations (Figure 8-2), and a reference page (Figure 8-3) for further help.

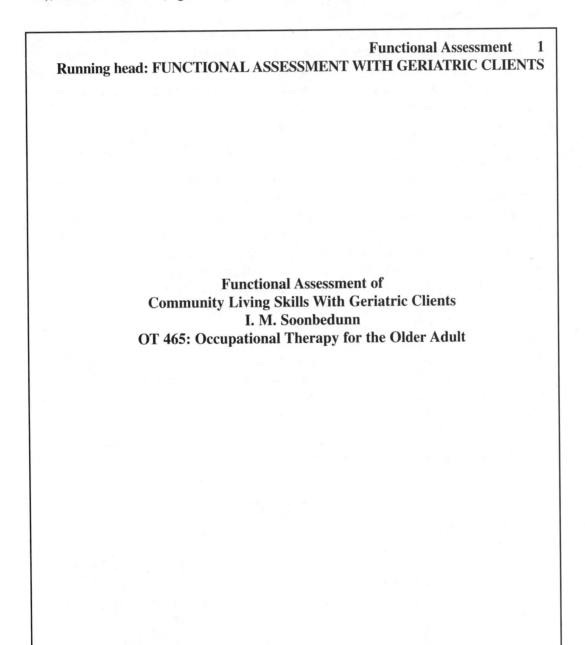

Figure 8-1. Sample title page.

Critical Thinking Vs. Clinical Reasoning

An important competency in occupational therapy is clinical reasoning. Mattingly (1991) argued that clinical reasoning involves more than the ability to offer explicit reasons to justify decisions. Mattingly noted that clinical reasoning was largely tacit, highly imagistic, and deeply phenomenological in thinking. Similarly, Rogers (1983) described clinical reasoning as a combination of science, art, and ethics. In 1991, Fleming presented clinical reasoning as thinking in three tracks: procedural, interactive, and conditional. Procedural thinking involves the therapist addressing the diagnosis and the treatment techniques. Interactive thinking involves the therapist and patient communicating with each other. Conditional thinking involves the therapist seeing the patient within the context of his or her own environment. According to Fleming (1991), expert occupational therapists use all three tracks of clinical reasoning in the smooth integration of treatment.

Cohn (1989) suggests theoretically based strategies to teach occupational therapy technique by simultaneously providing a foundation for clinical reasoning, reflection, and the facilitation of competency. Her outline includes: providing consistent patient population, using probing questions, observing the patient/therapist dyad, role modeling, telling stories, encouraging students to synthesize and summarize information, using journal writing, reviewing case studies, and videotaping treatments. These techniques encourage clinical reasoning skills and reflection that develop the more advanced learning skills and developmental competencies (Cohn, 1989). Specifically, the consistent patient population (not more than three different diagnoses throughout entire fieldwork) allows the student time to develop and practice skills and techniques needed to develop performance competencies. Probing questions, observing the patient-therapist dyad, role modeling, and telling stories are clinical reasoning techniques that require reflective interaction between the supervisor and the student. These techniques allow the student to work on transforming knowledge gained in classroom education to the clinic by looking at practice as deeper than the superficial application of treatment technique. Synthesizing and summarizing information, reviewing case studies, and viewing videotapes allow the student the opportunity to

Figure 8-2. Sample page of text with citations.

OT PROJECTS

OT students usually shine when it comes to special projects. Although many students do not believe they are creative, something about a love of activity brought you to the profession in the first part. It is only natural that OT educators will assign a variety of activity projects to their students.

The phrase "OT project" is loosely defined in this primer. Anything that is not a paper or a presentation is a project, even though projects might involve writing a supporting paper or presenting your project to the class. A project is an opportunity for the student to show he or she understands an academic concept in a creative way. This primer will discuss developing an OT project in a five-step manner (Table 8-2).

Performance in Occupational Therapy   18

References

Allen, C. K., Earhart, C. A., & Blue, T. (1992). <u>Occupational therapy treatment goals for the physically and cognitively disabled</u>. Bethesda, MD: American Occupational Therapy Association.

Bonder, B. R. (1995). <u>Psychopathology and function</u> (2nd ed.). Thorofare, NJ: SLACK Inc.

Burke, J. P., & DePoy, E. (1991). An emerging view of mastery, excellence, and leadership in occupational therapy practice. <u>American Journal of Occupational Therapy, 45,</u> 1027-1032.

Christiansen, C., & Baum, C. (Eds.). (1991). <u>Occupational therapy: Overcoming human performance deficits</u>. Thorofare, NJ: SLACK Inc.

Crepeau, E. B. (1991). Achieving intersubjective understanding: Examples from an occupational therapy session. <u>American Journal of Occupational Therapy, 45,</u> 1016-1025.

Crepeau, E. B., & Leguard, T. (1991). <u>Self paced instruction for clinical education and supervision</u>. Bethesda, MD: American Occupational Therapy Association.

Fleming, M. (1989). The therapist with the three track mind. In <u>AOTA Practice Symposium</u>. Bethesda, MD: American Occupational Therapy Association.

Fleming, M. (1991a). Clinical reasoning in medicine compared with clinical reasoning in occupational therapy. <u>American Journal of Occupational Therapy, 45,</u> 988-996.

Fleming, M. (1991b). The therapist with the three track mind. <u>American Journal of Occupational Therapy, 45,</u> 1007-1014.

Stein, F. (1989). <u>Anatomy of clinical research</u>. Thorofare, NJ: SLACK Inc.

Figure 8-3. Sample reference page.

The first step in developing a project is to outline the academic concept to be developed. Without the academic concept even the most creative project will get a failing grade. Look at the learning objective that the instructor has for the task. This often is found on the syllabus or can be attained from the teacher. The objective is usually something such as, "Demonstrate your knowledge of the human brain in a way that is not written" or "Using videotape, demonstrate your integration of the class material on psychosocial modalities."

The second step is to ask yourself "Will I be presenting the information or will the teacher view the project alone?" Each has its own benefits and problems. If the teacher will view the project alone, the academic concept must be presented clearly either in writing or in the project itself. If you will be presenting the project, there will likely be an opportunity for questions and answers to refine the presentation of the academic concept, but you will have to make a strong impact compared to other projects.

The third step is to develop a unique way to present the project. Some students spend too much time sitting and thinking of a modality to capture the project idea. The best way to get a project idea is to get up, get out, listen, and look. Visit museums, teacher supply

---

Table 8-2
Steps to Developing a Creative Project

---

1. Outline the academic concept that needs to be demonstrated.
2. Decide if the project is to be presented to the teacher or viewed alone.
3. Find the right modality for the project.
4. Build it.
5. Evaluate and refine it.

Table 8-3
Unique Project Ideas

- Museums. A display on rocks becomes a tactile exercise for pediatric class. A display on rain and lightning becomes a relaxation exercise for mental health modality class. A display on bones becomes a project on osteoarthritis. Added bonus: Museum gift shops have great educational ideas.
- Teacher supply store. Most major cities have a teacher supply store. Check the Yellow Pages. Browse the store for stickers that smell, posters, educational materials, overhead ideas, books full of ideas—all great for pediatric projects.
- Grocery store. Everyone loves a project they can eat as well as learn from. Find a cauliflower in the shape of a brain and label the lobes, an eggplant can be a giant pituitary gland. Bake a cake in the shape of a hand, a family system, a theory.
- Office supply store. Display boards become professional-looking poster presentations. Loose-leaf notebooks become activity card files. Assorted erasers are analyzed for prehension patterns.
- Craft supply store. Plaster of Paris becomes a tactile display of the cranial nerves. Friendly plastic is added to splints for decoration and increased compliance. Poster board becomes a reality orientation display for seniors.
- Department store. Clothes are analyzed for ease in dressing with arthritis. Blank videotapes can be used to record a treatment or make a MTV video on the parts of the digestive system. Buy a CD and change the words of a popular song.

---

stores, grocery stores, office supply stores, craft stores, and department stores. Try this exercise with some of your peers: Everywhere you go for one weekend, ask yourself "How can I turn this into a project?" There is a potential project in everything you see, hear, touch, taste, or smell. Review some samples in Table 8-3.

The fourth step is to build your project. A good supply of routine office supplies such as white glue, rubber cement, paper clips, assorted color paper, and poster paints will make the job easier. A hot glue gun comes in handy when trying to glue difficult things together (e.g., tree branches to cardboard to form a brachial plexus). If you have never used a hot glue gun before be aware that the glue can burn your fingers. Be particularly careful of toxic materials. Whatever the materials you use, it a good idea to read the directions before you start the project. Allow yourself plenty of time to make your project. Unlike studying all night, the supplies you may need may not be available to you after the stores close.

A few comments about humor in your project. Deciding to add "a funny" into a project depends on your evaluation of what the teacher will appreciate. Many OT faculty not only appreciate humor, but see the therapeutic aspect and encourage it. As the student, you must evaluate whether you can adequately meet the academic goal with humor or if the humor will lessen the academic concepts. Also, keep in mind that what is humorous to one person is not funny to another. As an example, students on campus often have answering machine messages that other students may find funny. When you leave your phone number for a professor to return your call and the professor is greeted by an offensive greeting or blaring rock music, your professional image is lessened. Do not add anything to your project that may negatively affect your grade or your professional image. In general, keep the humor clean, simple, and non-offensive. See the examples of safe humor in projects below.

Examples

In a mental health class, students were assigned to videotape themselves leading a group. Peers role-played the part of the patients. The students were required to integrate all the academic concepts covered in the class during the semester. Each student pulls a different scenario from a hat and has 2 weeks to prepare the tape. For the most part, students get scenarios that have really happened to the faculty in their practice. Below are some examples of how students met the academic challenges while adding humor.

- **Run a leisure awareness group with three nuns who have recently retired.** A male student pulled this scenario and instead of using female peers, he used his male buddies. He arranged for his peers to wear choir robes and each "nun" had a rosary. He lead the group with the most professional skill. There was no laughing or disrespect. He met the academic goals successfully.
- **Run a nutrition group with four overweight teenagers.** This student lead the group of teens who talked non-stop about junk food. Each peer had pillows stuffed in every possible place making them more than what might be expected in this type of group. Again, the student was professional. There was no laughing on the tape even when one teen tried to justify the orange powdered cheese on cheese puffs as nutritious. She led a successful group and met the academic criteria.
- **Run an assertiveness group with three pregnant teenagers who have not told their boyfriends that they are pregnant.** This student had the three teens sitting on a couch. Two students were "showing," one was at full term. The student ran an excellent group. As the teens were leaving the room, the full-term teen broke a water balloon and proclaimed "I'm in labor."

The last step before you hand in your project is to evaluate it. Review the grading criteria carefully. Remember that even great projects lose points if they fail to meet the academic criteria. Check the section on writing a good paper and compare any written aspects of your project against the written evaluation. If you are presenting the project, check the evaluation criteria in the next section. If the project is large or bulky, add extra travel time to class. When you are sure that the project is the best it can be, pass it in.

OT PRESENTATIONS

OT educators are likely to assign many presentations in your academic classes. Presenting is part of your job as a COTA or OTR. Whether you are presenting at team

---

Table 8-4
Steps to Developing a Creative Presentation

1. Outline the academic concept that needs to be demonstrated.
2. Find the right modality for the presentation.
3. Write it.
4. Evaluate and refine it.
5. Practice it many times.

---

meetings, in-services, or professional conferences, part of OT is educating others. Gaining presentation skills will make you more comfortable in dealing with other professionals. Presentations are just like verbal projects. Many of the same concepts outlined in the project section of this primer apply to presentations. Table 8-4 shows the five-step outline for effective presentations.

The first step in developing an effective presentation is to meet the academic challenges of the assignment. Just like the first step in a project, the academic aspect is the part of the presentation that will get the grade. Be sure you have reviewed the syllabus for the presentation objective and have met the grading criteria as you develop the presentation. If you have not done so already, review the section on OT projects in this primer for additional hints.

Finding the right modality for the presentation involves more than writing a script on index cards. Presentations are likely to be speeches but are not limited to talking. Consider incorporating audiovisual aids such as overheads, music, and videotapes. If you are extremely shy, you may want to make a video and show it in class. This way you can control some of your anxiety.

Writing out your presentation is an important step. Timing is the single most common problem students have in presentations. If the presentation has a time limit, stick to it. No one in class, especially the teacher, is happy about presentations that go way over the time limit. When you go over the time limit, you are projecting an image of "I am more important than any of you are" or "I am not smart enough to follow the directions." Either way, your professional image is lessened. Stick with the time limit and practice, practice, practice until you are within the time.

So why do students go over the time limit? They often try to present twice the information possible in the time limit. The solution to this problem is easy. Present everything possible within the time limit and prepare a handout with all the rest of the information you could not cover. This is a win-win situation. You stay within the time limit and you look brilliant to boot. Everyone likes handouts because they have the information for later.

In addition to the time limit issue, students should pay attention to content and delivery of the material. As mentioned in the OT project section of the primer, humor must be evaluated for adding to the presentation. If you are not familiar with humor's positive and negative effects, read the OT project section of this primer. In addition, students should try to avoid writing out the presentation speech and reading it. Write out only the first two lines and then outline the rest of the speech in detail. The first two lines will help you get over the initial anxiety, and talking instead of reading will make your information more enjoyable to listen to. If public speaking is a problem for you, consider a speech class or visit your school's learning center for a workshop on presentations.

After you have written out the presentation and practiced it until it is smooth, it is time to evaluate it. Review the presentation objectives from the syllabus. Ask yourself the following questions:

- Do I meet the academic goal of the presentation?
- Do I provide a smooth, easy-to-follow, clear presentation?
- Am I to the point (pithy)?
- Am I within the time limit?
- Do I have appropriate handouts, overheads, or other audiovisual aids?
- If I need equipment, such as a VCR, have I made arrangements?
- Have I practiced the presentation to the point that I am confident?

If the answers to all the questions are yes, then you are ready to do your presentation. Go out there and break a leg!

GROUP PAPERS, PROJECTS, OR PRESENTATIONS

OT is a social therapy because we work with human beings. For example, OT looks at how people function within their environment and what roles our clients take on. Everyone interacts with someone, a mother with her child, a student with his or her teacher, a worker with his or her boss. Just as it is natural for OT faculty to assign papers, projects, and presentations, it is natural that your educators will have you work in small groups. Working with other students will lead to new ideas and more flexible thinking.

There are positive and negative aspects to doing OT papers, projects, and presentations in groups. Group work can be totally fulfilling or a near disaster. Look at the positive and negative aspects listed in Table 8-5.

Group work can result in outstanding projects or ended friendships. This section of the chapter will focus on how to make group projects successful.

Table 8-5
Positive and Negative Aspects of Group Work

Positive	Negative
Everyone brings ideas to the table so the final result is a combination of the best ideas.	Hurt feelings if someone's ideas are negatively received by the group.
Work is shared so that the final results are much bigger than any one person could do alone.	Group members become angry when one person is not doing his or her fair share or when one person does poor work.
Working together allows for strengthening of social ties.	Groups formed from friendships often lose friendships when something goes wrong.
Working with other people develops team skills you will use later.	Some members may feel that others do not do good work, may say it's easier if I just do it myself. Loud group members overpower quiet members.

One of the most common mistakes a project group makes is to form out of friendship. The reason this may not be successful is that friendships are based on like interests not in success in OT school. For example, OT educators have found that "A students" typically hang around other students who get As. These are the students who generally sit in the front of the class and who form study groups on their own. Students who sit in the back of the class do not naturally interact with the students in the front row. When it comes time to form a project group, people join groups with others who are like them. The results are that groups may have an unequal distribution of creative ideas. Students start out thinking that friendship cannot interfere with work but generally it does.

To start, the key to a successful group is a clear mission statement from the beginning. Each member of the group should have a goal that is in common with the rest of the group. Values that are different can be respected but those in conflict should be allowed to find another group without embarrassment. For example, suppose an assignment is given to develop a new OT program in a local hospital. The OT teacher has already outlined the project and it is clear that it will take a lot of work. A group of friends agree to work on the project and during the first meeting it is clear the group members want to develop a hand therapy program. One member is not interested in hands but has an interest in pediatric OT. She says nothing, not wanting to leave her friends but she only puts half her interest into the project. Other members notice her half interest and become angry that their friend is not doing her fair share. Friendships are strained all because the group did not have a common mission.

When a group is formed to work on an OT paper, project, or presentation, an orientation meeting should be scheduled as quickly as possible. The first meeting should be no later than 24 hours after the assignment is given. The best meeting time is immediately after the class ends. This will allow the group members to form a mission and to find another group if the first one is not a good match. The focus of the first meeting is on developing group consensus on the focus of the group not on the project itself. Revisit the example above about developing a new OT program. The group began working on the task before establishing the ground rules. This led to a poor group structure before the task began.

The first question that should be asked of the group members is "What is our academic goal in this project?" Answers will vary from "I want nothing less than an A for a grade even though I'm involved in sports and other activities" to "I really do not have much interest in this type of project and just want to get it done with a decent grade." If the group members' values are close, see if compromise is possible. If compromise is not possible or if values are really different, majority rules and members may have to look for another group. Strong friendships can tolerate a member working in another group. Just remember that a friend switching groups is a sign that the friendship is important enough not to strain it by working in an unhappy group.

Once a consensus has been formed, the group members should elect one member as group manager. The group manager is responsible for maintaining the group mission and keeping everyone to task. In addition, the group manager schedules the meetings, arranges needed supplies, and speaks to members who are not doing their fair share. Everyone should agree to assist the manager when help is needed and to respect the authority of the role. The manager should remind everyone what the group has agreed to and provide support to anyone who decides to change to another group for whatever the reason.

After all the management functions have been decided, the group can then begin to focus on the task at hand. The group should then decide on how the task will be done and divide up the work. Keep in mind the "detail work" that comes at the end of the project such as how the paper will be typed or who will be responsible for making sure the typed paper is all in the same style and font. Agree on a deadline for the first goal and set the next meeting time. A short meeting might be arranged after a week to see how people are progressing and a full meeting arranged for evaluating the first goal. As a member of the group, you are responsible for meeting your assigned goals and attending all meetings. As an OT educator, I have seen groups fall apart because one member canceled because a "dating" opportunity came up. This leads to the group not meeting its goals and is irresponsible professional behavior.

So, if you are elected the group manager, how do you keep the group functioning and on task? One way is to set a formal agenda that lists everyone's names and what they will report on during the next meeting. This way everyone is heard. Use brainstorming techniques and make sure everyone participates. See Table 8-6 for helpful hints.

As the manager, you may have to speak to members about allowing others to speak. Review the section on assertiveness techniques found in Chapter 10 of this primer. Generally, you can say, "As the group manager, I've noticed that..." Use the word "I" more than you use the word "you." This way no one feels badly after the conversation. If you are still having problems with the group, consult your OT faculty for more advice.

Table 8-6
Successful Brainstorming

- The group manager reviews the rules before starting.
- No one is allowed to evaluate an idea before the evaluation stage. For example, no "good idea," "bad idea," "I like that," "wow," "no way," "let's do that." This is harder than you think. Everyone has an opinion but even good compliments can stop the flow of ideas. The manager must stop all evaluations.
- Someone should record all ideas, even the silliest ones.
- Silly ideas should be encouraged because they often lead to creative ideas.
- The more fun you have with brainstorming, the more creative the ideas.
- Separate the idea generating from the idea evaluating. Again, no evaluation allowed in the generating time period.
- After everyone has participated and the idea generating has slowed down, move to the evaluation phase.
- Before starting the real brainstorming, practice with something silly like: Parking is too far away from campus. How will we fix this issue?
  - Move faculty out of their spots
  - Arrange helicopter service
  - Have upperclassmen get priority

SUMMARY

This chapter addressed how to successfully manage OT papers, projects, and presentations. Attention is paid to balancing creative tasks with meeting the academic objective of the project. An important aspect of this is self-evaluation and making every project your best possible work. This chapter also contains practical guides to writing using APA format, using humor, and leading group projects.

BIBLIOGRAPHY

American Psychological Association. (1995). *Publication manual of the American Psychological Association* (4th ed.). Washington, DC: Author.

Apps, J. W. (1982). *Study skills for adults returning to school*. New York: McGraw-Hill.

Frender, G. (1990). *Learning to learn*. Nashville, TN: Incentives Publications.

Gardner, J. N., & Jewler, A. J. (1989). *College is only the beginning*. Belmont, CA: Wadsworth.

Gardner, J. N., & Jewler, A. J. (1995). *Your college experience: Strategies for success*. Belmont, CA: Wadsworth.

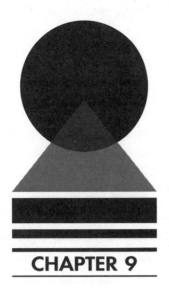

CHAPTER 9

WHAT TO DO IF YOU MAY NOT PASS

Lori G. Sladyk, MS, CSE

FIGURING OUT WHAT WENT WRONG

Many factors play into successfully meeting your academic goals. There are several reasons why you may not be making the grade. A common problem among college students is the lack of structure and clear expectations. The professor is seen as a resource and you are expected to be a self-directed learner. Another challenge is balancing studies with adult responsibilities such as work, budgeting, relationships, and community service. Most students are faced with additional challenges at one time or another. Difficulty or failure in a class may affect other aspects of your life including self-esteem and emotional stress. Before you can change problem areas into successes, it is extremely important to identify factors that may be inhibiting your progress. The purpose of this chapter is to help you recognize issues and to be aware of possible resources that are available to help solve or lessen challenges. Worksheet 9-1 is designed to help you determine those deterrents.

After you have identified some of the factors that inhibit your progress, make a plan to reduce these deterrents or at the very minimum, increase your ability to cope with these factors. Consult Table 9-1 for quick ideas or for information on where you may find other solutions.

Review the following sections for more detailed ideas on getting the help you need to succeed in your academic studies.

Worksheet 9-1

Inventory

Consider your current situation and check all that apply.

[ ] I have significant financial worries.

[ ] I am having difficulty dealing with stress.

[ ] My work schedule is horrible.

[ ] I think I have a learning disability.

[ ] I am experiencing medical problems.

[ ] I am having trouble sleeping.

[ ] I can't seem to find the motivation.

[ ] I have no place to study.

[ ] I am having difficulty gaining support from significant others.

[ ] Family responsibilities make it difficult for me to juggle school.

[ ] My activities/commitments take up a lot of time.

[ ] The instructors are unreasonable.

[ ] I sleep well, I just don't get enough of it.

[ ] I am in conflict.

[ ] I can't seem to get organized.

[ ] Time management is an issue.

[ ] I can't seem to focus/concentrate.

[ ] The professor doesn't like me.

[ ] I don't take tests well.

[ ] I "blank out" on a test.

[ ] I can't keep up on the reading.

[ ] My standards are very high.

[ ] The professor is boring.

[ ] There are too many things to memorize.

[ ] I am homesick.

[ ] I am having trouble meeting deadlines.

[ ] The teacher is inflexible.

[ ] I am having difficulty understanding the instructor due to his or her accent or vocabulary.

[ ] I am too shy to approach others for the help I need.

[ ] I often don't feel well.

[ ] I'm a procrastinator.

[ ] I don't know where/how to get help.

[ ] I am lacking the basic skills/experiences.

[ ] I don't seem to study the right material.

[ ] I don't attend every class session or I come in late.

[ ] I am distracted by other interests or side conversations.

[ ] I have difficulty applying what I learn in the classroom into practice.

[ ] I am not good at written expression.

[ ] I am disinterested and don't see the relevance.

[ ] I am experiencing personal problems (eating disorder, sexuality, suicide, etc.).

Table 9-1
Where to Start

Problem	Quick Resources	Other Relevant Chapters
Significant financial worries	Financial aid office	5
Difficulty dealing with stress	Counseling center	10
Work schedule is horrible	Campus employment center	12
May have a learning disability	504 coordinator, LD services office	11
Experiencing medical problems	Personal physician, campus health center	
Having trouble sleeping	Relaxation exercises	
Cannot find the motivation	Motivational tapes	10
No place to study	Unconventional places including the cafeteria	12
Gaining support from others	Support groups	
Family responsibilities	Goal review, nontraditional schedule, extended time	
Activities take up too much time	Personal planner	12
Instructors are unreasonable	Academic advisor, chair, dean	
Not enough sleep	Personal planner	
In conflict	Counseling center, hotline, RA, clergy	
Not organized	Personal planner	10
Time management	Personal planner, efficiency seminar	10
Cannot seem to focus	Focusing techniques	
Professor doesn't like me	Coping strategies	7
Don't take tests well	Study skills center	7
"Blank out" on tests	Study skills center, relaxation techniques	7
Cannot keep up with the reading	Speed reading course, study skills center	10
Standards are too high	Counseling center	
Professor is boring	Coping strategies, long-term picture	
Too much to memorize	Tutoring center, study skills books	7
Homesick	Counseling center, activity center, student union	

Trouble meeting deadlines	Professor	10
Teacher is inflexible	Support personnel and peers	
Teacher's accent/vocabulary	Teacher assistant, study group, classmate's notes	
Too shy to ask for help	Study group, study partner	
Often don't feel well	Personal physician, campus health center	
Procrastination	Self-help books, motivational speakers/tapes	10
Don't know where/ how to get help	Student handbook, library, student union	
Lacking basic skills/experience	Tutoring center, noncredit courses, computer lab	
Don't study the right material	Professor, study group, study partner	
Cut class or come in late	Set your watch ahead, commit to 100% attendance	6
Distracted by other interests	Personal planner, study partner	
Difficulty applying concepts	Tutoring center, private tutor	
Problem with writing	Computer lab, campus writing lab, peer tutor	8
Disinterested/lack of relevance	Motivational tapes, study partner	
Personal problems	Counseling center, RA, clergy	

RESOURCES

Resource Centers

Nearly all campuses offer some type of study skill center. These centers may provide walk-in tutoring or study skill workshops. Many schools offer writing centers and computer labs. Some centers offer a library of study aids, including books, videos, and cassette tapes. Some centers may help you analyze your study habits and your learning styles by administering individualized testing, interviews, and checklists. The purpose of a study skill center is to help you to identify your strengths and weaknesses and to provide helpful information regarding effective reading, writing, note taking, testing skills, etc. Consult your school catalog or phone directory to find out where your resource center is and what services they provide.

Self-Help Books

Self-help books are a major contributor to the publishing industry. There are books available to help deal with every problem imaginable. Since the college student has enough to read already, it is important to identify the area where help is needed, find the appropriate book, apply the suggestions, and get on with your life. Campus libraries hold many various self-help books. If the book you are seeking is not available, ask your librarian about interloan services. Not all problems can be solved by reading a book. A self-help book will provide general information, but a variety of resources may be needed to solve a problem, particularly if the problem is a serious one.

Counseling Centers

Difficulty with academics may stem from other issues. Relationships, depression, anxiety, eating disorders, drug involvement, family problems, and low self-esteem may make it difficult for you to concentrate on your studies. If you are concerned about this possibility, contact the counseling office on campus. Services may include peer counseling, support groups, hotlines, individual or group therapy, or a referral service. These services are confidential and are often offered free or on a sliding scale. Not all problems can be solved by yourself. Do not hesitate or wait too long to seek help. If your car needed repairs, you would not think twice about asking a specialist for help. You are more important than your car.

Private Tutors

Some classes are so large that it is impossible to ask the instructor a question. A minor question/problem can be solved by visiting an instructor during office hours. Many universities have teaching assistants who can work with small groups of students. If you feel you are in need of more individualized attention, you might consider hiring a tutor. The following is a list of places where a tutor can be found:

- **Another student in class.** Approach a student who appears to have a good handle on the material and ask if he or she would be willing to tutor you.
- **Department secretary.** Many offices maintain a list of qualified student tutors.
- **Campus newspapers or bulletin boards.** Often students willing to tutor will advertise their services for a particular class or a general subject area.
- **On-campus networking.** In most cases, it will be less expensive and more beneficial to hire an on-campus tutor rather than seeking help from an expert outside of the university.

Study Groups

Study groups can be extremely beneficial if they are used for the right purpose. The purpose of studying with others is to share information and insights, and to lend support. The intention is not to complain, become more anxious, or give each other the answers. Each member must be willing to come prepared and to participate constructively. Study groups are particularly popular around exam time but can be formed anytime. If your group meets more than once or twice, consider rotating leadership. The leader should arrange for a meeting place/time, keep the group on task, and make sure that everyone has an opportunity to contribute. If you are enrolled in a small class, ask a few responsible students if they would like to form a study group. If your class is large, ask the professor or teacher's assistant to make an announcement, or post flyers near the classroom.

DIFFICULTY FOCUSING

Most students have difficulty with focusing, remembering, or understanding material at one time or another. Assuming there is no medical reason for lack of concentration, there are several things that can be done to enhance your ability to sustain focus. Identify possible distractions and try appropriate solutions (Table 9-2). The following studying suggestions will also help you to focus:

Table 9-2 Tips for Overcoming Distractions	
Distraction	**Possible Solution**
Personal problems	Identify specific problem, determine what level of support is needed, work on changing things within your power, accept that you can't change everything.
Anxiety	Try relaxation techniques, use positive self-talk, dig in—getting started often reduces stress, break down task into manageable chunks.
Interruptions	Be firm! Utilize answering machines, go to the library, put a sign on your door, enlist others' support.
Distractibility	Minimize distractions by selecting a nonstimulating study environment, select a study cubicle, remove yourself from others, take frequent breaks, sit in the front row during class.
Mind wanders	Become a more active reader, underline, take notes, review and recite material aloud, ask questions like, "What have I just read? What is the main point and supporting details?"
You are in love	There is no known solution.

- Give yourself time to warm up. Get to class a few minutes early and expect the first 10 minutes of studying to be review.
- Change the time of day that you are currently studying. Morning seems to be the most productive part of the day for many people. Remember how you always had reading in the morning in elementary school?
- Do not lie on your bed to study, your brain will think it is time to go to sleep. Do not put yourself in the position where you are in competition with the TV, as the TV will likely win.
- Take time to be reflective. Rotate 10 minutes of studying/reading with 1 minute of thinking/processing.
- Position yourself by sitting in the front of the class and in a remote part of the library.
- Anticipate your studying needs. Gather supplies (i.e., snacks, highlighter, pens), clear your desk, and locate your notes before you attempt to study.
- If you have sincerely attempted to improve your concentration, but are still unsuccessful, it may be time to enlist the help of a professional.

DEALING WITH THE PROFESSOR

Sometimes, despite your efforts, you may feel that it is the instructor who is impeding your progress. Before you blame everything on the teacher, check to see if you need an attitude adjustment. Just because you are paying for your education, you are not guaranteed an A. If you are comfortable with your effort and you still are not meeting your goals, then you may need to confront the instructor or seek help from other sources. Although he or she may deserve it, consider the following suggestions before attacking the professor.

- Talk to the professor in a nonthreatening way. Don't be defensive and use "I" statements. Rather than saying, "You assign way too much reading," try saying, "I feel like I'm in over my head with keeping up with the reading." When making a suggestion, try, "I'm wondering if we might be able to..."

- For little problems, attempt to clarify in or after class. For larger or more personal concerns, think about and practice what you want to say beforehand. Anticipate possible responses and be prepared to express yourself in a clear, concise manner. If you are phoning the instructor, write out the major points you wish to make, particularly if you are nervous. Do not call late at night (9:00 p.m. is a good cutoff). Be prepared to tell the professor what steps you have taken to solve the problem on your own. Although there may be posted office hours, setting an appointment will be to your advantage. If in the event your problem is serious, seek help from your advisor or other appropriate personnel.

There are instances where you may need to negotiate with the professor. Taking a proactive approach is beneficial. For instance, ask for extra credit assignments early in the semester rather than waiting until the last week. Make sure that you really understand the grading procedure before you are in trouble. Refer to the class syllabus frequently throughout the semester. When faced with a disagreement on a grade, ask for advice on your incorrect answers. Start long-term assignments early to anticipate possible difficulties. Ask for an extension well before the due date, and not the night before. Get on the good side of the professor early in the course. Be a responsible student but don't kiss up so much that you alienate your classmates. After you have done your part, go after what you are entitled to. If you have exhausted all of your options, then know when to drop the course.

ACTIVE LEARNING

Many professors teach by the banking method. That it, students go to class and professors make a deposit of knowledge in the form of a lecture. Students often walk away feeling that they have no homework because all the professor did was talk. There are often surprises when the test comes along because some of the material was not discussed in class. Several things can be done to learn the required material. First, attend all classes and sit in the front. Attend all classes! Next, make a decision to become an active learner. Compare lecture notes with another classmate. Review your notes after each class session and then reread notes from previous lectures. Although you may feel this is time consuming, you will read previous notes quicker each time and you will begin to anticipate the end of each sentence. Be prepared for the next lecture by reading the syllabus and scanning the next reading assignment. Don't just read, but underline, highlight, take notes, write in the margin, photocopy, and ask questions.

Prepare for the test by finding out what is on the test and what the format is likely to be. Be prepared for essays by anticipating questions and outlining answers. If the test incudes multiple choice, then know what grading system will be used. Are you penalized for guessing? Look out for qualifying words such as *always, never, only, frequently,* and *often.* Overlearn the material by repetition. Use outlines to organize information. Try making flashcards and recopying your notes. See Chapter 7 for more information.

TIME MANAGEMENT

Finding the time to do everything you have to do is a constant challenge. It is particularly difficult when there are so many worthwhile activities to choose from. However, effective time management requires that you make a judgment regarding your participa-

Worksheet 9-2

Identifying Priorities

Rank the activities from 1 to 3 (1=very important, 2=somewhat important, 3=not as important). Then circle the appropriate response ("Y" or "N") for if you are currently meeting the goal of each activity.

Activity	Rank	Are You Currently Meeting Your Goal?	
Attending class	_____	Y	N
Reviewing notes/reading text	_____	Y	N
Spending time with friends	_____	Y	N
Sports (teams or exercise)	_____	Y	N
Chores (shopping, cleaning)	_____	Y	N
Sleeping (at least 7 hours)	_____	Y	N
Watching TV	_____	Y	N
Hobbies (sewing, art)	_____	Y	N
Spending time with family	_____	Y	N
Dating	_____	Y	N
Employment	_____	Y	N
Clubs/organizations	_____	Y	N
Church	_____	Y	N
Volunteer service	_____	Y	N

tion in an event. It is important to set priorities in order to accomplish your most important goals. The one great equality in this world is that we are all given 24 hours each day. The challenge is to use the allotted time to your best advantage. Begin by identifying your priorities (Worksheet 9-2).

Next, determine if you are spending the most amount of time on the things that you identified as priorities. If your priorities do not coincide with your current behaviors, then it is time to consider some changes. Some priorities are predetermined. In other words, some individuals must work in order to support themselves. However, some activities are negotiable. If you are not passing in your academic goals, a review of your time is needed. Fill out the time table in Worksheet 9-3 to identify your current schedule. Include time spent eating, getting dressed, showering, and commuting.

Examine your current routine and identify blocks of time that are available. Are there areas of time spent on activities that can be consolidated or reduced? Now complete the time table again, this time *planning* the upcoming week based on the tasks you must do and then the activities which you would like to do (Worksheet 9-4). Be sure to include time to work on long-term projects. Post this schedule or carry it in a planner and look at it frequently. Assess and modify your schedule regularly to monitor its effectiveness. Be realistic and expect the unexpected (e.g., no parking spaces, computer difficulties, long lines). Schedule in rewards for goals completed (e.g., phone call, ice cream, walk). Try to refrain

Worksheet 9-3

Time Log—Current Week

Day:			
Time:			
6:00-7:00 a.m.			
7:00-8:00			
8:00-9:00			
9:00-10:00			
10:00-11:00			
11:00-12:00 noon			
12:00-1:00 p.m.			
1:00-2:00			
2:00-3:00			
3:00-4:00			
4:00-5:00			
5:00-6:00			
6:00-7:00			
7:00-8:00			
8:00-9:00			
9:00-10:00			
10:00-11:00			

from feast or famine sleeping schedules. If after assessment and planning you are failing to complete your goals in a satisfactory manner, then you may need to make some decisions pertaining to your current goals. Perhaps it is not possible to do everything you want at this time. For additional guidance, see your academic advisor or another counselor to gain perspective and to see what options may be available. Read Chapter 10 for further ideas.

LACKING BASIC SKILLS

If you find that you are lacking background skills necessary to succeed in your coursework, you will need to make a determination as to the best way to cope with the deficiency. As stated earlier, most campuses offer remedial classes in basic skills. In addition, there are tutoring sessions where help is available on a short- or long-term basis. If your weakness is not too severe, you may be able to get by with a proofreader or by using a computer with a spell and grammar check. Determine where your difficulties are and to what extent they impact your ability to successfully meet the requirements of your current and future classes. Consider the extra time you may have to put into remediation or extra help compared to the possible outcomes. Is it worth the sacrifice, or are you comfortable taking a risk?

Worksheet 9-4

Time Log—Upcoming Week

Day:			
Time:			
6:00-7:00 a.m.			
7:00-8:00			
8:00-9:00			
9:00-10:00			
10:00-11:00			
11:00-12:00 noon			
12:00-1:00 p.m.			
1:00-2:00			
2:00-3:00			
3:00-4:00			
4:00-5:00			
5:00-6:00			
6:00-7:00			
7:00-8:00			
8:00-9:00			
9:00-10:00			
10:00-11:00			

STRESS

There is no doubt that expectations for OT students are high. Combined with the added responsibilities of employment, relationships, finances, and the competitive nature of the university experience, it is no wonder that stress is a common complaint of college students. Those suffering from severe anxiety or chronic stress need to ask for and accept help. There are a variety of resources available to help manage stress including counseling, group support, self-help books, and yoga classes. Do not let stress control you, rather, learn to control the stress. The following is a list of simple strategies to help cope with the demands you are meeting.

- Get sufficient sleep. When you are tired, you are less able to deal with challenges. You become more vulnerable and less in control. Let sleep be close to your top priority. Think of it as necessary for your health.
- Maintain a proper diet. How much evidence do you need? Although tasty, prolonged diets of candy bars and french fries wear on your body and your ability to feel and think well.
- Exercise regularly. This doesn't need to be an all or nothing activity. Often a 15-minute walk to class will relieve stress and help you to gain perspective and strength.

- Practice relaxation techniques. Deep breathing, visualization, yoga, positive self-talk, and putting your feet up are simple techniques to help conquer stress. Back and neck rubs are great if you can find a volunteer.
- Do not take on more than you can handle. A simple solution that is hard to implement. Examine your planner and reduce unnecessary or unprofitable activities. Tell people who invite you to do something that you regret that you cannot help at this time, as you would not be able to give the assignment the attention that it deserves.
- Avoid mind-altering substances. You have enough to accomplish without handicapping yourself.
- Schedule recreation. Your idea of recreation might be going to the mall or watching TV. By planning some down time, you will be less resentful of your responsibilities and less likely to feel guilty. Set aside time for something to look forward to and write it in your planner.
- Manage time efficiently. It is imperative to spend some time planning in order to fully utilize your time. Look for opportunities to double dip and to simplify. For example, study your flashcards while walking after dinner. Managing time does not necessarily mean squeezing as many goals into a day as possible. Managing time involves assessing current practices, modifying, consolidating, and reducing or increasing time on tasks as appropriate.

Stress is a natural and common occurrence. In many cases, it can serve as a motivator to accomplishment. If stress or anxiety is inhibiting your progress or the level of stress is too great, then it may be time to reevaluate your goals or to seek help from a qualified person.

MEDICAL CONCERNS AND DISABILITIES

There are times where academic failures are due to medical problems. In most cases, accommodations must be made for students with health limitations. However, your limitations may need documentation and only reasonable accommodations are required. You must still meet minimum qualifications. See Chapter 11 for more information.

MOTIVATION

It is impossible to accomplish anything without at least some degree of motivation. Since motivation comes from within a person, you must discover the things that trigger your desire to accomplish a task. Everyone has time periods where the urge to work on a goal wanes, but fortunately, the lack of motivation is temporary. The trick is to be somewhat productive despite your being glued to the living room couch. Sometimes reviewing past successes and accomplishments prompts you to continue working. Try finding a study partner who can check in on you and who is willing to hold you accountable. Promise yourself rewards for productivity. Review your goals and dreams. At the very least, start a task. Success breeds success and relieves anxiety. Break down assignments into manageable chunks. Write out a specific to-do list and make a ceremony out of checking things off. Prolonged difficulty with lack of motivation can be a symptom of another problem that may require attention.

FINANCIAL CONCERNS

Money problems and college students go together like pizza and pepperoni. Most people are aware that financial aid is available for those who qualify. Keep in mind that for the most part, financially struggling college students are in a temporary situation. Before financial frustration consumes you, investigate what options are available to ease your situation. At the very least, examine your current spending habits and work with a plan or budget. Beware of costly temptations that magnify your problem when the bill arrives. Be especially cautious of "special" credit card plans offered to college students because it is easy to max out a credit card without a job to cover the payments. A good rule of thumb is to set your budget at 10% less than your income, and then live within your means. Manage your resources and weigh your options.

WHEN ALL ELSE FAILS

Although many colleges, professors, and programs have some degree of flexibility, there are basic requirements which need to be met. Most OT programs have a minimum GPA for acceptance and even higher criteria for staying in the program. If you are unable to meet the standards set by your program, then you must ask yourself some difficult questions such as:

- Am I committed to this program?
- Are my priorities in order?
- Is this the right career for me?
- Have I done all that I can on my own?
- Have I asked for and accepted appropriate help?

If you have made a sincere attempt to correct the problem or difficulty and are still unable to perform at a level considered acceptable, then you must understand the consequences and alternatives. Perhaps there are related fields that you should consider.

SUMMARY

There are several factors that can contribute to impeding your progress. You are not alone if you have experienced stress, financial worries, health problems, unreasonable professors, or time constraints. This chapter attempts to aid you in identifying the factors that prevent you from succeeding in your coursework. The intent is to help you become aware of the possible options, solutions, and resources available for exploration.

BIBLIOGRAPHY

Farrar, R. (1984). *College 101*. Princeton, NJ: Peterson's Guides.

Jewler, J., Gardner, J., & McCarthy, M. (Eds.). (1993). *Your college experience: Strategies for success*. Boston: Wadsworth Publishing Co.

Kaye, E., & Gardner, J. (1988). *College bound*. New York: College Entrance Examination Board.

Mayer, B. (1981). *The college survival guide: An insider's guide to success*. Stokie, IL: VGM Career Horizons.

McCutcheon, R. (1985). *Get off my brain: A survival guide for lazy students*. Minneapolis, MN: Free Spirit Publishing Co.

Rowe, B. (1992). *The college survival guide: Hints and references to aid college students*. St. Paul, MN: West Publishing Co.

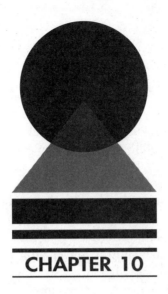

CHAPTER 10

SUCCESSFUL SELF-MANAGEMENT

Marijke Kehrhahn, PhD

INTRODUCTION

Learning to manage yourself as a student will be one of your biggest challenges in college and one of your most rewarding accomplishments. The work you do to develop ways of tracking your goals, managing your time, focusing your energy, and getting things done will help you develop skills that you will use for a lifetime. For most students, college is a stepping stone from the structure and supervision of high school to the demands of work and career. College is a great place to learn the many skills you will need to be successful as an OT professional: self-motivation, organization, time management, building professional relationships, and self-direction.

Stupka and Eddy (1992) of Sacramento City College listed some of the reasons why students have difficulty in college:

- Most students have little experience sustaining commitment to academic excellence and little experience managing their own learning.
- Many college students have not developed a support network and have difficulty resisting peer pressure against putting time and energy into learning.

Stupka and Eddy (1992) defined the role of the successful college student to include the following responsibilities:

- Knowing what is required
- Learning to be honest with oneself
- Identifying and using strategies that support learning
- Avoiding over-commitment

- Establishing priorities
- Planning and goal setting
- Developing personal support networks
- Attending classes regularly and on time
- Taking advantage of opportunities
- Speaking up in class
- Turning in assignments on time that look neat and sharp
- Being attentive in class
- Seeing your instructor before or after class
- Engaging the instructor in meaningful conversation

This chapter on self-management will address several of these suggestions and provide worksheets and strategies that you can use to become a more successful student. The following stories depict common challenges that college students in OT face. Each situation represents a learning opportunity—a chance to problem solve and develop new strategies for success.

KATE, A FIRST-YEAR STUDENT

Kate was an excellent high school student. She always completed her assignments on time and her grades were above average. Kate followed instructions to complete assignments and this approach worked well in the high school environment. Her teachers knew her and interacted with her regularly.

Now Kate is in her second semester of college. She is having difficulty keeping up with the work and her grades are not as good as she had hoped for. She often goes to class and is not familiar with the lecture content—she does not see the connection from one class to the next. Her teachers do not spend much time reviewing or linking information. Kate easily falls behind on reading assignments because her professors do not always remind the class about upcoming readings. Although she turns her assignments in on time and follows the assignment instructions, she gets comments on her papers that they lack insight and creativity. She sees her teachers only three times a week in class and she doesn't think they know who she is. Kate is feeling lost in a large group. She is discouraged by her average grades and the fact that her professors don't seem to know her. She really does not have any idea what she can do to turn things around.

Kate is experiencing the pressures and frustrations of the transition from high school to college. While she was a very good student within the rules, structure, and boundaries that teachers and administrators set in high school, Kate now needs to develop new skills for organizing and motivating herself. Kate is finding that, while in high school she stood out as a top student, in college she is one of many very capable students. In fact, for the first time Kate is feeling average rather than above average and she doesn't really understand why that has changed. The key to Kate's success will be in developing a better understanding of the academic demands of college and what she can do to become a better student.

MARK, A THIRD-YEAR FIELDWORK STUDENT

Mark did well his first 2 years in the OT program. He took five classes each semester and was able to get all of his work done. He was pleased with his grades. In addition to keeping up with his coursework, Mark participated in intramural sports, joined three clubs, served on the student Senate, and had a great social life.

This year Mark is struggling. He is completing his first semester of fieldwork which involves 40 hours a week on the job plus written assignments. Mark is also working part-time in the early morning in a cafeteria on campus. Mark has made many friends in college and never misses a good party. He plays volleyball in the early evenings and talks to his girlfriend every evening for at least an hour. They get together every Friday and Saturday night. Mark is falling behind on his fieldwork journal and has missed handing in two assignments to his fieldwork supervisor so far this semester. He is often tired when he arrives at his fieldwork site and is exhausted by the end of the day. Mark is worried that he will not be successful in his fieldwork and that his poor performance will be a problem when he is placed at a very popular children's hospital next semester. Mark hopes to work in the competitive field of pediatric rehabilitation when he graduates.

Mark is experiencing the transition from taking courses to the demands of fieldwork. While Mark was able to get his coursework done and had plenty of time for social and recreational pursuits, his entry into a 40 hour per week fieldwork assignment has really made it difficult for him to keep all of his interests going. In order to be successful, Mark will need to clearly define his goals and determine what is most important at this time to reach his long-term goals. Mark doesn't have to give up everything but his fieldwork, but he will need to structure his time well in order to balance the demands of the OT program with his need to work, socialize, and enjoy recreation.

KEISHA, A STUDENT WITH MULTIPLE DEMANDS

Keisha lives at home with her parents and younger brother and sister while attending classes. Her typical Monday includes classes at 8 a.m., 11 a.m., and 2 p.m. Between classes, Keisha hangs out at the student center and watches TV, talks to other students, and reads magazines. Keisha leaves school to go to her job where she works from 5 p.m. to 10 p.m. Monday through Thursday. Keisha has two classes on Tuesday and Thursday at 9:30 a.m. and 11 a.m. She usually spends Tuesday and Thursday in the library completing her assignments until she goes to work.

She is having difficulty finding time to read, study, and complete written assignments. Keisha often skips assignments or skims them and it seems as though her written assignments are always done at the last minute. Keisha is worried that she will fall behind in classes and settle for poor grades. Keisha usually goes out with friends on Friday and Saturday and will sometimes spend Sunday with her family or getting extra work done. Keisha's family give her the space and time she needs to get her school work completed, but they complain that they don't see much of her. Keisha's hometown friends complain that Keisha is not around much. Keisha has made friends on campus and she sometimes studies with them. Her campus friends, however, do not have jobs and spend much of their daytime hours working out, hanging out, and watching soaps. They get their school tasks done in the evening when Keisha is at work. Keisha is feeling left out of almost every social circle and is getting discouraged. She wants to have fun and be with friends, but she wants to do well in school and she needs to work to pay tuition. She is thinking about quitting school or cutting back on school hours to ease up her schedule.

Keisha is frustrated because she is trying to respond to a large number of demands, both from the outside and from within. The completion of her OT program will be one of the biggest challenges Keisha will ever face. If she can keep her "eyes on the prize" and connect herself to others who can share and encourage her commitment and hard work she will be successful. Keisha needs to recommit to her goal and build support for herself. In addition, Keisha may need to eliminate some activities during the school semester so she can do well.

These three stories about OT students illustrate the common challenges that you will face in managing yourself and your college career. As you read this chapter, ask yourself the following questions:

- What skills do I need to be a successful student in college?
- What transitions can I expect?
- How can I balance the demands of school, work, and social life?
- How can I keep my assignments in order and get things done on time?
- How can I make the best use of my time?
- How can I set and prioritize my goals so I am clear on what I am supposed to be doing?
- How can I set my schedule to help me meet my goals?
- How can I get to know my professors and help them get to know me?
- How can I build a social network that will support my goal accomplishment?

TRANSITIONS

Going to college requires you to engage in a number of transitions: the transition from high school to college, the transition from taking classes to doing your fieldwork, and the transition from college to work. Transitions are times in life when rules and expectations change. During a transition you may feel out of place, stressed, or frustrated because you are not fully aware of the new rules or expectations set before you. Be assured that you will adapt to your new situation, whatever it is, and move on.

While a transition may go smoothly for one person, it may be a rough ride for another. The difference between the smooth ride and the rough ride is related to whether or not you focus your attention on learning more about the transition, find and use the resources available to you, and build a support network that will help you work out problems.

Remember Kate? She was having a difficult time making the transition from high school to college. Table 10-1 shows some of the differences between high school and college that Kate is learning the hard way.

The transition from taking courses to completing your fieldwork is another common transition for OT students. The rules and expectations change when you work in a field setting and learn the practical side of being an OT.

Use Worksheet 10-1 to help you get a better understanding of the transition from coursework to fieldwork. Interview a few OT students who are currently engaged in the fieldwork part of their program and ask them to tell you all the things that are different. It helps if you ask them about both columns—rules and expectations in coursework and how they are different in fieldwork. Share Table 10-1 with them if you think it will help them understand the idea of changing expectations.

Remember, managing a transition means finding out about the new expectations, finding and using resources, and building a support network. Perhaps the fieldwork students you interview will be willing to be a mentor or support person as you advance into your fieldwork assignments.

TIME MANAGEMENT

A discussion about time management starts by remembering that there are only 24 hours in a day. No matter how many things you like or want to do, you will always only have 24 hours in a day to do them. Many time management problems begin when you underestimate the amount of time something will take, try to get too many things done at once, over-commit yourself, waste time, use time poorly, or fail to see the big picture of all the things that you are required to do.

Table 10-1
Differences Between High School and College

In High School	In College
Schedules are set and are the same for every student. The average school day goes from 8 a.m. to 2 p.m.	Each student sets his or her own schedule of classes. There are no bells or hall monitors reminding you to get to class.
Attendance is taken and teachers and administrators follow up on missing students.	Many professors do not take attendance after the first few classes and very few will actually follow up if you do not come to class. You are expected to be in class and to participate. There often is no penalty for not attending other than your grade.
Classes are conducted every day with incremental presentation of material and high amounts of repetition and overlap.	Classes meet two or three times a week. Lectures are distinct from class to class. You are expected to make the links and do the reading that will help you understand and process the material.
Teachers are responsible for seeing that students do well, for helping students who are falling behind, and for discipline.	Teachers are responsible for delivering the content of the course in a competent manner. It is your responsibility to seek help if you are not doing well in the course. All students are expected to show respect and to behave well in class.
Teachers know students because the high school is a closed environment and the number of students is fairly small.	Professors, especially those who are teaching introductory courses, may teach over 100 new students each semester. They have no idea who you are unless you make an effort to introduce yourself and become known.
Homework assignments are given at the end of every class and often are written on the board.	All assignments are printed in the syllabus that is given out at the beginning of the semester. Not all professors will remind you of the reading or written assignments that you are expected to complete.
The focus of assignments is on following the directions and structure. Students can get a good grade for completing the assignment according to the instructions and on time.	The stakes are higher in college. Students get good grades if they do the assignment according to the instructions **and** add creativity, analysis, and insight into the project or paper.
Students take classes in much of the same groups and come to know each other fairly well.	For the first year when you are taking required courses every class may have a completely different group of students. It's hard to get to know people unless you make an effort to learn more about them.
There is a wide range of student achievement—bright students stand out and become well-known to teachers and other students.	Everyone enrolled in college had to meet some standard of achievement in order to be accepted. You will find yourself more with your intellectual peers and competition is higher. You will have to work harder to stand out.

Worksheet 10-1

Transition from Coursework to Fieldwork

In Coursework	In Fieldwork

Hopson and Scally (1993) give you three key words to help you manage your time better: knowledge, choice, and time. They say you have to know clearly what you need or want to do, choose among all of those things, and schedule time to act on your choice. In this section, I will give you exercises and worksheets to help you manage your time better.

Getting a Handle on the Amount of Time Things Really Take

Multiple demands put many of us in a position of having to juggle lots of activities and to respond to a lot of different expectations in any given day. Some of our activities are routine and they are easy for us to estimate the amount of time they will take us. For example, most of us know exactly how much time we will need to shower, dress, eat, and get out of the house in the morning, and we set our alarm clocks accordingly. Most of use know exactly how long it will take us to drive to school, make a cup of coffee, or attend a biology class.

Estimating the time it will take to write a 10-page paper on home care OT for infants with cerebral palsy or to complete a project on schizophrenia is not as easy. Why is this? First, each of these assignments involve multiple tasks—you don't just write a paper. You have to develop a topic, develop an outline, research in the library, read several sources, take notes, write a first draft, refine and rewrite the paper, get feedback from a reader, and write the final document. Second, you generally do not complete all of these tasks at one sitting (unless of course you are a "last minute" person, which we will discuss later in this section). It is hard to step back and see just how much time you've put in. Third, you may not have enough experience at this set of tasks to have a good sense of how much time it demands. When you do not have a good handle on the many tasks involved in completing a project or the amount of time those tasks will take, you tend to underestimate the amount of time and energy that will go into completing the project. This is one reason why so many new college students do their assignments at the last minute—they just did not plan to spend enough time to get the assignment done.

Strategies for Better Time Management

Time Study

Select a specific schoolwork activity to analyze such as completing a project, writing a paper, or reading a textbook. Do your best to write down the tasks involved in completing the activity. As you work on the activity, log in the number of minutes you spend on each task. Some tasks may take several work sessions, so keep track of how many work sessions and the number of minutes you spend doing each. When you have completed the project and your time study, take a look at how much time each task took—you will probably be surprised.

Figure 10-1 is an example of a chart for doing a time study. You can use your computer to print out a chart using your word processing program or spreadsheet program. Put the chart in your notebook so you can log in your work time.

Available Time Chart

Make a chart of just 1 week in your life. Think about the time you have in three different ways:

Assignment: Spinal Cord Project for Neuroanatomy		
Task	**Time Spent**	**Comments**
Sketch out ideas	30 minutes	
Research in library	4 hours!	It took a long time to find books and articles—I stood at the copier forever.
Review/read books and articles	1 hour 1 hour 2 hours 1 hour	This took almost 2 weeks.
Nail down project ideas into actual model	1.5 hours	I also spent about 5 hours of "think time" over a week's time before I could sit down and work out the details.
Organize to-do list and materials list	30 minutes	
Buy/find materials	2 hours	
Build project	1 hour 1 hour 1 hour	
Write corresponding short paper for distributing at display	2 hours	
Make copies of paper	1 hour	
Prepare signs for display	1 hour 1 hour	It took some time to get this right. Had to choose a font that I liked.
Prepare entire display	1.5 hours	
Total hours	**23 hours**	**Grade on assignment: A-**

Figure 10-1. Sample time study worksheet.

1. Committed time: time you *must* be somewhere—class, work, appointments.
2. Necessary time: time you must spend but you have freedom to schedule it in—the 5 hours it will take you to complete reading assignments this week, you can schedule it into any uncommitted time.
3. Discretionary time: time that you can spend any way you want—you choose both the activity and the time.

Enter in all the things that you know you have to do and how much time those things take. Once you have all those activities entered, step back and take a look at how much time you have available in your schedule for your necessary time such as studying. Schedule that time in. Now take a look at how much discretionary time you have left. How will you use that time?

Figure 10-2 is an example of just a couple days in Keisha's life. Take a look at how much time Keisha actually has on these days to get schoolwork done once she has entered all her committed time.

Questions to think about:

• How many hours does Keisha have on Monday and Tuesday to get schoolwork done? Schedule in at least 2½ hours of study time into Keisha's schedule.

Time	Monday	Tuesday
6:00-7:00 a.m.	Get up, get ready	Get up, get ready
7:00-8:00	Drive to school (7:15)	
8:00-9:00	Biology class	Drive to school (8:30)
9:00-10:00		Math class (9:30-11:00)
10:00-11:00		Math class
11:00-12:00 noon	English class	Sociology class (11:00-12:30)
12:00-1:00 p.m.		Sociology class
1:00-2:00		Library
2:00-3:00	Intro to OT class	
3:00-4:00		
4:00-5:00	Leave for work (4:30)	Leave for work (4:30)
5:00-6:00	Work	Work
6:00-7:00	Work	Work
7:00-8:00	Work	Work
8:00-9:00	Work	Work
9:00-10:00	Work	Work
10:00-11:00	Home from work (10:20)	Home from work (10:20)

Figure 10-2. Keisha's routine.

- How much discretionary time does Keisha have left once she has scheduled in her necessary time?
- Is there anything Keisha can do to make her schedule work better for her?
- What times do you think would be best for Keisha to use for getting schoolwork done?
- Do you think Keisha is trying to do too much?

Use Worksheet 10-2 to chart 1 week for yourself. Ask yourself the same questions about your own schedule. If you find that you have too much to do and not enough time you will need to actively reflect on these questions and come up with solutions to the problems you uncover.

How Do You Use Your Time?

Each of us has a time-use style and our own favorite ways to waste time. Wasting time can be a lot of fun and has no particularly bad consequences when your time schedule is open and you have a lot of free time. When you are busy and have to use your time well, your time-use and time-wasting styles can really get in the way! One of the most useful ways of learning to manage your time more effectively is to recognize the things you do that keep you from using your time well, take responsibility for your own style, and do what you can to manage your tendencies to your best advantage.

Your Time-Use Style

There are several ways that people have learned to take advantage of time (or have time take advantage of them). Each time-use style has its own strengths and limitations. You might recognize yourself in one of these descriptions:

Worksheet 10-2

Day: _____

Time:			
6:00-7:00 a.m.			
7:00-8:00			
8:00-9:00			
9:00-10:00			
10:00-11:00			
11:00-12:00 noon			
12:00-1:00 p.m.			
1:00-2:00			
2:00-3:00			
3:00-4:00			
4:00-5:00			
5:00-6:00			
6:00-7:00			
7:00-8:00			
8:00-9:00			
9:00-10:00			
10:00-11:00			

- **The procrastinator.** "Never do today what you can put off until tomorrow." The procrastinator comes up with 100 or more reasons why he or she should not work on something right now. A really good procrastinator comes up with reasons that even seem to make sense like, "I can't work on this report right now because the library is closed today." While procrastinating can help if you need time to mull an idea over, it can leave you with too little time to complete a project and the feeling that you are not getting anywhere.

- **The marathoner.** "I'll just stay up for the next two nights and get this project finished." The marathoner does an entire project at one time rather than plan out a project over a period of weeks or months. He or she usually underestimates the amount of time the project will take and forgets to factor in exhaustion. Being a marathoner can really work if you have overlooked a project or need to cram for an exam, but it doesn't help when you are juggling multiple priorities and end up running yourself into the ground.

- **The busy-bee.** "I really like being busy—I've got a million things to do." The busy-bee is involved in many activities and does have a lot on his or her plate. The busy-bee tends to have a lot of energy and is good at tracking and working on multiple tasks. He or she is spread so thin, however, that most projects don't get the attention they deserve. The busy-bee over-commits and has to cancel things at the last minute to devote enough time to a project that is due.

- **The last-minute energy burst.** "I do my best work under pressure." The last-minute burster depends on the pressure of deadlines and expectations to generate a kind of panic energy for getting a project done. There are times when all of us benefit from a last-minute energy burst, particularly toward the end of a college semester. Unfortunately, the last-minute burster often leaves things until the last minute and does a poor quality job or misses the deadline and has to turn projects in late.
- **The planner.** "I schedule all my time so I know exactly what I need to do. If you want to talk to me you will need to make an appointment." The planner is very good at listing and scheduling all anticipated assignments and activities and does a fairly good job of estimating how much time each will take. The planner's major limitation is in the area of flexibility. He or she leaves little discretionary time in his or her schedule and has difficulty being spontaneous or responding to a last-minute change or a surprise assignment.
- **The shotgunner.** "I work on everything all at once. If I do a little work on each job every day I will eventually get them all done." The shotgunner is good at juggling a lot of different projects and making progress on each. He or she is probably the best of all the styles at sustaining his or her commitment to several different projects over the long haul. The shotgunner can get stuck when a specific project demands extra time and attention because he or she has to put other projects on hold and feels constrained.
- **Alfred E. Newman.** "What me worry?" Alfred E. tends to let everything go and doesn't seem to have any attention on planning or even worrying about the tasks he or she needs to accomplish. Interestingly enough, while Al may not pay in emotional terms, he or she almost always trades off quality and grades for style. He or she is a mediocre student at best, but doesn't worry about it—or at least that's what Alfred E. says!

Hopefully you have recognized yourself in some of these style descriptions. Each style is an advantage in certain situations but is a liability in others. In order to be a successful student you will need to flex your style and develop new styles that best match the demands on your time.

Wasting Time

College campuses are full of good ways to waste time. No matter where you go on campus there are always plenty of opportunities to spend your time doing things other than studying or keeping up with your work. Here is just a short list of ways that students waste time:

- Spreading your classes out over the course of the day and not using the time in between to get work done
- Using the library as a social hub
- Procrastinating—putting things off until tomorrow and finding other things to do with your time today
- Long phone calls
- Driving home or going back to your dorm between classes
- Reading materials for a paper before you have a good outline
- Hanging out at the student center watching TV or playing video games
- Worrying or complaining about how much work you have to do

- Overdoing certain activities or getting over-involved
- Partying—particularly if you party so hard that you can't work the next day
- Scheduling all your classes later in the day so you can sleep late
- Piling books, papers, and assignments all over your room and spending a lot of time looking for things

Avoiding time wasters takes honesty and discipline. First, be honest with yourself about the ways you waste time. Take a hard look at the ways you are using your time. Are they the best ways to reach your educational goals? If you don't know if or how you are wasting your time, do a time study similar to the one explained earlier in this section. Map out a week and write down what you are doing every hour. Note where you are wasting time or where you could use your time better. Develop specific ways to avoid time wasters and to use your time to your advantage.

Second, develop the discipline you will need to avoid wasting time. Much like any change effort, such as losing weight, starting an exercise program, or bettering your tennis serve, changing the way you manage your time takes a strong commitment to your goal, a plan, and the self-discipline to follow through on your plan (Table 10-2).

GOAL MANAGEMENT

What is a goal? A goal is a future state, a dream of the future, a place you want to get to. If a goal is strong and clear it can motivate you, direct you, guide your actions, help you make decisions about your time and energy, and propel you toward the life you want. Goals are particularly important in times when you feel discouraged about your ability to be successful because they help you refocus on what you are working to accomplish.

When you decided to go on to college to pursue a degree in OT you probably did so with a specific goal in mind: to be an OTR or a COTA. If this goal is strong for you, it will serve as a guiding star for all your work in college. To strengthen your sense of your ultimate goal, spend some time visualizing what it will be like when you achieve your goal. Generate an image of yourself graduating, passing your qualifying exam, receiving your official credential, and working in a job that you enjoy. See Chapter 2 to record your progress. This visualization idea may sound funny to you, but it works! In fact, many OTs use this very same technique with their patients to help motivate and speed rehabilitation.

Your ultimate goal of being an OTR or a COTA will translate into shorter term goals that are important in helping you reach your long-term goal. You should ask yourself the question: What do I need to accomplish in college, in this semester, in this class, to help me reach my goal? Short-term goals are usually closer to now and more action-specific. Some examples of short-term goals are:

1. Present the best project in Advanced Anatomy.
2. Be fully successful in my nursing home fieldwork.
3. Receive an 85 or better on my qualifying exam.

Of course, each of these short-term goals implies a number of objectives, focused action steps that, if accomplished, will guarantee that the goal is reached.

Let's take the second goal: "Be fully successful in my nursing home fieldwork." Imagine a student who understands and appreciates the value of fieldwork in learning about the specific area of OT and building good on-the-job skills. What specific focused action steps should the student take to achieve this goal? In order to answer this question you will need to think about the expectations for a fully successful fieldwork student from

---

Table 10-2
Helpful Tips to Reduce Time Management Stress

- **Goal setting.** Set measurable objectives for your career, family, finances, fitness, and social life. Written goals provide a framework to help you assess your use of time. What gets measured gets done.
- **Setting priorities.** List all pending activities, including paperwork, meetings, and telephone calls, in priority order. Assign the letter A to tasks that *must* be done, B to those that *should* be done, and C to those that *might* be done. Tackle items on your A list first.
- **Bunching.** Cluster similar activities together. Schedule blocks of time for returning phone calls, writing reports, meeting with other students, and doing desk work.
- **Strategic scheduling.** Schedule classes to your advantage. Do not spread your classes out over an entire day or an entire week. Cluster them together so you have bigger chunks of time to study or work.
- **Chunking.** Break down complex or unpleasant tasks into smaller, more manageable parts. Complete one chunk first (e.g., a one-page outline of a lengthy report) and another chunk (e.g., write the introduction) later.
- **Closure.** Condition yourself to complete each task the first time you start it. For example, ask a drop-in visitor to wait outside your room until you finish the memo you're working on. Emphasize completion.
- **Deadlines.** Set personal due dates that precede the stated deadlines, or create a deadline when one is not given. Submit reports before due dates. Be an early bird.
- **Elimination.** Get rid of the time wasters—long lunches, going nowhere meetings, long telephone calls, trips—and anything that distracts you from your goals.
- **Planning.** Anticipate future events. Planning time saves operating time, so prepare weekly plans and daily to-do lists. Each morning, review your game plan for the day.
- **Saying no.** Avoid over-committing yourself. Success depends on knowing what not to do. Be firm but gracious in rejecting tasks unrelated to your goals and reject time wasters whenever possible.
- **Hiding out.** Schedule quiet time. Take a walk, close the door, smell the roses, reflect. You need time for thinking and relaxing each day.
- **Fitness.** Exercise increases energy. To charge your battery, schedule time to jog, play golf, play racquetball, or take a walk. Invest time in yourself. Your capital gain will include higher energy levels, renewed desire to work, a more positive self-image, better health, and increase productivity.

Adapted from The University of Connecticut Advance. *(1996, May). Storrs, C. 1-8.*

---

the point of view of how students are evaluated and from the student's point of view (Worksheet 10-3).

Hopefully you wrote things such as:
- Meet with my supervisor to get feedback and suggestions on improving my performance once a week.
- Meet and talk to three OTs who work in this specific field to find out what they see as the critical knowledge and skill areas.
- Develop excellent rapport with all patients—get to know four patients very well.

Worksheet 10-3

Action Steps and Ideas _____

_____

_____

_____

_____

_____

_____

_____

- Be on time every day—no matter what.
- Write in my journal every other day for 20 minutes.
- Complete all written assignments 24 hours before they are due.

Notice how each action step has two specific characteristics: an action and a quantification. Your action steps must be actions, something you can do, and they must have a quantifying feature. Whether your quantifiers are "by when" dates, the number of times you will do something, how many minutes you will spend, or the grade your will receive, numbers and actions make your action steps measurable. Either you are meeting with your supervisor once a week and getting feedback or you are not. Either you are on time every day or you are not. Action steps such as "Be on time," "Get my fieldwork supervisor to like me," and "Do a good job on my written assignments" are not good action steps because they are not measurable, are very subjective, and leave quite a bit of room for interpretation, which may leave you less than successful. Use your semester-long planning calendar to write in action steps that must be completed on certain dates or action steps that should be completed every week. For example, it might make the most sense to set up a weekly meeting time with your fieldwork supervisor at the beginning of the fieldwork and write it on your calendar. The reminder on your calendar will give you time to prepare questions for the weekly meeting.

The list of possible objectives for this goal will be related to the specific expectations of your college and on-site supervisor in relation to fieldwork. Your list may look different from someone else's. You want to make sure to include your personal objectives for the fieldwork along side those of your supervisor and program. For example, this student wanted to meet and talk to other OTs working with elderly people so she wrote that objective in. This activity was not required by her program but she thought it would be a good way to learn about this particular career path.

What good do all these goals and action steps do? No good if you don't use them. There are many ways to use goals and action steps to help you be successful. First, you have to write them down. A goal or an objective in your head is not effective. I suggest that you reserve the first 5 to 10 pages in your notebook for writing down your goals and action steps. You may want to put all your goals and action steps in your computer, print them out, and post them near your desk.

This suggestion leads to the second tip: Keep your goals and action steps where you can see them and refer to them. Goals and action steps are a good way to remind yourself what you are in college for. If you find yourself sitting at your desk wondering what to do, you can refer to your list to determine your next step. Your list can also help you plan out your week. For example, the fieldwork student whose action steps are listed earlier reviewed her action steps and made a plan for the week that included meeting with her supervisor with specific questions that she had written, contacting one OT who worked in another nursing home, visiting with a patient and her daughter, and leaving her dorm by 7 a.m. every day.

Third, well-developed action steps will help you get a very good picture of how you are doing and a way to correct your actions for better success. For example, what if you review your progress at the end of a week and determine that you have been a few minutes late to your fieldwork twice in one week. Even if no one else noticed you have not followed your action plan, now you can figure out what went wrong: Did you leave late? Did you run into traffic? Did you stop for coffee both days? Did you have trouble finding a parking space? Did you stop to talk with a friend on the way out of the dorm? Figuring out what kept you from being on time allows you to make a correction and get back on track (Table 10-3).

Prioritizing Your Goals

You have goals related to school and career, but you may also have goals concerning romance, relationships, family, fitness, work, financial stability, and other areas. To be successful in college you must recognize and take all these other important goals into account. Many college students have difficulty because they let their unwritten goals concerning recreation or relationships take precedence over their educational goals. Begin each semester with a thinking exercise around the question, "What is important to me this year?" Make sure that you write down everything you think of, not just education-related goals. Once you have this list, step back and take a look at the whole picture. Make a decision about what is most important to you at this point in time and what deserves the most attention from you. Label your priorities. You may be labeled a "serious student" or even a "geek," but making your studies your priority will help you make those tough decisions like whether to study for a test or head out to a party on a Thursday night.

Remember Mark in the story at the beginning of this chapter? His school life is packed with all kinds of activities, studying, and now his fieldwork assignments. In order to resolve his concerns about being successful in his fieldwork, Mark will have to set some priorities. If a career in OT is important to Mark and successful fieldwork experience is critical to his finding a good job in the field, Mark will probably have to give up a few of the ongoing activities he has been involved in, limiting the time and energy he spends on other activities to focus on a successful fieldwork experience. It will help Mark to keep in mind that his fieldwork will not go on forever, that cutting back on his extracurricular activities is a time-limited task, and that developing self-discipline around the use of his time and energy will be of great benefit to him in his career as an OT.

It takes some soul-searching to decide where you are going to put your energy. It helps to remember that you have a whole lifetime ahead of you, but you only have this time in college. At risk of sounding like your mother, your college career will set the stage for the rest of your life and it is something that you will want to look back on and be proud

---

Table 10-3
Questions to Consider When Developing Goals and Action Steps

- Do I know what my ultimate goal is?
- Do I have my ultimate goal written down or recorded in a way that I can see it and use it for inspiration and motivation?
- Do I have goals for this semester that are related to my classes or fieldwork experience?
- Does each goal have a list of action steps that, if followed, will lead to success?
- Is each action step written as an action, as something I can do?
- Does each action step have a way to measure it—a by when date, a number of times, or a how often?
- Do I have a specific time for reviewing my goals and action steps on a regular basis to evaluate my performance and make corrections?

---

of. If you manage yourself well, work hard to reach your goals, and make good decisions, you will be able to say with pride that you did your best.

Rewarding Yourself for Reaching Your Goals

All this goal-setting and action-planning may make doing college work sound like a real grind. On the contrary, if you become a good planner and follow your plans you will find yourself with more time for having fun, not less, because you will learn to use your time well. In the spirit of fun, don't forget to build in ways to reward yourself for completing your action steps and reaching your goals.

Here are some ways that students rewarded themselves for a successful semester:
- An entire weekend with no books
- A new outfit
- Time with best friends
- A new book
- Sleeping until noon on Saturday
- A romantic evening out
- A decadent dessert
- An all-day hike
- A new CD

Building Support for Reaching Your Goals

One of the most powerful things you can do with your goals is to share them with the people who will help you reach those goals. None of us can complete a degree program successfully without the support of our family, friends, fellow students, and faculty. When those people hear you speak your goals powerfully and intentionally, they will line up to see how they can help you.

Imagine what might happen if you sat down with your family, close friends, or roommates and shared with them your goal to receive an 85 or better on your OTR exam. Speaking the goal will build instant support for you to accomplish this goal. Be prepared to say what you need from your family or friends in the way of support: a break from doing dishes, encouragement, quiet time, a strict adherence to no invitations to do something fun on Saturdays (your prime study time), or dinner delivered to your room so you can study. In my experience, people who care about you always listen and support your goals, and they are more than willing to do what you ask so they can help you accomplish them. Remember Keisha who was having trouble with her hometown friends because they complained that she wasn't spending enough time with them? Perhaps if Keisha shared her goal to be an extraordinary student with her hometown friends, and asked them to support her by only asking her to do things with them on Friday night, Keisha would feel better and her friends would stop bugging her about not seeing her as much. If you have friends who don't respect your goals and the hard work you will need to do to get there, it may be time to break ties with those friends and find new ones who can support you.

FOR ADULT LEARNERS

As an adult student—someone who is going to college after having had a chance to hold down a full-time job, respond to life changes, live independently, and perhaps raise a family—you have had many experiences that have helped you develop good skills for succeeding in a college OT program. In all likelihood, you have an advantage in terms of time management, goal management, and relating to professors because you have had to rely on those skills to be successful in your own life. You will be better at assessing your strengths and limitations because you have more experiences to evaluate. Although adult learners are not necessarily more motivated than traditional students, you probably have a clearer picture of why you are pursuing an OT degree and what you will be able to do with it. This clearer picture will serve you well in discouraging moments.

On the other hand, being an adult student brings with it various hurdles to being successful in college as well. You will probably have to respond to more financial, work, and family demands than your younger counterparts. You may have hidden attitudes that will get in the way of your learning such as, "I never did well on tests" or "My reading and writing skills are rusty." You may feel out of place with traditional students and will have to bridge the gap or find a group of adult students with whom you can feel comfortable. While traditional students continue from one academic setting to another, you will have to change your routine and behavior in order to readjust to being in an academic environment. You may hit barriers with your employer, such as missing an important project deadline, or with your family, such as leaving them to cook dinner for themselves, that will demand good problem-solving skills on your part. Finally, while you are working toward your degree, as one adult student put it, "Life happens." The time it takes you to finish your degree may include the death of a loved one, divorce, sending your child off to kindergarten, unemployment, or a serious personal illness. Fortunately, your experiences with change and adjustment as an adult will help you through these challenges. In addition, there is increased attention in recent years on how to help adult learners succeed in college and your college or university is bound to have special supports for adult students like you. As a fellow adult student, I wish you much success.

ORGANIZING YOURSELF

One sure way to succeed in college is to organize yourself. Organizing yourself means setting up systems to help you reach your goals. There are many products available to help you organize yourself: semester calendars, personal organization software that even gives you warnings a week before a paper is due, personal filing boxes, goal-setting manuals, desk organizers, and book-marking self-sticking notes to name just a few. Visit your college bookstore or your local office supply store to see what they have. This section will describe three ways to organize yourself: a semester-long calendar, your desk, and action plans.

Semester-Long Calendar

Each of your professors will give you a plan for the entire semester called a syllabus. The syllabus will list class topics, class readings, and class assignments with due dates. If you are taking five classes it is up to you to coordinate the syllabi from each class so you don't get stuck doing four projects at one time. Mapping all of your courses out during the first few weeks of classes is a good habit to get into. It gives you an overview of the highs and lows of the semester and helps you plan out your efforts on bigger projects.

A semester-long calendar is good and many college bookstores sell calendars that start in September and end in May. Mark the beginning and end of the semester in your calendar. Use a highlighter to color in mid-term week and final exam week. Sit down with the syllabus from each of your classes and note the due dates for papers, projects, and reading assignments in brightly colored ink. Use the syllabus from each of your courses to map out the following information on your semester-long calendar (Worksheet 10-4).

- Circle due dates of papers and projects in red ink
- Highlight mid-term and final exams
- Star important events

You can see at a glance where you will have to be disciplined to accomplish tasks. There may be a cluster of mid-term exams in mid-October, a cluster of papers and projects due in November, and final exams in December.

Other events you may want to write in your semester-long calendar include:

- Work hours
- Big social events
- Backward time lines: plan backwards from a due date to figure out when you need to start working on a project or paper (this is especially important when you have a bunch-up of papers or projects due at the same time)
- Schedule study time right into your calendar
- If you buy a daily calendar you can write in your action steps related to your goals or to a project or paper

One word of caution. Once you write in all the specific things you must accomplish over a semester you may feel overwhelmed. Working through a semester of classes is a lot of work and takes a lot of juggling on your part to make sure that everything gets done. If you follow the suggestions in this section, don't be surprised if your calendar is packed with deadlines and tasks.

Organizing Your Desk

In order to stay organized, you need to have a work place that is set up to make you efficient and effective. Here are some suggestions for organizing your work materials and work space:

- Have all books handy.
- Post a weekly calendar of assignments and action steps.

- Keep extra supplies on hand, such as paper, pencils, pens, staples, even a printer cartridge. You don't want to have to find a printer cartridge right in the middle of printing a final paper that's due tomorrow.
- Have all your reference materials handy—dictionary, medical terminology reference, phone list.
- Hang up a bulletin board so you can post notes, reminders, and goal posters.
- Set up a notebook or a file box in which to keep class handouts and information. Office supply stores have desktop files with four or five slots that you can label for each class.
- Set up folders for organizing projects and papers. Closing accordion files work well. Keep all your materials and references in your folder until the project or paper is completed and turned in. Then clean out the folder and keep only the references and materials that will be helpful to you later.
- When you sit down to study, have a supply of high energy snacks and drinks on hand. Getting up to get something to drink or eat is one of the most popular time wasters of all time.

Action Plans

Action plans can help you map out and complete big assignments. Writing a paper or doing a project will involve many different steps. The only way to get the assignment done well is to anticipate the amount of work that will go into it and to plan out the time you will need. Figure 10-3 is a sample action plan for writing a paper. Use Worksheet 10-5 to create your own action plan.

Use action plans for all kinds of projects. Be sure to transfer the "by when" dates from your action plan to your calendar. Don't forget to check off tasks as you complete them. There is nothing more satisfying than marking a task done—it not only makes you feel good, it gives you a little burst of energy to move on to the next task.

SUPPORTIVE RELATIONSHIPS

Other people can help you reach your goals by supporting you to do your best and helping you use your time well. Having good relationships with your professors, particularly those in your field of study, is an important part of being an effective student. In addition, you may want to develop a student study group with other OT majors.

Building Relationships With Professors

Most professors choose to teach on the college level because they love their subject and want to share it with interested people. One of the best ways to form a good relationship with a professor is to show a genuine interest in his or her subject. Most professors wince when they hear a student say, "I'm only taking this course because I have to." Although they know that their course is required, professors don't really appreciate hearing how you could care less about how much work they have done. On the other hand, if you show an appreciation and interest in the course content by discussing issues, asking questions, demonstrating curiosity, and writing provocative papers, a professor will notice.

Most OT professors are registered OTs who teach students because they love the field and want to share their enthusiasm and knowledge with new professionals entering the field. Unfortunately, many college students miss the opportunity to learn everything they

Worksheet 10-4

Month:

Sunday	Monday	Tuesday	Wednesday	Thursday	Friday	Saturday

can from their professors because they are shy, don't know how to start a conversation, or don't want to look like they are kissing up to the teacher. Use them to your best advantage and learn everything you can from them. The vast majority of professors are happy when a student makes the effort to meet them, converse, and inquire.

The best way for you to develop a good relationship with your OT professors is to build on your common interest in the field—share your enthusiasm with your professors, use their expertise to learn more, find out where they worked in the field, and what they think about changes in the field. Use your OT professors to sharpen your professional skills and get feedback on your performance as it relates to a future in OT.

Here a some specific ways to build solid relationships with your professors:

- Follow the syllabus. Know the topic of each class and keep up with your reading. Be sure to let your professor know that you have done the reading and what you thought of it.
- Participate fully in class. Arrive early, join in discussions, be attentive, ask questions, be prepared, and lead group projects. Give your best effort. Not everyone can be up for every class, just make sure that your participation level far outweighs your "down" days.

Action Plan		
GOAL: Write teenage pregnancy paper **DUE DATE: March 13** CLASS: Social Issues		
Task	**By When**	**Completed**
Choose a topic		☐
Outline main ideas for the paper		☐
Research main ideas by finding articles, books, and papers on the topic		☐
Read one third of the materials to make sure that topic will work		☐
Read remaining materials and keep good notes*		☐
Write first draft of paper		☐
Revise first draft		☐
Get someone to read second draft		☐
Incorporate feedback into third draft		☐
Polish draft for submission		☐
Have someone read final paper		☐
Make final corrections in spelling, punctuation, and format		☐
Print out paper		☐
Turn in paper		☐

*You may want to break reading materials down into clusters (e.g., "Read three articles or chapters by Friday," "Read five articles by Tuesday," "Review Ray and McKenna book by Monday"). This is particularly helpful if you have a lot of reading to do for a paper. Even if you read just one article a day you can get your reading for a paper done within a few weeks.

Figure 10-3. Sample action plan.

- Ask for feedback. Whether you are submitting an exam, a paper, or a project, ask your professor specific questions to which he or she can respond. For example, Which of these references do you think are best to use for my paper? Can you add to my outline? Is there anything that I have missed? Do you have any suggestions for making this project better? Do you know of a conference or meeting where I could present this project?
- Set up a time to meet with each of your professors at least once, preferably early in the semester. Don't just drop in. Schedule a time to talk during the professor's office hours. Arrive at the meeting prepared to ask questions or discuss a particular lecture, reading, or project.
- Turn in high quality work and avoid excuses (Ellis, 1985). Every professor's ultimate goal is to have his or her students do well. Submitting excellent work will let a professor know that you are engaged in his or her course and you are working your hardest. Giving lame excuses for not completing your work on time or without

Worksheet 10-5

GOAL:	DUE DATE:	
CLASS:		
Task	By When	Completed
		☐
		☐
		☐
		☐
		☐
		☐
		☐
		☐

regard for quality is disrespectful of yourself and the teacher. Take responsibility for foul-ups and work with the professor to negotiate a new time line or needed improvements. Along these same lines, whining, complaining, and defending poor work will do nothing for your image in the eyes of an instructor.

- Establish expectations. Read materials and instructions that are distributed by the professor. Clarify any misunderstandings you might have about instructions. Some students don't do well on papers or projects because they thought they understood the instructions but didn't.
- Finally, remember that professors are people, too. It sounds trite, but many students don't see professors as adults, like themselves, in a learning career that is built around the sharing of knowledge and ideas. Educators are motivated and encouraged by student success. The best foundation for a good relationship with a professor is to be a strong, enthusiastic student. Share your knowledge and enthusiasm with others.

BEING ASSERTIVE

Many students say that, at times, they do not know how to approach a professor or another student about a problem. Some students say nothing and suffer the consequences of passive behavior. Some students wait until they get really angry and just yell. This is called aggressive behavior. Somewhere between passive and aggressive is the state of being assertive. Assertive students make their needs known without stepping on the rights of others.

Being assertive takes practice. It means being able to say no and feel guilt-free. It means getting the help you need without making the other person feel angry or guilty. Being assertive starts with listening to the words that come out of your mouth when you are trying to get your needs met. Look at the examples below.

Passive: "Sara asked me to give her all of my notes from psychopathology and I said sure. I could kick myself for saying it, but I couldn't say no."

Aggressive: "Are you crazy? You must be insane if you think that test was fair. At best, your questions were unclear!"

Assertive: "I have some concerns about my paper. I am not pleased with the work I did and I want to do better next time. Can I get some help?"

Notice how the assertive person takes responsibility for his or her behavior while initiating his or her need for help. The assertive person used the word "I" five times. In the aggressive statement, the person uses "you" four times. An assertive person takes responsibility for what has occurred and actively seeks to rectify a situation, using "I" statements more than "you" statements. A passive person uses "I" statements but in a negative, self-defeating way. For example, "I could just kick myself."

When it is time to approach a professor or peer about an important issue, remember to be assertive.

- Practice using "I" statements before you sit down to talk.
- Listen carefully to the other person's statements.
- Recognize any traps around wanting to blame the other person. Assertiveness is about generating power by claiming responsibility, not being a victim.
- Be respectful and avoid "you" statements.
- If you feel yourself getting out of control, or the other person says something sur-

prising, say "That's very interesting. Let me think about it and get back to you." Always follow up later so you don't act passive about the issue.

ESTABLISHING A SUPPORT GROUP

Successful students associate with successful students. There is nothing you could do that would be more harmful to your successful college career than to join the study group that meets Monday through Friday at the local pub. On the other hand, if you join a study group that meets at the library twice a week you will be that much closer to success. Learning groups provide a rich resource to support your success, offer friendship, fill in missing information, and provide encouragement (Smith & Walter, 1995).

Study groups do not generally exist as something you can join—you have to initiate a study group and form it with others. Find students in your program who seem to be serious and seem to be doing well. Organize a group meeting to figure out how you might work together to benefit each member of the group. Here are some suggestions of things a study or learning group might set as regular activities:

- Split up class readings and share notes. Discuss the readings as a group.
- Study for exams together.
- Do group projects together.
- Use e-mail to communicate with each other.
- Share second-to-last drafts of papers for feedback.
- Share and discuss notes from class.
- Cover for each other and share notes when a member can't attend class.
- Clarify assignments and instructor expectations.
- Share your goals and action steps with each other and support each other to reach them.
- Go to a movie together when you've all completed your final papers and turned them in.
- Celebrate each other's successes.

Establishing a learning group with fellow students within your program might be one of the smartest things you can do to further your college career. If you find the right match of people and really commit yourself to each other's goals, you will have a strong source of support and will probably become lifelong friends.

SUMMARY

A college education is a tremendous source of information and knowledge that will build the foundation for your career in OT. The focus of the formal activities in college center around the development of specific knowledge and skills that can be translated into your future work. Less obvious, however, is the opportunity as a college student to develop self-management skills that will be invaluable to you as a working professional.

Particularly in the OT field, you will need well-developed self-management skills that include time management, goal management, building professional relationships, and developing lifelong learning habits. Many in OT work independently and the field is increasingly demanding that OTRs and COTAs perform their jobs without direct supervision, responding to a variety of demands and situations efficiently and effectively. I encourage you to take the opportunity that being a college student presents to set and work toward goals to develop your ability to manage yourself, your learning, and your future.

BIBLIOGRAPHY

Ellis, D. B. (1985). *Becoming a master student* (5th ed.). Rapid City, SD: College Survival, Inc.

Hopson, B., & Scally, M. (1993). *Time management: Conquering the clock.* San Diego, CA: Pfeiffer & Company.

Schlossberg, N. K. (1984). *Counseling adults in transition: Linking practice with theory.* New York: Springer.

Smith, L. N., & Walter, T. L. (1995). *The adult learner's guide to college success* (Rev. ed.). Boston: Wadsworth Publishing Company.

Stupka, E., & Eddy, B. (1992). *The right to succeed: Making it happen in your classroom.* Sacramento, CA: Sacramento City College.

The University of Connecticut Advance. (1996, May). Storrs, C. 1-8.

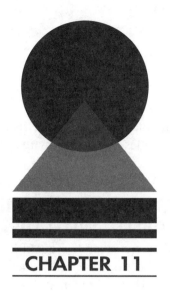

CHAPTER 11

OT STUDENTS WITH DISABILITIES

Kimberly D. Hartmann, MHS, OTR/L, FAOTA

INTRODUCTION

Individuals with disabilities have rights to equality as protected by the Americans With Disabilities Act (ADA) signed into law by President George Bush in 1990. This law is a civil rights legislation that prohibits discrimination against individuals with disabilities in all institutions that receive federal funds. The Rehabilitation Act of 1973 set the foundation for the ADA. Section 504 of this act established requirements and procedures that institutions of higher education, colleges and universities, follow in order to provide an equal educational opportunity for individuals with disabilities. The law is not a guarantee of success but a promise that the students will be provided with an opportunity to try. This chapter will provide an overview of the law, a listing of the rights and responsibilities of students with disabilities, discussion of why OT school may be more difficult than high school, methods to follow for communication, and tips for becoming a self-advocate and an independently responsible OT student.

OVERVIEW

A student with a disability may use reasonable accommodations to assist him- or herself in meeting the essentials of the program. Reasonable accommodation is a term that includes alterations, accessibility tools, auxiliary aids or equipment, flexibility of scheduling, or a variety of other items that have as their purpose to educate and assess learning without the disability being a hindrance. These reasonable accommodations should allow the student's individual potential to be activated without deterrence from the limitations of the disability. The establishment of reasonable accommodations is an interactive process between the student with a disability, the Section 504 coordinator on the campus, and appropriate members of the OT faculty. It is the utilization of these accommodations that often provides the student with a disability a tool for meeting the essential requirements of the program.

RIGHTS AND RESPONSIBILITIES OF STUDENTS WITH DISABILITIES

Students who believe that they are otherwise qualified but have a disability have both rights and responsibilities under Section 504. The student must be the one who self advocates and seeks out advice, as college or university life is very different than high school where parental involvement and control are accepted. The Rehabilitation Act of 1973, its amendments, and in particular Section 504, are to protect the student's rights. However, as with most rights comes responsibilities that the student must also consider in order to become in control of his or her educational experience and learning.

If the student wishes to benefit from these rights, then the student must assume certain responsibilities (Worksheet 11-1). These responsibilities mean that the student may need to seek out information, ask clarifying questions, follow college or university policies, communicate with the proper people on campus (504 coordinator and OT chairperson), and self-disclose that a disability does exist. See Appendix A for further resources.

MAKING IT THROUGH THE TRANSITIONS

When, Why, and How to State "I Have a Disability."

The Rehabilitation Act of 1973, Section 504, and the ADA state that if an individual with a disability would like academic adjustments or reasonable accommodations, then that individual must self-disclose the disability and request the adjustments or accommodations. This is a dramatic change over of responsibility that the student with a disability must become accustomed to. In the law that covers students with disabilities in the public school (Individuals With Disabilities Education Act [IDEA]), the professionals are responsible for seeking out, assessing, and identifying students with disabilities. After high school, the responsibility for identification and disclosure of a disability belongs to the student.

This switch over to student-driven responsibility may make the transition to college education very difficult. The issue of self-disclosure by the student with a disability may be emotionally sensitive, frustrating, and fear generating. Therefore, the student with a disability should be well prepared and have carefully planned how to self-disclose to professors, fieldwork supervisors, clinicians, and peers. Self-preparation can help reduce emotional anxiety, promote self-esteem, and lead to self-empowerment while minimizing possible stereotyping. Table 11-1 was developed from interviews with OT students who experienced both success and failure in college. The table can be used by students themselves or by educators to prepare students for fieldwork or work interviews.

Many students may have entered college or the university feeling very confident from

---

Worksheet 11-1

"Am I Ready to Assume These Responsibilities?"

Check off those responsibilities that you understand and are ready to assume. If you are ready to assume the majority of these responsibilities, then prepare yourself to self-disclose to the 504 coordinator on your campus and your OT chairperson.

[ ] Responsibility for explaining my strengths, weaknesses, and needs.

[ ] Responsibility for providing appropriate documentation of these strengths, weaknesses, and needs according to the procedures of the college or university.

[ ] Responsibility for following institutional policies and procedures.

[ ] Responsibility for obtaining and meeting the technical and academic standards of the institution and the program.

[ ] Responsibility for requesting reasonable accommodations.

[ ] Responsibility for working with appropriate staff and faculty to determine reasonable accommodations.

[ ] Responsibility for utilizing reasonable accommodations to meet the educational requirements of the program.

[ ] Responsibility for the self—evaluate the effectiveness of reasonable accommodations and share that information with appropriate faculty.

---

their high school experiences and successes and may believe that the disability is no longer an interference. Other students may be filled with anxiety that their disability will cause continued problems. In both situations, and despite whether a student decides to self-disclose or not, it is important to understand why transitioning to an OT program and eventually fieldwork may be difficult.

Transition from High School to College

Developmental transitions can be difficult for all students, and can be especially difficult and anxiety provoking for students with disabilities. Transitions are necessary to develop independence and empowerment. Transitions that are particularly difficult are from high school to college and college to fieldwork.

There are two basic reasons why transitioning may be difficult and create new hurdles to learning for the OT student with a disability. First, as the student moves from a high school environment to a college or university, the primary law that determines services a student receives moves from IDEA (originally P.L. 94-142, Education for All Handicapped Children Act) to both Section 504 of the Rehabilitation Act and the ADA, respectively. IDEA places the responsibility for identification of a disability and providing services on the public school personnel. When the student moves from the auspices of IDEA into a college or university environment, the responsibility for seeking services and advocating for accommodations and answers becomes the sole responsibility of the student. The parent has involvement only as the student allows, according to the Buckley Amendment, and in fact the student must be the one to initiate the reasonable accom-

Table 11-1
Preparing to Self-Disclose to Others That You Have a Disability

Know Yourself: Self-Analysis
- Develop your skills
- Be ready to demonstrate your skills and abilities, despite your disability
- Develop and practice techniques to build self-confidence, self-control, self-independence, and empowerment
- Know about your disability and be ready to educate others
- Learn to express yourself with ease
- Practice your interview skills frequently with a trusted peer who can give you input

Know OT (the requirements of the college, the program, the fieldwork site, and the job for which you are applying): Program Analysis
- Read the college catalog, OT student and fieldwork manuals
- Write an analysis of the standards, functions, and competencies that may pose difficulty to you secondary to the limitations imposed by the disability
- Write an analysis of the academic adjustments, aids, and reasonable accommodations that you currently use that will allow you to successfully meet the standards
- Establish a volunteer work history in OT using your adjustments, aids, and accommodations; use school vacations and summer breaks to volunteer in a therapy department and practice your skills
- Seek a mentor or a supportive peer who has a similar or a related disability, share frustrations and accomplishments, seek out valid, honest feedback
- Be prepared to deal with peers, faculty, and clinicians in a non-threatened, positive manner

modations. In the short time between high school and the beginning of college, the student moves from being supported by a team of professionals with parental input to the role of college student with the primary role of self-advocate and a user of services and accommodations (Brinkerhoff, Shaw, & McGuire, 1993). Being prepared for such a significant shift in responsibility can make transition very difficult.

Second, transition may be very difficult for OT students with disabilities due to new learning requirements. The primary difficulty is managing the freedom and lack of structure found in college while maintaining the grades that the students achieved in high school. The student with a disability is very use to imposed structure or structure systems that were developed in high school as a compensatory strategy. However, in a new learning environment, with a lack of structure, or new structures and definitely new freedoms, the student with a disability often discovers that old, familiar patterns of behavior no longer lead to success. The role of the parent, now missing, increases the frustration and anxiety of the student which can enhance his or her disability limitations. The drastic change in the learning environment may be minimized by discussion of the change in requirements and demands of college life and how reasonable accommodations should be implemented to assist the student (Table 11-2).

In order to effectively meet and cope with this array of possible transition difficulties, and to avoid the possible panic frequently encountered when students with disabilities pass through transition periods (Aase & Price, 1987; Aune & Ness, 1991), a

Table 11-2
Differences Between High School and OT School Requirements

Requirement	High School	OT School/College
Entry	Mandatory, by law	Must apply, be accepted
Graduation	Minimal hours in broad subject areas	Core college curriculum subject areas in liberal arts and sciences and mandatory OT courses, with few waivers or substitutions, and required OT coursework, fieldwork I and II
Grades	Passing grades needed	Minimum grade of "C", with minimum GPA, may be asked to leave program if grades, fieldwork evaluation, or professional behavior drops below acceptable levels
Class time	6 hours per day for 180 days per year	12 to 18 hours per week for 28 weeks plus lab time and fieldwork time
Schedule	School and parents design, attendance mandatory	Diverse schedule, student is responsible to attend
Teaching style	Teachers check work and book is often what is in lecture, emphasis on facts	Lecture may be nonstop, books may be additional to lecture, emphasis on knowledge, application of facts, and creative and critical thinking
Exams	Homework, quizzes, tests, notebook checks	Lab sheets, lab practicals, quizzes, tests, papers, projects, fabrication of products and clinical competence
Responsibility	Student is structured, limits set by parents and teachers, must comply or face a regular, daily consequence	Student makes own structure, requirements are set but the student can choose to comply often or not comply, with no significant consequence until end of semester, can withdraw
Environment	Sheltered, structured with most variables or distracters known and can be controlled by parents or adults	Open, decisions on what to eat and when and how much to sleep or party up to student, multiple choices often without control or input from parents or adults

transition plan is strongly recommended (Brinkerhoff et al., 1993). A transition plan should be developed, in writing, involving the faculty and the student with a support person or mentor if the student feels it necessary. The roles of the faculty, fieldwork educators, and student may be different depending on the type of transition. The primary roles remain the same. The faculty are to educate the student about the next environment about to be entered and to provide reasonable adjustments, aids, and accommodations when requested. The student is to understand the requirements, and be proactive and assertive in trying to articulate needs for the new learning or working environment. A transition plan with delineated tasks, activities, and persons who will be accountable for meeting the plan will best ensure the most effective transition possible. Even with such a plan, people's needs change, the environments undergo change, and the student may always have to deal with issues of acceptance. A structured plan will attempt to control and circumvent those entities that can be changed or altered within the new environment.

Transition from OT College to Fieldwork

Fieldwork is an essential requirement in all OT programs. Both fieldwork Level I and fieldwork Level II provide the student with the necessary interaction with practicing therapists, team members, and most importantly, with the individuals whom OTs serve. Many students with disabilities may succeed in the classroom and the lab environments but may experience near or actual failure in the fieldwork experience. Although there is only limited research on why this occurs, there are some key elements of the fieldwork environment that can be identified as being very different from classroom learning that may contribute to difficulties for students with disabilities.

- Fieldwork requires the merging of the art and science of observation, which often calls upon the accurate use of all senses to gather information, information processing to associate, differentiate, and formulate questions or activities that will clarify and enhance information gathered by observation. This may be difficult for students with sensory deficits or learning disabilities.
- There is always a critical element of the therapeutic use of self that includes social interactions, personal reflection, self-assertion, and rapport with the client. This may be difficult for students with social-emotional disabilities.
- The fieldwork environment is usually not only one location but requires the therapist to work effectively and efficiently in the clinic, the community, the school, the hospital, or the client's home or room. This may be difficult for students with mobility problems or for students with difficulty changing environments.
- The fieldwork environment usually has multiple supervisors from several professions with possibly different teaching and personal interaction styles. This may pose difficulties for students with learning or social-emotional disabilities.
- The fieldwork environments require critical thinking, immediate application of knowledge in adaptive activities, and clear documentation of the outcome of the activities all within a specified time period. These activities may exacerbate the limitations of students of all disability areas.

Fieldwork is a critical and an essential element in OT education. Yet by its nature and requirements, fieldwork may actually exacerbate the limitations of a student with a disability unless the fieldwork placement is carefully matched to the student's strengths and can allow for reasonable accommodations in difficult areas that will not compromise the standards of the fieldwork program. This matching process requires collaboration between the clinical supervisor, the academic fieldwork coordinator, and the student with a disability. This transition is critical, challenging, and exciting for the student with a disability and should be planned at least 6 to 12 months in advance of the fieldwork placement. The transition plan should again be written and checked frequently. This plan must be initiated by the student as in this transition period the ultimate responsibility for success is that of the student. Therefore, the student must initiate the request for academic adjustments or accommodations for fieldwork and the

OT educators must be ready and willing to provide a process for this transition. This may include:

- Encouraging the student with a disability to read the fieldwork file on placement sites and formulate questions to be answered
- Encouraging the student with a disability to talk with students who previously succeeded at the site
- Encouraging the student to visit the site and have all questions answered
- Having the academic clinical coordinator meet with the student to discuss learning needs for the particular placement site, encourage the student to interview, dicuss self-disclosure, delineate strengths, and identify accommodations
- Encouraging the student with a disability to sign a release of information so that when appropriate the academic clinical coordinator and the clinical supervisor can discuss the student's progress; always include the student in the discussion to facilitate direct communication and decrease misinterpretation as this will increase self-awareness of the student
- Encouraging the student with a disability to work with a student mentor
- Writing a transition plan and a plan for academic adjustments, auxiliary aids, and reasonable accommodation for specific activities at the fieldwork placement site
- Evaluating the effectiveness and the impact of these adjustments, aids, and accommodations; the academic clinical coordinator, the fieldwork supervisor, and the student meet to evaluate both the learning activity and plan for the next fieldwork experience

Developing a transition plan for the OT student with a disability to move successfully from the classroom into the clinic will facilitate open communication and the development of realistic, effective, and efficient accommodations. The learning of effective communication can then be used to transition successfully future fieldwork sites and to future employment environments.

THE FOUR "Es" TO ENSURE EXCELLENT COMMUNICATION

OT students with disabilities often have to spend more time than other students in various types of communication with faculty, administrators, academic fieldwork coordinators, and fieldwork supervisors. The four "Es" may help ensure excellence in communication.

Engage

Become an active participant in all interactions. Set up appointments when necessary, don't wait for faculty to chase you down. You should actively engage in the communication process. Ask the faculty for assistance in formulating questions. Discover how to recognize when you may need to seek assistance, how to seek assistance, and how to evaluate advice and suggestions without playing the game, "Well, he said this and she said that and now you are telling me what?" Actively engage in effective communication and decision-making processes.

Efficient

Working at an efficient and effective rate may be difficult for any student with a disability. The nature of the disability is often compounded by the extra time it may take to complete work due. The use of assistive technology, academic adjustments, or the extra time to check work may leave the student with a disability very short of time.

This shortage of time may also contribute to a poor or inadequate balance of work, play, leisure, and exercise that may contribute to increased fatigue, lower self-esteem, and frustration. Develop strategies to become more effective and efficient such as:
- Strategies that are personally developed
- Strategies that are developed by the student, faculty, and clinical supervisors as a team
- Strategies that are simple and can be used in a variety of different environments or situations
- Strategies that are based in reality of the true requirements of the program or fieldwork environment
- Strategies to evaluate the effectiveness of other strategies and reasonable accommodations

Enthusiasm

Select a role model for a mentor. Often it is the enthusiasm of the mentor that motivates the student with a disability to persevere, eventually overcome, and compensate for difficulties that lead to success in OT education. Encourage faculty to interact with you as an individual and with enthusiasm. Accept the mentor's praise and enthusiasm for your work. Often the mentor relationship has to be cultivated over a period of time so that the belief that you can succeed as an OT is a true and genuine feeling.

Empowerment

Lastly, empower yourself with the same skills and the same independence as all other OT students. Become a self-advocate in an assertive yet non-aggressive manner. In order to feel this empowerment, the faculty and fieldwork supervisors should not lower standards or requirements, nor should the faculty and fieldwork supervisors assume that because a student has a disability the standards or the quality of care will be diminished. Instead, the student, faculty, and fieldwork supervisors should work collectively to enhance the student's individual strengths and to develop academic adjustments, prescription of aids, and institution of reasonable accommodations that will ensure quality performance and build a true sense of empowerment within the student.

Becoming engaged, efficient, and enthusiastic will lead to self-empowerment. Collectively, these four skills will help develop communication skills and a positive self-esteem that will last a lifetime and enhance your skills as an OT student and eventually a practitioner in OT. Keep this list of "things to do" in order to keep your empowerment growing and developing (Worksheet 11-2).

Worksheet 11-2

Checklist for Empowerment

Check these off as you develop the skills, and review this list whenever you are attempting to solve a new challenge in your life.

[ ] Communication (engage, active listening, participatory, clarify, answer by self)

[ ] Socially responsible behavior (on time, respect, sensitive to others)

[ ] Develop self-awareness (strengths, weaknesses, needs, styles)

[ ] Maintain ADLs independently (cook, clean, manage money)

[ ] Balance work, school, and leisure

[ ] Develop personal relationships (give to others, reflect on self, identify needs)

[ ] Seek counseling when needed (friends are friends, family are family)

[ ] Seek a mentor (possibly someone with a disability who has made it)

[ ] Be willing to work harder than others

[ ] Be willing to take risks

[ ] Set appropriate goals (reflect on the goals, redesign those goals)

[ ] Use learning strategies (go to the learning center)

[ ] Use assistive technology (use reasonable accommodation devices)

[ ] Use compensatory skills (accept long-term problems and work around them)

[ ] Learn to manage time (don't let time run your life)

[ ] Be your own best advocate (learn about your strengths)

[ ] Update your skills in test-taking strategies

[ ] Volunteer in OT (know what you are in for)

[ ] Educate others about who you are (while educating them about the disability)

[ ] Recognize that you can't change others, but you can change yourself

SUMMARY

OT is a profession of challenge, growth, diversity, and opportunity. These rewards are within the grasp of students with disabilities who are otherwise qualified due to the civil rights protection of Section 504 of the Rehabilitation Act and the ADA. These laws provide the student with the right to an equal opportunity to participate in the programs and activities of colleges and universities. Along with these rights come responsibilities that may pose new dilemmas and probably new solutions that the student did not experience in high school. In order to meet these new challenges, and to discover the new solutions, the OT student with a disability must become a proactive self-advocate. The student must always be reflective, always working harder with newer strategies and methods to meet with success. Success may need some support, guidance, and new ideas. This chapter has presented some methods to develop new ideas and seek support and guidance, while becoming empowered and independent. Hopefully, this chapter has already empowered you with facts about the laws that protect you, self-assessment tools for personal reflection and growth, ideas for enhancing communication skills, and understanding of why the strategies that worked in high school may be challenged by the difficulties involved in any transition process. Use these tools to move you along the path to becoming an empowered, independent OT student and with success, in time, a therapist.

BIBLIOGRAPHY

Aase, S., & Price, L. (1987). Building the bridge: LD adolescents' and adults' transition from secondary to postsecondary settings. In D. Knapke & C. Lenderman (Eds.), *Capitalizing on the future* (pp. 126-149). Columbus, OH: Association on Handicapped Student Service Programs in Postsecondary Education.

Aune, E., & Ness, J. (1991). *Tools for transition: Preparing students with learning disabilities for postsecondary education*. Circle Pines, MN: American Guidance Service.

Brinkerhoff, L. C., Shaw, S. F., & McGuire, J. M. (1993). *Promoting postsecondary education for students with learning disabilities*. Austin, TX: PRO-ED.

Dalke, C., & Franzene, J. (1988). Secondary-postsecondary collaboration: A model of shared responsibility. *Learning Disability Focus, 4,* 38-45.

Goldhammer, R., & Brinkerhoff, L. C. (1992). Self-advocacy for college students. *Their World,* 94-97.

Madaus, J. (1994, Spring). Transition: Tips for students with learning disabilities. *Postsecondary LD Network News,* 4.

National Joint Committee on Learning Disabilities. (1994, March/April). Secondary to postsecondary education transition planning. *LDA Newsbriefs*.

Shaw, S. F., Brinkerhoff, L. C., Kistler, J., & McGuire, J. M. (1992). Preparing students with learning disabilities for postsecondary education: Issues and future needs. *Learning Disabilities: A Multidisciplinary Journal, 2,* 21-26.

Trapani, C. (1990). *Transition goals for adolescents with learning disabilities*. Austin, TX: PRO-ED.

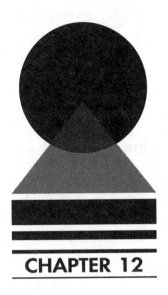

CHAPTER 12

LIFE BEYOND OT SCHOOL

Andrea Passannante, OTR/L

LIFE AS A STUDENT

You have been accepted into the OT program and you have an exciting career ahead of you. Getting through OT school is not going to be easy; it takes a lot of time and effort. But you can, and should, have a life outside of OT school. Getting involved in other activities is an easy way to meet people as well as being a great getaway from school work. It is your opportunity to discover other talents, develop leadership and socialization skills, and problem solve with other people, and it's a great addition to your résumé. Many times out-of-class activities will force you to explore new places, learn to be organized, and can even be good exercise. This chapter is a guide to what is available for clubs, work, partying, money management, and staying in shape. It will also offer insight into dorm life, family responsibilities, dating, and development of personal and career goals. There is a lot available to you out there, be daring, jump in, seek, and discover!

SETTING GOALS OF BALANCE

Time management will be crucial in having the "total college experience." By the end of your college career, you will have developed a new reflex—it's called the "reach into your bag and grab your schedule book reflex." So go ahead...yes, right now, take out your schedule book. Fill in your class times and also blocks of study time. Refer to your learning style in Chapter 6 to figure how much time you'll need for studying. Do not continue reading until you have done this. After all, if you are not planning on going to classes or maintaining your grades, you will not be in college to enjoy the things we're going to talk about. Now you can see a general outline of your available time. Of course, there are other responsibilities that will take up some of that time such as work, family time, time with a significant other, etc. Before choosing additional activities, you will need to know how much time you truly have available, how much time is needed for each activity, and whether it is meaningful to give up that time. Refer to Chapter 10 for time management tips.

In order to get a true idea of available time, you will need to identify all time commitments, prioritize your wants and needs, and come up with an acceptable balance of work, rest, and play. As an OT, you will be developing treatment plans with goals for your patients. Writing out goals is a forceful way to organize yourself. Let's start by formulating long-term goals outside of OT (Worksheet 12-1). Write them in the order that is most important to you. Not easy, but do it because if you should ever have to cut out something, it will be a lot easier if you have prioritized these before other circumstances may taint your decision.

The next step is to break these down into short-term goals (Worksheet 12-2). Once you have come up with your short-term goals, you can then develop methods to reach these goals. Following the example of short-term goals (in Worksheet 12-2), let's examine each goal and briefly discuss possible methods of reaching the goal.

The first short-term goal, maintaining your GPA, is one of the most difficult but definitely achievable goals. Prioritize your time so that study time comes first. Refer to Chapters 7 and 8 for more in-depth information on study skills. Be realistic about how much time you need for studying, do not be chintzy, especially during your first semester. It takes a long time to bring up a GPA destroyed in the first semester. You will find there is a big difference in the time you have to allow yourself to complete college-level work than for high school work. You can always find something to do if you do not need all of your study time, but you are stuck if you have not set aside enough time. It is best to give yourself set times throughout the week as if studying were a scheduled class. Make it steady throughout the semester; this will help you to spread out your learning, helping you retain much more information.

BALANCING YOUR FINANCES

Between nighttime pizza binges, party cover charges, and phone bills, it is very difficult to maintain a monthly budget and to control the flow of money, and this can be very stressful. Give yourself monetary guidelines. If you are not worried about where you are going to get money for your next phone bill, you will be a lot less stressed. Allow yourself a few months to adjust your budget. Keep track of what you are spending and then determine where you need to make cuts (Worksheet 12-3). Save on your phone bill by writing letters, everyone enjoys receiving a letter and you'll find it actually takes less time than a phone call. You can get a lot of satisfaction from it and probably a full mailbox of your own, too.

If you are a full-time student, think about getting a small job; it is really nice to have that little bit of income. This leads us into the goal of getting a job. Try not to balance a full-time job with school, it's just too much. Of course, some people have to and those people will have to be extremely organized with their time. If this is you, remember that rest and play are also integral parts to maintaining your sanity.

WORKING WHILE STUDYING

Finding the perfect job requires some research. Take into account travel time, scheduling flexibility, stress on the job, and whether you will take that stress home with you. Try

Worksheet 12-1

Formulating Long-Term Goals

Example	Long-Term Goals
By graduation day I will:	By graduation day I will:
Graduate from the OT program.	
Have fun!	
Be in a sport/keep up an exercise program.	
Maintain family obligations.	
Maintain relationship with boyfriend/girlfriend.	
Hold a part-time job.	
Get involved in outside organizations.	

Worksheet 12-2

Formulating Short-Term Goals

Example	Short-Term Goals
In the next year of school I will:	In the next year of school I will:
Maintain GPA needed to stay in OT program.	
Maintain a monthly party, food, and phone allowance of $150.00 each month.	
Join soccer intramurals or go to the gym three times each week.	
Go home once a month.	
Spend 20 hours with significant other per week.	
Get a part-time job.	
Join one OT-related club.	
Join one non OT-related club.	

to look for on-campus jobs, they are the easiest and safest to get to, and are usually very flexible, especially around exam time. Because of this, on-campus jobs are also typically hard to come by, so try to get one before classes begin. If you are not close enough to go for an interview before school starts, ask if you could have a phone interview. If you're an early bird on getting papers done, a great job for you may be typing papers. Other students panicking to get their papers done will pay big bucks to get their papers typed. Remember to stand your ground regarding how many hours you want to work. Do not let an employer push you to work extra hours, simply express to him or her that you are also going to school and that it is your first priority.

Worksheet 12-3

Monthly Budget

	Month 1	Month 2	Budget	Month 3	Month 4
Income	$	$	$	$	$
Food	$	$	$	$	$
Parties	$	$	$	$	$
Phone	$	$	$	$	$
Supplies	$	$	$	$	$
Clothes	$	$	$	$	$
Misc.	$	$	$	$	$

KEEPING FIT

Maintaining your physique can be just as much fun and easy as it can be dull and difficult. It is a great stress reliever and motivator. Investigate what is available on-campus, as well as off-campus, by talking to upperclassmen, reading the school and local papers, and inquiring at the school information desk. Team sports are a great way to meet people. If you have never been involved in a team sport, give the intramurals a try. Intramural teams are usually made up of people who have played the sport for years, as well as those just starting out. If you would rather go more of an individual route, ask a friend to accompany you to the gym; you can motivate each other to go on those not-so-motivated days.

Also, buddy-up on watching what you eat. Eating with someone can help the temptation to pig out on those fried foods. Give each other the push to pick up some fresh vegetables. A common problem experienced by most freshmen is called the "Freshman 15." This is when adults gain weight when they go away from home. To help keep off those Freshman 15, plan ahead. If you are planning on studying, pick up some low-fat snacks or fruit rather than opening a jumbo bag of chips, which can have over 500 calories.

MAINTAINING RELATIONSHIPS

Spending quality time with your loved ones is important to your mental health and relationships. With time being so sparse during school, make a conscious effort to give your family and boyfriend or girlfriend quality time. This means setting aside a certain amount of time or visits without expecting yourself to study or work on a project. If one of your planned visits happens to land just before a big exam, either make your visit short or postpone your visit for another time. You will not be very pleasant if you are worrying about getting your work done and you usually won't get in quality study time at home. You may even wind up resenting the person you are visiting, which is nonproductive and can be hurtful to your relationship. If you start to see that your grades are falling and you are spending a lot of time at home or with your boyfriend or girlfriend, then you need to reevaluate your priorities and change your schedule accordingly. Some people can have their significant others help them study by quizzing them or come up with memory techniques. If you do try this, be honest with whether or not you are getting anything accomplished and whether or not your significant other can understand the information in the context that you need to know it.

Family responsibilities can get pretty hefty. Talk to your family about what is expected of you and how much you can realistically handle while going to school. Look ahead to what may be busy times for you and ask family members to try to help you out ahead of time so there will not be resentment. Ask them to do the same as an even exchange. Write down in their calendars when your midterm and final weeks are so that they are forewarned. There really has to be commitment on both sides for this to work out.

FINDING THE RIGHT ACTIVITIES

Now that you have considered most of the "known" and less flexible time commitments, we can discuss choosing additional activities that will help you reach your "have fun" goal. Choosing the right activities requires good research. Investigate clubs on- and off-campus (Table 12-1).

Attend introductory meetings to find out about the clubs. Do not just join a club on a whim; college clubs require much more effort then your high school organizations. Talk to current members and find out the time, work, and money commitments required of you (some have pricey dues, especially sororities and fraternities). Consider off-campus organizations as well. On-campus activities versus off-campus activities is not a transportation issue. Just because you do not have your own car, off-campus activities are not off-limits (Table 12-2).

Whether you walk, jog, bike, or rollerblade, here are a few important safety hints:
- Bring a friend with you, especially if you are going in the evening hours
- Wear a safety helmet if biking or rollerblading
- Always bring a few dollars (for a cab if you're just too tired or too scared to take the trip back home alone)

If you are planning on using the public transit system, look in the front of the Yellow Pages in the community services section for the system that services your area. Call and request a schedule. Some schools have a mini-van that is available to students for cheap and sometimes at no cost. You can find out about this through the Student Affairs/Student Life office.

Generally, on-campus groups require less time commitments and are much easier to get other friends involved in. When making a decision as to which club to join, or even which club to be involved in at a higher level such as an officer, look carefully at the time commitment you will be making (Worksheet 12-4).

Table 12-1
Where to Learn of Activities

Off-Campus Activities	On-Campus Activities
Local papers, school paper, *Pennysaver*	School admissions packet
Church bulletins	School catalog
Posted bulletins in shopping areas, school mail area, on the Internet	Student Affairs bulletin board
Pamphlets from area parks, community centers	School newspaper
	Word of mouth, especially upperclassmen

Table 12-2
Transportation

Method	Pros	Cons
Walk, jog, bike, rollerblade	Exercise, stay in shape	Takes more time, can be tiring if not used to it
Beg a ride from someone	Easy, minimal cost	Minimal cost (always offer gas money or some other favor, do not take advantage as this can cost you a friendship)
Public transit system (bus, train, subway)	Relatively easy, minimal to moderate cost	Time constraints of transit schedule, cost
Carpool (yes, even if you do not have a car)	Inexpensive, social	Offer a service in exchange for your turn driving (money for gas, bringing a snack each meeting, type the minutes)
School mini-van	Cheap, social	Usually need a minimum amount of people being transported, need to reserve it ahead of time

Once you have this kind of information, you can look at the whole picture including schoolwork, family obligations, and other interests to determine whether or not you can handle this commitment. Some groups that may be available to you at your campus are listed in Table 12-3. In addition, you may chose to join the more than 25% of college students in giving your time to volunteer work, a very rewarding prospect. Suggestions for volunteer work are listed in Table 12-4.

If you are thinking about what looks good on a résumé, here is what people are looking for: diversity and some further interest in OT beyond your academic schoolwork. Employers want to see that you have other interests besides your degree, but also that you will go the extra mile to do something toward the beliefs and values of your profession. This does not mean you have to be president of the student OT association. If you are a natural leader, then by all means, you should go for those positions if you feel you have time for the commitment. Keep in mind that if it does become too much, you will have to make a decision between getting good grades and keeping that position. It is a good idea to become a regular member of the group for a year, become familiar with the positions that you are interested in, and talk to the persons who are in those positions to get the real dirt as to what is actually involved. Remember that once you make this type of commitment, it not only gives you the title of the position, but it also says that you are willing to put work into this group and that you are going to extend yourself so that the group can depend on you to get things organized and done.

Being a leader of an organization is a wonderful experience because it gives a person confidence, power to make changes, and the opportunity to develop people skills. To be an effective leader, you must remember the purpose of the organization and the needs of its members. Of course, being charismatic helps, but this wears down if members feel you are wasting their time or if they do not feel involved enough. Therefore, use your creative

Worksheet 12-4

Time Commitment

Project/Event	Preparation Time	Event Time	Independent Time
1.			
2.			
3.			
4.			
5.			

Table 12-3
Student Groups

- Student government
- Sororities/fraternities
- Student advisory board
- Student OT association
- Pi Theta Epsilon (OT honor society)
- Hiking club
- Intercollegiate sports
- Karate or tae kwon do
- Kick line
- Debate club
- Marching band/jazz band
- Drama
- Religious organization
- Biking club
- Hiking club
- Historical society
- Creative writing
- Campus radio station
- Campus paper
- Yoga
- Yearbook
- Photography club
- Chess club
- Aerobics
- Intramural sports
- Student life
- Special Olympics

energy to make meetings productive and short. Always have a prewritten agenda with time set aside for discussion. Do not let discussions get out of hand. Remember you are the mediator and should guide people back to the main issues. Do not gather all the members if the topics are really only for the board members. Make yourself available to the members; give them your phone number and do not delay in getting back to them as energy and motivation dies quickly. Finally, delegate responsibilities to prevent burnout. If you start delegating right at the beginning, you will not get to the point when "no one else

---

Table 12-4
Volunteer Work

- Counseling (rape victim hotline, AIDS)
- Soup kitchens
- Handing out educational pamphlets
- Tutoring
- Adopting a child for a day
- Being a "Big Brother" or "Big Sister"
- Teaching English as a second language
- Tending to HIV-exposed babies
- Peer advising
- Reading to hospitalized children/adults in nursing homes
- Weekend volunteer programs
- Environmental protection

---

could possibly do it because I'm the only one who knows what is going on." Following these simple guidelines will make you an effective and well-liked leader.

THE GOOD TIMES

So what about the fun part? It will be all around you, beckoning to you at every turn. Again, give yourself a set of rules regarding partying and make sure they are reasonable and reachable. For example, if you plan on going out Saturday night, don't plan your study time to be Sunday morning as this would not be reachable. If you wind up exhausted from the party, it may prevent you from studying the next morning. Make plans to meet friends later and accept that you have to do your work first. This way you get the best of both worlds—you will become disciplined in your work and will enjoy the party as well. Do not expand the weekend to include Thursdays and Mondays, it is hard enough to get up for morning classes.

Let's talk a little more about partying. It is important to be aware of the risks of excessive drinking and the danger it imposes on others. Here are some figures based upon a survey of 140 U.S. colleges by the Harvard School of Public Health for you to consider. They speak for themselves.

- 61% of "frequent binge drinkers" had problems missing classes
- 41% of "frequent binge drinkers" engaged in risky behavior
- 23% of "frequent binge drinkers" were injured
- 87% of students had experienced at least one serious problem caused by another student's excessive drinking (Gorman, 1994)

Looking to have a different kind of party that is good to your body and mind, as well as being a lot of fun? Have a "New Games" party by gathering a lot of people (anywhere from 20 to 100), borrowing one of those parachutes you used in elementary school gym and/or an earth ball, and playing a few of the many New Games. You can find books on New Games in your local library. This is a really interactive party and a great stress reliever, especially during finals week. It could also give you some ideas of short games to play with your study group to get you started working as a team.

DATING

Dating during college is just as much an emotional roller coaster as it was in high school, except that the roller coaster now is due to more serious sexual issues and societal pressures than the hormonal changes of the good old high school days. Every person is so different in his or her values and intentions regarding dating that it is impossible to give a general guideline regarding this issue. Here you must examine what you are looking for, whether it be a non-committing relationship or a long-term relationship, determine whether the person you are interested in has the same outlook for the relationship as you do, and go on from there if your outlooks are compatible.

ROOMMATE WORRIES

Your roommate can be your best friend or your worst enemy. Don't panic if you and your roommate seem to be opposites, you may in fact be very compatible. Opposites often can learn a lot from each other, hopefully sharing their good qualities with each other. Some hints that will make your dorm life a little easier:
- Draw up a contract with your roommate addressing issues such as acceptable sleeping and studying hours, use of personal belongings, and phone use
- Give a copy of the contract to your RA in case any issues arise
- Speak to your roommate about visitors at least a couple of weeks in advance
- Try your hardest to compromise no matter how unreasonable your roommate seems to be, that way you will not be blamed for being stubborn yourself

When there is a problem, approach your roommate as soon as possible. Let your roommate hear about the problem from you first, not from someone else, and it will be more easily resolved. If you have a hard time approaching your roommate, refer to Chapter 10 on assertive techniques.

THE BALANCING ACT

At times you will feel that you've taken on too much. It is OK, everyone feels that way at least once a semester. You need to stop the whirlwind of thoughts going through your head and determine whether you have taken on too much or you are just at a very stressful time of the semester. If you determine that it is just a stressful time, try to do some relaxation techniques such as deep breathing or progressive muscle relaxation. Go for a walk, take in a movie, or visit the pet store to play with the dogs. If you feel as if you are caught up in a tornado, envision yourself going toward the eye of the storm. In other words, take 5 or 10 minutes to calm down in whatever way works best. Once you have calmed down, take a pen and paper and write down exactly what needs to be done, and then number it in priority (include the little things, they take time too). Usually when you do this, you can figure out a way to fit everything in, even if it is putting a few things off until the next day or if you have to ask your roommate to help you out (like buying him or her dinner if he or she cleans the bathroom for you).

If you find that you are getting into this situation pretty often, then it sounds as if you have taken on too much overall and you need to make a change. How do you choose what to cut down or cut out? Well, that will be based on your priority list we discussed earlier. It is important to use this and not base your decision totally on emotion. Of course, if something is making you incredibly unhappy, that is probably the thing to dump. But do not automatically get rid of the thing that is giving you the most grief, because that same thing could be very fulfilling to you if you were able to dedicate more time to it. It is pretty hard to decide that you have to drop something, and harder yet to decide what to drop, but face it, you cannot do everything. Talk to your peers, supervisors, family, and significant other for different perspectives. Again, refer to your priority list. It will direct you toward your long-term goals. You are not a failure if you drop out of something, instead you are a person who has made an intelligent decision that you cannot dedicate enough time to the things you value most. Notice I say "most." You probably value those other things but you have learned to prioritize and that is something you will have to do every day of your life. Not only will you have to prioritize for yourself, but you will have to prioritize when coming up with treatment plans for patients, and you will have to teach your patients to prioritize. It's a good habit to get into and, just like any habit, it gets easier the more you do it.

Sometimes things are just too much for you to handle on your own; professional guidance and support may help. All colleges have counseling services for many different levels of need. Don't be afraid to use these services. They are there for your benefit and are usually free.

And finally, as you embark on the most wonderful endeavor of your life, constantly remind yourself why you are in OT school. Some people sacrifice what they want most of all in life for what they want at the moment—be cautious that this does not happen to you. Stay true to your long-term goals. Do not forget that you are investing thousands of dollars and several years of your life toward starting a career that will support you for the next 50 years. OT is an incredible career. Go to it, get that degree, and have fun!

SUMMARY

This chapter addressed various methods to balance OT school and outside activities. Highlights include personal and professional goal-setting exercises, simple budgeting hints, options for on- and off-campus organizations, suggestions for time management, and troubleshooting techniques for roommate difficulties, lack of time, and inefficient self-direction.

The chapter also reviewed leadership skills and self-discipline guidelines to assist the OT student in having a successful and exciting college experience.

BIBLIOGRAPHY

Bradman Knight, E. (1994, Aug. 24). Telltale signs brand the frosh. *Tribune News Service.*

Gorman, C. (1994, Dec. 19). Higher education: Crocked on campus. *Time,* 66.

Hardigg, V., & Nobile, C. (1995, Sept. 25). Living with a stranger. *U.S. News & World Report,* 90.

Shapiro, M. (1994, March 24). Don't call me a slacker. *Rolling Stone,* 85.

Wright, A. (1995, Sept.). Hooking up: Creative and fun ways to meet people. *Essence,* 118.

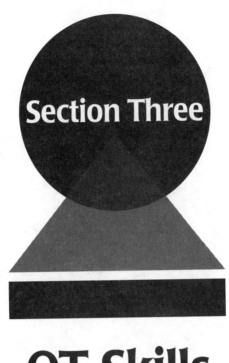

Section Three

OT Skills

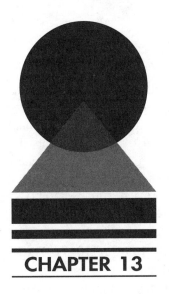

CHAPTER 13

UNIFORM TERMINOLOGY AND ACTIVITY ANALYSIS

Beth O'Sullivan, OTR/L

INTRODUCTION

Many careers have specific tools of their trade, OT included. This chapter will discuss two specific tools that are used constantly by practicing COTAs and OTRs. Both are very helpful in your career as an OT student and professional. This chapter is not designed to teach you everything you need to know but as a starting base for further understanding. There are several ways you can master the use of these specific tools. However, the practice and use of them is the best way to make them the heart of your OT career.

UNIFORM TERMINOLOGY

In order to understand the importance of uniform terminology one must know the history behind the document. Previous to the adoption of the uniform terminology document there was concern that not all OT personnel were practicing from the same baseline and were not using the same terminology to report their procedures and treatments. A solution to this problem was originally requested by the AOTA executive board. That board charged a Commission on Practice to form a specific task force to review the existing OT terminology and relative value reporting systems and to develop a proposal for a national OT product reporting system. The document as developed provided an outline of OT services, such as assessment, OT treatment, patient/client-related conferences, patient-related travel, service management, and education. Besides providing individuals with an outline of OT services, the document gave complete definitions of each item related to OT. It also established uniform terminology and language for AOTA, textbooks, and college curricula. The first draft of the document was adopted in March 1979 by the Representative Assembly of AOTA.

Following feedback from the profession, uniform terminology was revised in 1988 to include current practices and any further developments of theory utilized by the profession. The revision task force also suggested the document should be periodically reviewed and updated when necessary. This second document described "OT Performance Areas. These included activities of daily living (ADL), work and productive activities, and play or leisure" (AOTA, 1994, p. 1047). It also outlined "OT Performance Components which include sensorimotor, cognitive, psychosocial, and psychological elements of performance that OTs assess and, when needed, in which they intervene for improved performance" (AOTA, 1994, p. 1047). The second edition of uniform terminology remained in effect until the third revision in 1994. The latter continued to utilize performance areas and performance components but added performance contexts which "are situations or factors that influence an individual's engagement in desired and/or required performance areas" (AOTA, 1994, p. 1047). Performance contexts consist of temporal aspects such as chronological age, developmental age, place in the life cycle, and health status. Environmental aspects such as physical, social, and cultural considerations are also included (AOTA, 1994).

HOW TO USE THE
UNIFORM TERMINOLOGY DOCUMENT

Before you continue reading this chapter, I suggest you get a copy of the November/December 1994 issue of the *American Journal of Occupational Therapy (AJOT)*. Review the article on uniform terminology and become familiar with the grid presented. When OT personnel initially start using this document it can become overwhelming, but with patience and practice you will become very familiar with it. In order to familiarize yourself with the whole, first look at the parts of the grid and the specific meanings of each part. On the top of the graph you will see the term performance areas, which include subcategories of ADLs, work and productive activities, and play or leisure activities. The performance areas are the general broad categories that OT personnel use to evaluate how an individual functions within his or her environment. When you look down the side of the grid you will see a category called performance components. These skills or components are evaluated but are also looked at to see if any deficits in the performance components could be the root of the problem in ADLs, work, and play or leisure. "These micro abilities or performance components are the building blocks that support occupational performance and are necessary to normal functioning" (Punwar, 1988, p. 11). Performance components are also divided into several subcategories, such as:

- Sensorimotor components, those that require the central nervous system to receive and compute sensory stimuli
- Neuromuscular functions, those that require the body to move and function accordingly
- Cognitive components are the functions that are needed in order to learn and problem solve
- Psychosocial skills and psychological components include the ability to understand oneself and others realistically, to express one's feelings, and to understand the feelings of others (Punwar, 1988)

The last area along the grid is performance contexts which include temporal aspects and environmental concerns. This area must also be evaluated by OT personnel to see if any factors such as age, disability status, or cultural values will impact upon the client's ability to be independent. Performance contexts allow OT practitioners to choose the most appropriate intervention for each client.

THE DEFINITIONS

What do some of these words mean? As stated previously, this document was originally created to provide a uniform language pertinent to OT and it did just that. Still, some of the terms used can be very confusing to a layman or a beginning student. In the November/December 1994 issue of *AJOT,* the article definitions are located on pages 1051 through 1054. In order to become more familiar with these terms, it is suggested you first review the formal definition and then find an everyday example to match that definition. Many of the everyday definitions may seem very simple, but their simplicity makes an obscure term understandable. Here are some everyday examples for some performance components.

- **Stereognosis**—Being able to get a quarter out of your pocket by touch only
- **Form Constancy**—A tube of toothpaste is still a tube despite the size or label difference
- **Praxis**—Being able to move oneself through a maze or obstacle course

STUDY TECHNIQUES

Remember when you are just starting to utilize uniform terminology some of the terms may seem very foreign. Relax! With practice and thinking of everyday examples uniform terminology will become very useful and be part of your everyday therapy language both verbally and in written form. Including uniform terminology with activity analysis will also become very beneficial in your career in therapy. See Chapter 7 for ways to memorize initially difficult information.

THEORY BEHIND ACTIVITIES UTILIZED IN OT

Activities are the tools that OT personnel use daily. Many times you will see the terms *media, modality,* or *medium,* which also relate to the term *activity.* The many options of activities available could confuse the beginning therapist, while, at the same time, offer a multiplicity of aids for his or her client. A wide background of knowledge and skill will be required to make the best use of all options available. The selection of the appropriate activity or medium is very important and must be carefully thought out, tailoring the goal, the objective, and the client who is in need of intervention (Reed & Sanderson, 1992). Unfortunately, many therapists make several mistakes in choosing an appropriate task. For beginning practitioners, it is easy to utilize the same activity over and over again without careful consideration to each case. Another common error of new therapists is made when one does not engage the client in the task selection. If the task does not have meaning to the patient, then the activity can seem useless and can easily lead to the client becoming disinterested in therapy. A client who needs to improve fine motor control could benefit from tip-to-tip pinching as provided by a small pegboard. However, if the client does not see a value in this activity, he or she will not be as interested in the therapy process. Upon interviewing the client, OT personnel can find activities the client likes to do that will accomplish the goal of improving fine motor control, including the ability to pinch. A small arts and crafts activity such as origami might be substituted for the pegboard. "OT differs from many medical fields because it depends on the client's active participation in the process through the medium, rather than passive participation" (Reed & Sanderson, 1992, p. 165).

ACTIVITY ANALYSIS

Another important factor in activity selection is using a tool called activity analysis or task analysis. This process is particularly helpful when specific tasks involve several steps or units of behavior (Reed & Sanderson, 1992). By completing an examination of each step involved, in order, and examining what is needed for each step, one can identify which step a client can or cannot perform. Treatment is at its best when therapists have a thorough understanding of an activity and the ability to identify the skills required to complete the task (Lamport, Coffey, & Hersch, 1993).

There are several ways one can perform an activity analysis. When you are just starting the analysis it will seem very difficult. However, with practice, the steps of completing an activity analysis can become second nature. One suggestion is to complete an activity analysis on common activities you utilize in your OT department and record them so you have them for future reference. OT personnel also frequently link uniform terminology and activity analysis and identify performance components involved in the task. By doing so, you can determine if the activity will help address some of the deficits your client is exhibiting.

EXAMPLES OF ACTIVITY ANALYSIS

Analyzing a task by range of motion (ROM) can provide you with information that will assist you in knowing if the task is appropriate for your client. Let's look at an example of a simple task and analyze the movement involved (Figure 13-1).

Task: Brushing Your Teeth

Steps Involved	Movements Involved
1. Reach for toothbrush	1. Shoulder flexion, elbow extension, forearm pronation, wrist extension, finger extension
2. Grab toothbrush	2. Finger flexion, thumb opposition
3. Bring toothbrush to toothpaste tube	3. Elbow flexion, horizontal shoulder adduction
4. Squeeze toothpaste onto brush	4. With other hand—slight shoulder flexion, horizontal abduction, elbow flexion, wrist neutral, fingers flexed
5. Raise toothbrush to mouth	5. Elbow flexion, forearm neutral, wrist flexed, fingers flexed
6. Brush teeth up and down	6. Elbow flexion, forearm neutral, wrist flexion and extension, fingers flexed
7. Rinse toothbrush	7. Shoulder flexion, elbow extension, forearm pronated, wrist ulnar and radial deviation, finger flexion

Adapted from Lamport, N. K., Coffey, M. S., & Hersch, G. I. (1993). Activity Analysis Handbook (2nd ed.). Thorofare, NJ: SLACK Inc.

Figure 13-1. Sample of activity analysis.

In looking at this activity analysis, you can see the ROM that is involved in each part of the task. Granted, this is but one way of completing the task and individuals may perform some of the movements differently, but the task will require these general motions. In applying this task to patient performance, you can see brushing teeth would be difficult for someone who has lost elbow flexion. A plan for such a client would require some type of adaptation. Using this task as therapy can assist in developing several upper extremity movements.

Now that you have seen a task analyzed according to the movement involved, try this everyday task analysis yourself (Exercise 13-1).

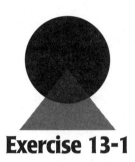

Exercise 13-1

TASK: GETTING A DRINK OF WATER

Steps Involved	**Movements Involved**
1.	1.
2.	2.
3.	3.
4.	4.
5.	5.

Analyzing the task by performance components can provide you with specific information about an activity and how you can relate the activity to your client's specific areas of weakness. Let's look at a task frequently used with children to increase fine motor coordination. Keep in mind this task addresses many areas. When working with school-aged children an important performance area is that of play/leisure. Children spend many hours playing and developing peer relationships, competition, and friendships. A common playground game is jacks, initially seen as a fine motor activity. There are many other strengths or benefits addressed by this game. Below are the performance components utilized while playing jacks.

- **Tactile**—Feeling the jacks
- **Proprioceptive**—Feeling the position of your upper extremity by feedback from your shoulder joint
- **Visual**—Locating the jacks and ball
- **Auditory**—Hearing the ball bouncing on the ground or table
- **Kinesthesia**—Throwing the ball and grabbing the jacks
- **Depth perception**—Determining the distance between the jacks
- **ROM**—Using the upper extremities
- **Strength**—Moving your upper extremities against gravity when throwing the ball
- **Crossing the midline**—Picking up the jacks
- **Bilateral integration**—Picking up the jacks and putting them in your other hand
- **Fine motor coordination**—Manipulating the jacks (Adapted from Lamport. N. K., Coffey, M. S., & Hersch, G. I. (1993). *Activity Analysis Handbook* [2nd ed.] Thorofare, NJ: SLACK Inc.)

Through this analysis, one can see the many performance components that are addressed by the simple game of jacks. It answers the need for fine motor control, speed, and dexterity. It may be your game of choice, solving a child's need and providing fun— a perfect base for therapy.

SUMMARY

Adding activity analysis and uniform terminology to your package of skills will be helpful and gratifying. However, proficiency in service will take time, patience, and practice. We recommend that you try to analyze many simple activities that you complete every day. Analyze for both ROM and for performance components. Once having practiced this you can link the activity to therapeutic goals you have set for a client. Uniform terminology and activity analysis will then become the heart of your career in OT.

BIBLIOGRAPHY

American Occupational Therapy Association. (1994). Uniform terminology for occupational therapy (3rd ed.). *American Journal of Occupational Therapy, 48*, 1047-1059.

Breines, E. B. (1995). *Occupational therapy activities from clay to computers: theory and practice.* Philadelphia: F.A. Davis Company.

Lamport, N. K., Coffey, M. S., & Hersch, G. I. (1993). *Activity analysis handbook* (2nd ed.). Thorofare, NJ: SLACK Inc.

Punwar, A. J. (1988). *Occupational therapy principles & practice.* Baltimore: Williams & Wilkins.

Reed, K. L., & Sanderson, S. N. (1992). *Concepts of occupational therapy* (3rd ed.). Baltimore: Williams & Wilkins.

Royeen, C. B., Cynkin, S., & Robinson, A. M. (1990). Analyzing performance through activity. *AOTA self study series: Assessing function* (No. 5). Rockville, MD: American Occupational Therapy Association.

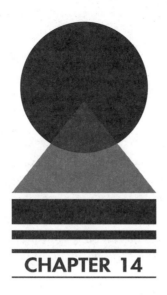

CHAPTER 14

UNDERSTANDING FRAMES OF REFERENCE

Marilyn B. Cole, MS, OTR/L

INTRODUCTION

Frames of reference are the unique ways in which OTs put theory into practice. Concepts from theory must be reformulated (Mosey, 1981) in order to provide the profession with useful guidelines for practice. Frames of reference are hard to explain, because often we are not aware that we are using them. To the experienced therapist, the process of applying theory just comes naturally, so it may be difficult to put into words. This chapter will begin to explain frames of reference so you can build a deeper understanding later.

If you have ever looked through a pair of rose-colored glasses, you noticed at first that everything looked different. But as you continued to wear these glasses, you became accustomed to the way everything looked, and the change was no longer noticeable. Yet the tinted glass colors everything you see, and affects how you interpret it. Rose-colored glasses make everything look "rosy," and you may interpret things as brighter than they really are. Wearing dark-colored glasses on a cloudy day may have the opposite effect. Both will affect how we interpret what we see, and will also affect our decisions and our responses. It is the same with a frame of reference, but more complex, because it involves all of our sensory and cognitive experiences.

To further illustrate the nature of a frame of reference, let us use an example. Imagine yourself asleep in the upstairs bedroom with no one else home. You are suddenly awakened in the middle of the night by a loud noise. You are lying alert, but motionless in your bed, listening intently. What could it be?

Option 1: Thunder. You keep listening but the sound does not repeat itself. You look out your window from your bed, and stars twinkle back at you. The moon lights up the sky, but there is no lightning or rain. Using your knowledge of the nature of a thunderstorm, you eliminate this option.

Option 2: A nearby explosion or car crash. You listen for sirens, signs of fire engines, flashing lights. There are none. You try to remember more about the sound you heard. It was blunt and muffled, with a tinkling after sound. You then realize the sound must have been close by.

Option 3: A burglar. He or she has entered your house by breaking a window. This is the option you fear the most, and thus do not want to believe it. To eliminate it, however, you must get out of bed and investigate. You get up quietly and put on your bathrobe and slippers. Then you open the bedroom door silently, still listening intently...Nothing. Now that you are more awake, you become more anxious. What if it is a burglar?! Do I really want him or her to see me? I might be in danger. You quietly close the bedroom door, lock it, and begin making your way to the telephone next to your bed. You pick up the receiver: "Hummmmmmm..." a dial tone sounds, and the night light lights up. You remember from the movies that when a burglar enters a house, he or she usually cuts the phone cord and the power. It now seems less likely that it's a burglar, so you quietly replace the phone, and continue sitting on the edge of your bed, listening intently. "Meow." Scratch, scratch, scratch. "Meow."

Option 4: Your cat, Mittens. Cats are nocturnal, you recall, and while you are sleeping, a cat will prowl, investigate the surroundings, maybe even jump onto forbidden surfaces. You unlock your door, open it, and sure enough, there is Mittens, purring and rubbing against your legs. Encouraged, you step outside the bedroom into the hall, and peek around the corner and down the stairs. There at the bottom, clearly lit by the moon, is a broken vase on the floor, surrounded by water and scattered long-stemmed roses. Relieved that the mystery is solved, you go back to sleep, Mittens at your feet. Clean-up can wait until morning.

During this experience, you have imagined four different scenarios, formulated four different theories, and done the necessary research to test them. Based on your findings, you have changed your perceptions, your emotions, and your behavioral responses. You have essentially changed your frame of reference four times. It is the same when OT practitioners encounter patients in the clinic. They analyze what they see, formulate theories, mentally contemplate different approaches to test the theories, and act on the interpretation that makes the most sense. This example also illustrates why we need more than one frame of reference, and why it is necessary to use different frames of reference in different situations.

ORGANIZATION OF A FRAME OF REFERENCE

Anne Mosey, one of our best-known OT theorists, says that theory cannot be applied directly to practice. Theory must be combined with an action component. A frame of reference is defined by Mosey (1981) as a set of interrelated concepts from a variety of disciplines that are compatible, combined with a plan of action. The parts of a frame of reference include: domain of concern, basic assumptions, function-dysfunction continuums, postulates of change and motivation, and assessment and treatment techniques (Table 14-1).

Table 14-1
Parts of a Frame of Reference

- Domain of Concern
- Basic Assumptions
- Function-Dysfunction Continuums
- Postulates of Change
- Motivation
- Assessment and Treatment Techniques

Domain of Concern

This part identifies the focus of the frame of reference. Some frames focus on psychological aspects of the patient, others focus more on physical aspects. The domain of concern also identifies those functional activities best addressed by a particular frame of reference. For example, the spiritual and emotional side of a person is better addressed with the *humanistic* or *psychoanalytic* frames, while perception and practical problem solving are better addressed with the *cognitive perceptual* frame.

Basic Assumptions

If you have ever wondered why you are required to take all those science, psychology, and philosophy prerequisites for OT, here is one of the reasons. The concepts we use come from many areas of related knowledge. For example, the *biomechanical* frame of reference deals with physical range of motion (ROM), strength, and endurance. The concepts needed to apply this theory come from physics, chemistry, anatomy, and physiology. In order to help our patients recover from the physical aspects of illness or injury, we need to understand how the human body works (physiology), its anatomical make-up (anatomy), the effects of body chemistry (chemistry), and the role of gravity and movement in human activity (physics). In the humanistic frame of reference, many basic assumptions come from existential philosophy and neo-Freudian psychology. These concepts often help OTRs and COTAs treat the more spiritual and emotional aspects of illness.

The concepts or ideas that we borrow from other disciplines or areas of study may be quite diverse, but they must be compatible with one another. OT draws upon these concepts to form a unified view of the effects of illness on the functioning of patients and clients.

Function-Dysfunction Continuums

This is the part of a frame of reference that applies theory to human beings with specific illnesses and in specific situations. It is a fancy way of saying that illness and injury have varying effects on how people function in everyday life. In order to assess the functioning of our patients, we must first define what healthy functioning is and establish a baseline. Then when an assessment is done, we can see how our patient's functioning compares to the "norm," and this will help us set realistic goals for treatment. For example, in the *sensory integration* frame of reference, function is defined by several parameters. One of them is that the brain functions as a whole. Sensory information, sights, sounds, smells, movement and position senses, and tactile sensation are processed subcortically (i.e., without having to think about it). Integration of sensation is necessary for balance, posture, and automatic movements (i.e., walking). This enables the brain to free itself for the higher cortical functions (i.e., learning, reasoning, and problem solving). Through this understanding of function, we know that the ability to be a successful student or worker, which requires learning, reasoning, and problem solving, depends on the subcortical sensory processing. We also know that every sensory system has norms, and that integration of each sense occurs at different ages, and in a predictable sequence. When a patient fails as a student or worker, one of the things we may do as an OTR or COTA using this frame of reference is to assess the sensory systems to see where the problems might be. If sensory deficits are found, the OT practitioner will know exactly which senses are not working correctly, and will be able to apply treatment to correct the problem.

Postulates of Change and Motivation

This part of the frame of reference is the most important for treatment, because it provides concepts about how it is possible for therapeutic change to occur in a given individual. The easiest one of these to explain is *behavior modification*. In the behavior modification frame of reference, change is always motivated by external reinforcement. B.F. Skinner demonstrated this by teaching a pigeon to turn around. The pigeon was given food rewards every time it made progress in the direction of the turn. This is called "shaping" behavior. OTs may use rewards to encourage patients to try new behaviors, especially when it means enduring some pain or overcoming their fears and anxieties. Behavior modification is not used widely in OT because, according to the philosophy of our profession, we believe that our patients are internally motivated to recover, and that they are sufficiently rewarded just by the experience of success. However, the behavior modification frame does give us a good fall-back position, so that we will be prepared when encountering patients who are not very motivated.

The term *postulates* describes the relationship between two or more concepts. For example, concepts could have a temporal relationship. In the *developmental* frames of reference, change occurs in a predictable sequence, over time spans that relate to chronological age. In the sensory integration frame of reference, the more primitive sensory systems, tactile and proprioceptive, develop first, followed by the auditory and visual systems. This predictable temporal sequence gives OT practitioners a guideline for planning treatment. Many treatment procedures in the sensory integration frame of reference focus on stimulation of the tactile and proprioceptive (position) senses, with a goal of laying the foundation for further development of higher level sensory systems.

Assessment and Treatment Techniques

This part of a frame of reference can be somewhat confusing. It is rare that a specific assessment or treatment technique is used exclusively with only one frame of reference. A highly developed and defined frame of reference does tend to have its own exclusive assessment and treatment techniques. In *Sensory Integration*, for example, Ayres (1989) and her colleagues developed the Sensory Integration and Praxis Tests (SIPT), which assess the sensory systems and their effect on various behaviors. This battery of tests has been standardized on thousands of children, and has well-established age-equivalent norms for children from 4 to 8 years old. Treatment is based on a computer-generated profile of the status of a child's sensory integration test scores, clinical observations, information from others, and available specialized equipment (e.g., scooter boards, hammocks, and bolster swings are commonly used in the sensory integration frame of reference).

Another example of a specific assessment and treatment format occurs in the *cognitive disabilities* frame of reference. Claudia Allen and colleagues have done extensive research on developing and defining six cognitive levels in patients with brain dysfunction (1992). Several specific tests are designed to measure cognitive levels, including the Allen Cognitive Level (ACL) test and the Routine Task Inventory (RTI). Craft activities such as woodworking and leathercrafts are used extensively in this frame. Problem-solving abilities observed while the patients are doing crafts are generalized to everyday life tasks. The cognitive disabilities frame of reference is one of the best developed, giving us very specific guidelines for predicting a patient's functional level after discharge.

TYPES OF FRAMES OF REFERENCE

Frames of reference in OT seem to be multiplying each year. There are more than 12 published and defined, and probably more by the time this book is published. For this reason, it is useful to group them into categories, according to their similar features. This was first done by Mosey (1981) in the area of mental health practice. All of the OT frames of reference at the time fit, more or less, into three distinct categories:

- Psychoanalytic
- Behavioral
- Developmental

During the 1980s and 1990s, our profession has minimized the distinction between the mental and the physical areas of practice, and other frames of reference have been added to Mosey's original list. However, the same categories have remained. The following is a brief explanation of the categories and the frames of reference currently included in each (Figure 14-1).

Psychoanalytic

The term psychoanalytic comes from Freud's psychoanalysis, a form of therapy most of us think of as lying on a couch and saying the first thing that comes into our head. The idea behind this type of "talk therapy" is to find out more about our unconscious thoughts and to get a better understanding of ourselves. Insight or self-understanding is the goal, and that goal is achieved through a therapeutic relationship with the therapist. While psychologists and psychiatrists practice psychoanalysis by talking, OTs use a wide variety of creative media to help patients explore their unconscious and achieve greater self-understanding. The OTR or COTA using the psychoanalytic frame of reference may use drawing, painting, or sculpture to produce symbolic representations of the inner thoughts and feelings of patients. We may ask patients to write stories or poems, and discuss the meaning of these. Drama, dance, and music are other expressive media which may be useful in accomplishing self-understanding.

Freudian psychoanalysis has come a long way since Freud. Many schools of psychology have begun with Freud and taken off in various directions. One of those that is most useful to OT is the *ego-adaptive* approach. This frame of reference focuses on the functions of the "ego" or the "self." The goal is still self-understanding, but the focus is on practical, everyday skills such as self-control, reality-testing, and the use of rational thought to solve problems. The idea is to help the patient to "adapt" his or her self-concept so that recovery from illness is possible.

A frame of reference that has always been central to OT is the humanistic frame. The

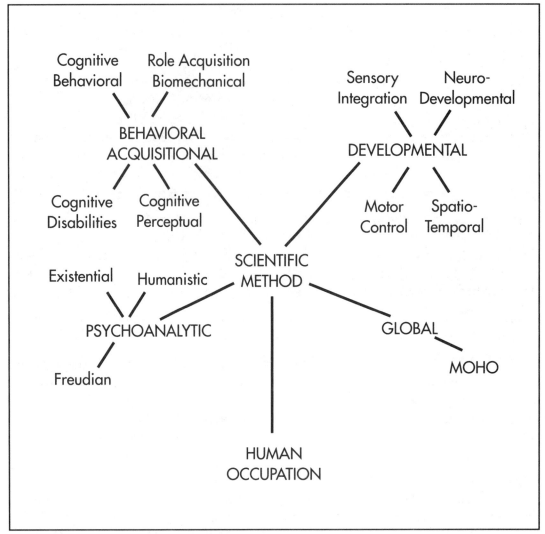

Figure 14-1. The frames of reference branches.

focus of this frame is also the self, but takes a more holistic perspective. In this frame of reference, change occurs through relationships with others. Feedback from both the therapist and other patients is vital to the patient forming a realistic self-image. Motivation is assumed to be internal, and a basic assumption is that all people have a tendency to strive for self-actualization. OT uses this frame of reference often in combination with others, especially when dealing with emotional or motivational issues. The therapeutic relationship is seen as vital to compliance with treatment, and ultimately, to successful rehabilitation.

Behavioral/Acquisitional

The common element in the behavioral frames of reference is that they are all based on the scientific method. Some of them are biomechanical, behavior modification, cognitive behavioral, cognitive perceptual, cognitive disabilities, and role acquisition. Mosey (1981) used the term *acquisitional* to describe all of these frames because they are based on the acquisition of skills. One of the earliest of these frames is behavior modification, and the concepts of learning implied in that are basic to all of the others. Activities are broken down into small steps to make learning easier. Each step is reinforced, either externally or internally. Problems are specifically and narrowly defined, solutions systematically applied. Homework, repetition, and practice are fundamental.

Another important element of behavioral frames is the way in which they were developed. Behavior must always be "observable and measurable." Thus, all of these theories use specific, standardized assessment techniques and base their hypotheses on the results of these. In the cognitive disabilities frame, for example, Allen's (1994) six cognitive levels are based on carefully observation of behavior in patients with brain damage or chronic mental illness. The ACL test consists of standardized observations of patients in doing progressively more difficult types of leather lacing.

The biomechanical frame of reference is, perhaps, the most scientific, in that it is based on measurements of ROM, strength, and endurance. Instruments for testing these physical functions include goniometers, which measure degrees of joint motion, dynamometers, which measure grip strength, and the Baltimore Therapeutic Work Simulator (BTE), which simulates work tasks and is widely used in the field of work hardening.

The cognitive perceptual frame is one of the newest of the behavioral frames. It was developed as a rehabilitative approach to brain injury, and uses theories of information processing. This frame looks at recovery of brain function as a series of steps, from simple to complex, using cuing as reinforcement. On the lower end of the hierarchy is the ability of the brain to focus attention and orient oneself to time, place, and person. Visual processing, motor planning, memory, and problem solving are progressively higher level skills.

A commonly used *cognitive behavioral* approach in OT, is the *psychoeducational* approach. This approach to rehabilitation resembles classroom teaching. Patients are "taught" socialization skills or coping skills for managing stress or how to identify side effects of their medication. Internal motivation is assumed in this frame, and because of this, it is mostly used with patients who are functioning at a fairly high cognitive level, and are capable of abstract thinking and reasoning.

Developmental

Developmental frames have one major element in common: they assume what Mosey called "recapitulation of ontogeny," which means that recovery from illness parallels the normal developmental process. Concepts from the *neurodevelopmental (motor control)* frames tell us that stroke patients, who are paralyzed on one side of their body, must relearn movement on that side, just as an infant does, beginning with primitive reflexes and working toward voluntary movement and eventually, walking again. Therefore, the OTR or COTA plans therapeutic movement sessions based on the known predictable sequences of normal child development.

Many of the developmental frames of reference we use in OT were created from concepts of child development. In creating the theory of sensory integration, Ayres applied what was known in the neurosciences about normal development of the brain to better understand and test her ideas about how sensation develops and becomes integrated. Using these concepts, Ayres was able to identify several specific types of sensory integrative dysfunction in children. Another OT theorist, Lorna Jean King, used the same concepts Ayres developed to identify and treat sensory integrative dysfunction in adults with dementia, autism, and chronic mental illness. *Spatiotemporal adaptation* is a frame of reference which has helped us understand the importance of stress and the external environment in motivating a child to master new skills. Research is now underway to explore how this frame of reference can be applied to adults who are dysfunctional. Theories of psychosocial (Erikson), psychosexual (Freud), moral (Kohlberg and Wilcox), and intellectual development (Piaget) are helpful in guiding the OTR and COTA in using concepts from normal child development to better understand and treat dysfunctional adults.

Global

There is only one frame of reference in this category, and that is the *Model of Human Occupation*, or MOHO as it is currently known. This frame of reference was first described by Gary Kielhofner, Janice Burke, and Cynthia Igi in 1980 (Kielhofner, 1992). Historically, this frame of reference comes from the "occupational behavior" approach which was developed by Mary Reilly at the University of Southern California. Reilly, in turn, based her theories on the historical roots of OT, which were articulated by Adolf Meyer and others back in the 1920s and 1930s. To fully understand this frame, the student must look more deeply into the history of OT as a profession. The basic idea behind both occupational behavior and MOHO is that any human activity, or "occupation," is in itself health-producing. The therapeutic value of everyday activities, whether work, leisure, or self-care, is the one of the most important founding principles of OT. This is why the MOHO frame of reference is considered "global," and some of our practitioners use it exclusively. This issue will be discussed later in this chapter. What is new about the MOHO frame, which makes it different from all others, is that it is partly based on systems theory, borrowed from business management. MOHO defines every person as a "human open system," that is, one that takes in material/information (input), and generates a response, hopefully adaptive (output). In addition, the human open system is capable of changing itself as a result of feedback from the environment (Figure 14-2).

HOW FRAMES OF REFERENCE GUIDE OUR PRACTICE

For the purposes of illustration, let us assume a patient, who is female, age 40 with chronic osteoarthritis and depression is referred to OT. Without knowing anything else about her, what kinds of thoughts come to mind about this patient? What is her position in life, her occupation, family roles, leisure activities, and accomplishments? Or, maybe you'd like to know about her emotional state, whether she's had some disappointments lately, or lost someone close to her. Her physical state may concern you also, the kinds of limitations she experiences because of the arthritis. Finally, you may want to consider her level of mental ability, how capable she may be of rational thought, and how she uses her mental strengths to cope with the problems she encounters. Any of the four types of frames of reference could be useful with this patient, depending on the area of dysfunction on which you choose to focus treatment. Even before you meet the patient, your frame of reference has already begun to guide your thinking as a therapist. Joan Rogers (1983), another one of OT's prominent theorists, called this the "pre-assessment image," a beginning stage in the process of clinical reasoning. Now try Exercise 14-1.

The next way that frames of reference guide our clinical thinking is in selecting the assessments we will use. When we assess and measure the extent of dysfunction in various areas, we will confirm or refute our original hypothesis. This means, the original

PSYCHOANALYTIC	BEHAVIORAL/ACQUISITIONAL
Emotions	External Reinforcement
Art, Music, Drawing	Biofeedback
Sculpture, Pottery	Pain Management
Psychodrama	Work Hardening
Creative Writing	Cognitive Levels
Poetry	Attention, Visual Processing
Projective Techniques	Memory, Problem Solving
Self-Actualization	Rational Thought
Therapeutic Relationships	Psychoeducational
	Self-Management
	Role Acquisition
DEVELOPMENTAL	**GLOBAL**
Ages and Stages	Holistic
Adult Developmental Stages	Occupational Behavior
Adaptive Skills	Human Open System
Maturing Nervous System	Volitional Subsystem
Internal Drive Toward Mastery	Personal Efficacy
Growth Facilitating Environments	Values and Beliefs
Just-Right Challenges	Roles and Habits
Calm Alertness	Performance Subsystem
Sensory Integration	Everyday Activities
Voluntary Movement	Temporal Adaptation

Figure 14-2. Four types of frames of reference.

ideas we had about the patient could have been right or wrong. The only way we'll really know this is to ask the right questions, and take the right measurements to find out.

When we have a realistic definition of the problems this patient encounters, the next step is to select appropriate treatment. We want to develop a treatment plan that has some chance of working; therefore, we need to summon all that is known about the patient's problem, and what treatments have worked for others with similar problems. The OTR or COTA should keep up with the published research on various treatment techniques, so that he or she can select the approach that stands the best chance of working. Frames of reference help professionals organize a vast array of knowledge, so that it can be recalled at the very moment we need it, or can be found quickly in a file or textbook. Each frame of reference, as we discussed earlier, gives us guidelines about how change occurs, and this tells us which techniques are likely to make a difference for our patient. Perhaps it is time for an example.

Suppose the OTR or COTA chooses to deal first with depression in our 40-year-old female patient, and selects the psychoanalytic frame of reference. We will want to know more about her feelings of sadness and hopelessness, and where they are coming from. We may ask this patient to do some drawing, say a picture of herself with her family, or

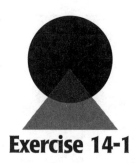

Exercise 14-1

Develop 10 questions you'd like to ask your client (40-year-old female with chronic osteoarthritis and depression) before you begin your assessment and treatment.

1. _____
2. _____
3. _____
4. _____
5. _____
6. _____
7. _____
8. _____
9. _____
10. _____

Once you have done this, organize your questions into the following categories.

A. Questions dealing with her job, her family, or other life roles and responsibilities: _____.

    A global approach, such as MOHO, or a more specific behavioral approach, such as role acquisition, may be your preference.

B. Questions dealing with her beliefs, feelings, and emotions: _____.
    These may best be dealt within the psychoanalytic, humanistic, or cognitive behavioral frames.

C. Questions concerning physical condition, fitness, amount of pain, or fatigue: _____.

    These may best be dealt within the biomechanical frame.

D. Questions about her mental ability, sensation, concentration, thinking, and prob lem solving: _____.
    Sensory integration, cognitive perceptual, or cognitive disabilities frames are most helpful here.

The road your thoughts have taken as you contemplate this case will give you a good sense of your own frame of reference as you approach the OT profession.

in a situation that is meaningful to her, and use the drawing as a focal point for discussion. The MOHO would lead you in another direction. You would look at the patient's roles and activities associated with them. In depression, we know that persons often lose interest in normal daily activities, and their routines need to be re-established. The MOHO frame would also guide us to strengthen our patient's sense of personal efficacy, so that she will see herself as capable of controlling her life and having a positive effect on her environment. Assessment and treatment will follow the clinically tested strategies for the frame of reference being followed.

ONE FRAME OF REFERENCE VS. MANY

In the late 1970s and early 1980s, Kielhofner proposed that MOHO be established as a "paradigm" for the profession of OT. A paradigm is defined as a group of core assumptions, values, and a focal viewpoint that unifies the field and defines the nature and purpose of OT (Kielhofner, 1992). Many OT leaders, being the diverse, creative thinkers they are, disagreed. Mosey was one of the OT leaders who opposed most vehemently. She argued that a variety of frames of reference are needed to keep the field dynamic and adaptive. This issue is still a source of controversy.

When an OTR or COTA becomes too fond of one frame of reference, that therapist is at risk of making that frame of reference into an "ideology." This means that he or she uses only that one frame for all patients and all situations. For example, when sensory integration was first developed as a form of assessment and treatment, some OT practitioners embraced it as the answer to any and all problems encountered in our pediatric patients. We now know that this is not the case. Different children respond to different approaches, leading one to believe that their problems arise from a variety of sources. Using an ideology is not making the best use of our knowledge. Different frames of reference have much to offer in the way of guidelines for all aspects of our practice.

HOW FRAMES OF REFERENCE ORGANIZE KNOWLEDGE

Picture your brain as a giant filing cabinet. Frames of reference help us create a filing system for all the knowledge we will gather during our courses and fieldwork experiences. Taking the time to understand frames of reference early in your education will help you learn and remember information later on. The office worker who stacks up a new file folder each time he or she learns about a new subject quickly loses track of the information at the bottom of the pile. Organizing the subjects into categories, labeling them carefully, and placing them in correctly labeled file drawers will make it much easier to recover information as it is needed. Create one file drawer for each frame of reference. Then, as you go through your coursework and fieldwork, make the connection between what you are learning and the frame of reference with which it is associated. This method may also prevent you from becoming overwhelmed when the stack of files becomes too high.

The OT knowledge base begins with the philosophy of OT. This contains the profession's fundamental beliefs, and is similar to Kielhofner's definition of a "paradigm." I prefer to think of this central core as a shared vision of our profession that is accepted without question. Around this central core are the frames of reference. Kielhofner calls them conceptual models of practice, but they are really the same thing. The OT frames of reference gather concepts from many diverse areas and use them in forming a unique vision of the patient and of treatment (Figure 14-3).

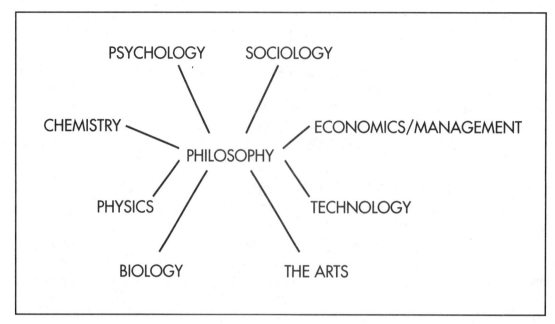

Figure 14-3. Frames of reference: the OT's vision.

Throughout this chapter, you may have observed that there are alternate terms to describe similar concepts. *Paradigm*, for example, is Kielhofner's term describing the core of the OT profession. Mosey uses the term *model* of our profession to mean something similar. For this reason, it is important to connect the term with the person who defined it, so that confusion can be avoided. It must be accepted from the start that the leaders of our profession do not agree on how the various parts of our knowledge fit together. This is the price we pay for being a part of such a creative profession.

LEARNING FRAMES OF REFERENCE

The best way to learn the frames of reference is by creating a giant poster grid. Across the top, list the frames of reference. Down the left side, list the structural parts defined earlier: domain of concern (focus), basic assumptions (interdisciplinary base), function (order), dysfunction (disorder), change and motivation (therapeutic intervention), and assessment and treatment (technology for application). Fill in the squares under each frame of reference by summarizing the information from source references (Worksheet 14-1). In this way, you will learn how the frames are similar, and how they differ. You will be able to distinguish between them by asking discriminating questions, such as "How do these two frames of reference explain how change occurs?" The subtle differences will become clear.

In addition, each frame has its own theorists, its own terminology, and its own research. You will note in Worksheet 14-1 that these have been added to the study guide. It is important that you associate the concepts or ideas of each frame with the names of the theorists who developed them. Kielhofner and Mosey are good examples of two OT theorists who have opposing views. Understanding a theory from the perspective of its author or developer, will always give you a deeper appreciation for the interpretation and application of the theory. Whether you are reading a journal article or on a fieldwork visit,

Worksheet 14-1

Frames of Reference Study Guide   (continue on your own)

	Biomechanical	Cognitive Disabilities	Sensory Integration	MOHO
Domain of Concern				
Basic Assumptions				
Function				
Dysfunction				
Change and Motivation				
Assessment and Treatment				
Theorists/Contributors				
Terminology				
Research				

you will be able to recognize the frame of reference being used by its unique vocabulary. It will help to make a list of terms that are common to each frame of reference and write out their definitions. Just making these study aids for yourself will help you keep the frames of reference from becoming confusing or overwhelming. You will then be able to impress your teachers and fieldwork supervisors, and later, your administrators and your patients, with the clarity of your clinical thinking.

SUMMARY

This chapter introduced the concept of frames of reference, and explains how they are used in OT. A frame of reference was compared to a pair of tinted glasses, coloring all that we see and affecting our thoughts and behavior. The parts of a frame of reference discussed included a central focus or domain of concern, definitions of function and dysfunction, explanations of how change occurs and how people are motivated to change, and approaches to assessment and treatment. Frames of reference were divided into four general categories: psychoanalytic, behavioral, developmental, and global. We learned why it is better to know and use a variety of frames of reference, and how different frames are used for addressing different types of functional problems. Finally, some strategies were suggested for identifying your own frame of reference, for using frames of reference to organize your professional studies, and for discriminating between the different frames used in OT. What exactly is a frame of reference? As depicted in Figure 14-3, it's gathering compatible concepts from many areas of study and using them to form a unique vision of our patients and a plan of action for treating them.

BIBLIOGRAPHY
Allen, C., Earhart, C., & Blue, T. (1992). *Occupational therapy treatment goals for the physically and cognitively disabled.* Bethesda, MD: American Occupational Therapy Association.

Ayres, A. J. (1989). *Sensory integration and praxis tests*. Los Angeles: Western Psychological Services.

Kielhofner, G. (1992). *Conceptual foundations of occupational therapy.* Philadelphia: F. A. Davis.

Mosey, A. (1981). *Occupational therapy: Configuration of a profession*. New York: Raven Press.

Rogers, J. (1983). Clinical reasoning: The ethics, science and art. *American Journal of Occupational Therapy, 37*, 601-616.

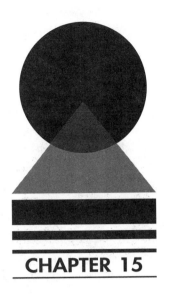

CHAPTER 15

WORKING WITH MEMBERS OF A TREATMENT TEAM

Ellen Berger Rainville, MS, OTR/L, FAOTA

When good jazz musicians improvise together, they...manifest a "feel for" their material and they make on-the-spot adjustments to the sounds they hear. Listening to one another and to themselves, they feel where the music is going and adjust their playing accordingly...As the musicians feel the direction of the music that is developing out of their interwoven contributions, they make sense of it and adjust their performance to the new sense they have made. (Schon, 1983, p. 55)

Like musicians, therapists have many opportunities to "improvise" with other caregiving persons. You will hear this referred to as communication, collaboration, teamwork, or other names. Without doubt, working with others can be one of the most frustrating, satisfying, motivating, supportive, and complex aspects of practice that you will encounter. However, from the perspective of our clients, there is nothing more important than coordinated, meaningful services from competent professionals. This is the goal of caregiving.

You can and will participate in many types of both planned and improvised care coordination during your career as an OT or OTA. You have the ability to not only contribute to, but also to benefit from, the experience.

THE MYTH OF THE INDEPENDENT PRACTITIONER

Before you began your education in OT, and even now, you may have dreamt about what it might be like after graduation when you are finally free. Many students believe that they will someday have a private practice and there they will practice completely independently. They imagine that in independent practice they will have complete control over their work life, their clients, their colleagues, and their finances. To some extent, this may be true. If you become the administrator of an organization, you will have the authority and the responsibility to make choices about these matters. You may be self-employed or employed by others. You may or may not become an administrator. Regardless, you will not be alone.

You probably chose a career in OT, at least in part, because it is a people-oriented profession. Likely you enjoy and are skilled at interacting with others. This is fortunate because in OT practice there really is no such thing as truly independent practice. You will have independent responsibility, independent knowledge, and work that you will do independently of others, however, the very nature of therapy involves interaction with people— our clients—and with the other professionals involved in what can be very complex care.

The interactions among professionals and clients are integral to the efficiency and effectiveness of care. COTAs and OTRs rely heavily on others for information, cooperation, and assistance to achieve shared goals. Others rely on them for the same. Truly *independent* practice is a myth. *Inter*dependent practice is perhaps a better way to describe our interactions with others.

BECOMING A THERAPIST

As a practicing OTR or COTA, you will continually be developing knowledge, skills, and attitudes unique to OT. Your individual expertise will reflect your personal and professional interests, values, and, of course, experience. If you work in hand therapy, for example, your expertise will more likely be in orthotics and prosthetics. However, a colleague of yours who works in the public schools will likely develop special expertise in learning and development. Your respective areas of expertise are reflective of OT's breadth and scope.

As a new graduate you will make unique contributions—different than those of the more experienced therapist. As a group, new graduates are thought to possess the most current theoretical and technical knowledge. In addition, new graduates are enthusiastic, inquisitive, and really facilitate quality care. Be proud of that interest and energy. Use it to learn about your patients and clients, your colleagues, and your work setting.

Over time, you may practice in a variety of settings, perhaps with different clinical populations and service philosophies, or you may stay in the same setting for many years. Both time and experience will influence your individual expertise and hence your potential contribution to the care of your clients, especially if you take the time to reflect on your clinical experiences.

WORKING WITH OTHERS

As you develop expertise, you will learn from books, journals, magazines, television, film, video, and many other media. You will also learn from others. If you share your musings with interested colleagues, they can help you make sense of your experience. You will have shared experiences that will shake you up, will distress or delight you, or will leave you feeling immobilized. There is nothing like the help of another to make sense of the situation, to imagine alternatives, and to move forward. Working with others gives us the kind of support, acceptance, and understanding in our work that friends and families can in our personal lives. Through shared experience we can learn and grow.

On the other hand, working with others can be difficult. Like personal relationships, professional relationships require attention, care, and work in order to be satisfying. Without this, they can be downright unpleasant. There may be personality or style differences between people that may seem insurmountable. There may be conflicts in values, goals, and beliefs that make interactions feel strained and unpleasant. Some people are more skilled at interpersonal interaction than others and some value it more. If people do not wish to work together, yet their jobs require them to, there may be discomfort and discord. Some people feel "threatened" by others who they perceive to be more knowledgeable, more skillful, or more personable than they are.

As previously stated, it is unlikely that you will work alone in the field of OT. Thus, it behooves you to be prepared to make your experiences working with others the very best they can be. This involves special knowledge, skills, and attitudes related to communication and collaboration. These will benefit your personal experience and your practice of OT.

SERVICE DELIVERY MODELS

There are numerous formal mechanisms by which you will work with others. You may attend case conferences or team meetings regarding clients you see. You may send copies of your written reports (with your clients' permission) or talk on the phone with the other professionals involved in their care. There will also be informal mechanisms, a casual conversation over lunch, a shared discussion during a cotreatment, or an unplanned observation.

There are also various models or ways of organizing service delivery. These each provide different mechanisms for working with others. Direct and indirect service delivery models will be discussed here. *Direct* therapy involves those activities that are individually designed by the OT and implemented by the OTR or COTA because they cannot be safely carried out by any other person (Dunn, 1991). For example, certain sensory integrative treatment techniques are best done by a therapist who has been specifically trained in this frame of reference for therapy. Direct services may be provided on a one-to-one or group basis. In this model, however, the process and content of therapy is directly experienced by the therapist and his or her clients. Relevant information about what occurs during direct therapy must be communicated to others on the caregiving team. For example, the sensory integrative approach to treatment will have the most impact if the child's performance in therapy can be related to his or her performance in the classroom or at home.

Indirect services involve either consultation or monitoring (Dunn, 1991; Gilfoyle, 1981). Consultation is a process, often collaborative, where a problem is defined and resolved within the context of a mutually respectful, trusting relationship. (Jaffe & Epstein, 1992). Consultation may be time limited, being related to a specific problem or situation, or it may be ongoing. The therapist uses his or her expertise to help another person address an issue identified by that person. Unlike in direct service, the consultant is not immediately responsible for the outcome (Dunn, 1991).

Monitoring is where the OT practitioner is fully responsible for conducting the evaluation and developing an intervention plan, but a person in the client's natural environment is trained by the OT personnel to carry out the plan. The OT then *monitors* the actual implementation of the plan, providing supervision, support, and assistance, and making changes as necessary.

In practice, you will likely encounter a mix of these service delivery models. As you can see, each model of service is appropriate for different clinical situations and each requires different interpersonal communications. You will need to adapt to each.

BEING A TEAM MEMBER

Communication of relevant information improves understanding and hence coordination of care. If one person does not know what the other is doing, of course there will be confusion, misunderstanding, and negative feelings. Not only is this embarrassing, it is also disrespectful. In order to minimize potential communication problems, many organizations establish teams. A team is defined as "an organized body of individuals that share goals and interests" (Case-Smith & Wavrek, 1993, p. 131). Essential to effective team functioning are member skills and knowledge, commitment to team goals, good communication, a common language, stability of membership, effective leadership, and clearly delineated member roles and responsibilities. All teams experience developmental changes over time as illustrated in Table 15-1 (Blechert, Christiansen, & Kari, 1987).

Teams are also characterized by the ways in which the members interact with each other. These interactions fall along a continuum from intradisciplinary to transdisciplinary as illustrated in Table 15-2.

Teams generally adopt the interactional model that best fits their overall goals. However, most teams actually function at varying points on the interactional continuum, depending on the individual situation(s) they are dealing with. For example, a team may be able to function at the transdisciplinary level when members are working with a client who is familiar to and with them. They may need little outside input. On the other hand, a team may function at a more multidisciplinary level with a new client, especially one who receives services from multiple outside agencies who are not regular team members.

WHAT IS COLLABORATION?

Collaboration is the most cooperative level of professional interaction. It is a dynamic, ongoing process where collaborators share responsibility for data collection, data analysis, decision making, program planning, development, implementation, and evaluation. Mutual respect and trust are the foundations of effective collaboration and communication skills are essential. In today's world, collaboration is emphasized as the interactional style of choice both in the professional literature and in public policy (i.e., laws and regulations).

Using the same qualities which are essential for good teamwork, any number of people can collaborate. However, there may be some problems. For example, if the people involved in an interaction are not clear about its purpose, about the roles and responsibilities of the participants, and/or are not certain about their own potential contributions, it is unlikely that they will be able to effectively collaborate. Therefore, it is helpful to ensure that this information is communicated at the outset of the interaction.

KNOW THYSELF AND KNOW OTHERS

As a caregiver, it is essential that you know and carefully examine your own experiences, values, and beliefs (Davis, 1994). The work of caregiving can evoke powerful feel-

Table 13-1
Developmental Team Chart

Stage of Team Development	Characteristics	Supervisor's Tasks	Team Members' Issues	Communication
I. Initiation Stage Exploration and definition of member roles and responsibilities within the context of team and work settings.	Prior to and in the beginning phase of team formation, individuals may experience self-doubt, lack of trust, role ambiguity, and a degree of powerlessness in the work setting.	Promote atmosphere of acceptance and trust: • State expectations openly • Encourage discussion of members' expectations Encourage commitment to team building by helping members to: • Identify skills, areas of strength and interest • Provide opportunities to increase self-esteem Provide general definition and direction for newly formed team: • Define the situation and resources available • Define roles and responsibilities for team members	Learn and explore role expectations. Begin to share resources, identify own areas of expertise and interests.	Express anxieties and insecurities of new relationships. Verbalize support for team efforts. Demonstrate acceptance and begin to develop trust.
II. Transition Stage Adjustment and rearrangement of roles to create a team.	Team members experience increased anxieties, defensiveness, and struggles for control. Reclarification and adjustments of roles are evident. Group norms are forming. Relationship issues are important at this stage.	Provide encouragement. Manage conflict openly. Provide structures for team to make decisions, solve problems, and set priorities. Effectuate intervention strategies if needed. Reclarify roles, team goals.	Develop skills, gain confidence. Learn about the organizational structure. Commit self to teamwork.	Begin to identify and deal with conflicts openly. Verbalize group norms and values. Encourage team affiliation by engaging in community building activities.
III. Working Stage Tasks are identified and achieved.	Team members experience cohesion and productivity. Conflicts are dealt with openly and are effectively managed.	Refine leadership skills. Allow team members more autonomy and support development of their professional skills. Provide liaison functions for team with the external organization. Help team members find solutions to difficult problems; provide resources and support services. Assess and evaluate work done relative to the team's overall performance.	Participate fully as a team member in the planning, decision making, and execution of tasks. Clarify personal goals. Ask for needed direction/support from supervisor. Participate in evaluation of task completion. Develop sense of mastery.	Communicate support and challenge members through feedback. Discuss how methods of problem solving, decision making, and conflict management occur in the team.
IV. Interdependence Stage Team members are effective in their work and achieve interdependence in their working relationships.	Team members are mutually supportive, take pride in the team, value each other, and experience the successes of the interlocking roles.	Model collegial relationships. Become a mentor; empower others. Continue to develop personal and professional skills.	Reflect on self as a professional, reassess goals, offer peer evaluations. Learn to think about issues form multiple points of view. Take risks; achieve greater competency.	Express valuing of team members and demonstrate support for each other's achievements.
Separation Team separation may occur at any stage; however, characteristics and tasks will be different depending on the maturity of the team.	Team members experience anxiety as they anticipate separation. There is an awareness of the successes and failures of the team.	Ensure opportunity for and assist members in summarizing, integrating, and interpreting the team experience. Provide a framework that will help members evaluate the team effort and individual roles. Allow time for members to resolve unfinished business and express feelings about the separation.	Summarize the team experience and the attainment of personal and professional goals. Evaluate personal and team performance. Define tasks for new members.	Express feelings about separation. Avoid withdrawal or distancing of members. Give and receive feedback; discuss the application of current experiences to future teams.

Ministration →

Mastery →

Maturation →

From Blechert, T., Christiansen, M., & Kari, N. (1987). Intraprofessional team building. American Journal of Occupational Therapy, 41, 580-581. © 1987 by the American Occupational Therapy Association, Inc. Reprinted with permission.

Table 15-2
Team Interaction Continuum

Intradisciplinary

One or more members of one discipline provide treatment to the individual. Generally, other disciplines are not involved. If other disciplines are involved, communication is limited.

Multidisciplinary

A number of professionals conduct assessments and interventions independent from one another. Some formal communications occur between involved professionals. Resources and responsibilities are individually allocated between disciplines.

Interdisciplinary

Several disciplines agree to collaborate for decision making. Evaluation and intervention is still conducted independently, within defined areas of each profession's expertise. Formal communications, such as treatment planning meetings, do occur to exchange information, prioritize needs, and allocate resources and responsibilities.

Transdisciplinary

An interdisciplinary team whose members are committed to ongoing communication, collaboration, and share decision making for the patient's benefit. Evaluations and interventions are planned cooperatively. Programs are often the responsibility of a primary interventionist, but treatments are often shared. Ongoing training, support supervision, cooperation, and consultation among disciplines is important to this model.

ings that, if left unrecognized and unresolved, are not helpful to our clients. There are many mechanisms to increase self-knowledge. These include self-exploration workshops (i.e., Outward Bound, values workshops), personal psychotherapy, and self-study guides for helping professionals (i.e., *Patient Practitioner Interaction: An Experiential Manual for Developing the Art of Health Care* [2nd ed.] by Carol Davis). Keeping a journal, writing, or other creative activities also help with self-knowledge and expression. Physical activity, particularly if it is both challenging and enjoyable, can help to improve one's self-confidence and spirit.

As you get to know yourself better, you will find that you not only accept your short-comings but that you also like yourself more. This feeling is contagious to others. The most well-liked people seem to be those who project an image of liking themselves. These individuals appear to have an easier time engendering cooperation from others as well. So, knowing and feeling the best that you can about yourself will likely make others *want* to work with you.

As you interact with others, it is important to get to know them as well, not just as professionals or clients, but as unique individuals. Spend time learning about your colleagues' educational backgrounds, professional experiences, and interests. Start off slowly, building trust and rapport as you become more familiar with each other.

As your interactions progress, you may want to inquire about personal matters. Of course you will use good judgment and keep your conversation at an appropriate level. For example, it is appropriate for colleagues to know some general information about each other's personal lives, such as their marital status, who is in their family, perhaps where they live. In most cases, it is not appropriate, however, for colleagues to know the intimate details of each other's family or romantic relationships.

With clients or colleagues, it is best to let each individual decide how much personal information to share. In all cases you will need to be sensitive to what information is relevant to your work together.

The level of interaction between people is mutually set, usually informally, although some companies have very specific policies about interactions among employees and between employees and clients. You will need to be familiar with these. In any case, be sensitive to the feelings and comfort levels of others. Be polite, friendly, and interested, but not intrusive. Knowing yourself and knowing others will help your interactions flow as smoothly as they can. It will also increase your investment in each other and hence your investment in the outcomes of your work together.

VERBAL AND NONVERBAL COMMUNICATION

Perhaps the most important tool we have for successful interactions with others is our ability to communicate. Think about how effective a great speaker can be at using verbal communication to engender interest in a subject or how powerfully an infant can communicate without words or even gestures. Both verbal and nonverbal communication are powerful tools. Mastering the use of these through understanding, practice, and reflection will make you feel more competent in your interactions with others at work and at home.

Verbal and written communication, the use of words, helps us to exchange information. This includes professional "lingo," medical jargon, for example. The interpretation of that information is influenced by our understanding of the language used; our values, beliefs, and attitudes; and our ability to listen. Successful verbal communication depends on the actual words used, the organization of expression, vocal tone, clarity, volume, and the attitudes of both speaker and receiver (Purtillo & Haddad, 1996).

You will find that humor is used rather extensively in the workplace. This can be very effective at reducing stress, anxiety, tension, and can sometimes be a way of expressing difficult thoughts or feelings (Navarra, Lipkowitz, & Navarra, 1990; Purtillo & Haddad, 1996). It can also be cruel, inappropriate, and destructive. Making fun of others is simply not appropriate for adults. Sexual and other forms of verbal harassment are no longer tolerated in the workplace. Enjoy good humor but do not allow yourself to participate in or tolerate verbal misuse of people.

Nonverbal communication, or metacommunication, is wordless communication made up of gestures, body postures, physical appearance, facial expressions, etc. It may or may not accompany verbal communication. Regardless, it is a very powerful means of expression, perhaps more powerful than verbal communication.

Sign language is an example of nonverbal communication that has very clear rules and patterns. Pantomime, or imitation of an act, such as demonstration of a physical technique, is another form of intentional nonverbal communication. For example, when an OT practitioner observes a nonverbal client performing ADLs they are receiving important information through nonverbal communication channels. Not only are the physical actions used by the client important, but the facial expressions may also tell an important story. If he or she is relaxed and smiling, one message is received. If he or she grimaces, grits his or her teeth, and sighs, a very different story is told.

In our regular communication, we convey a variety of emotion and information through facial expression, eye contact, posture, and touch. It is helpful for therapists to understand the nonverbal messages that they may be sending to clients and to colleagues, as well as those they are receiving. At a team meeting, for example, a person who sits facing the others, leaning slightly forward, indicates interest. If the therapist sits facing away from the group with crossed arms and legs, this indicates disinterest and an unwillingness to participate. A client may say he or she wants to be at this meeting with words, but his or her nonverbal messages tell the truth more often than not.

OT personnel can help others to better understand nonverbal communication. For example, individuals with certain types of central nervous system or psychiatric dysfunctions may have difficulty both encoding (expressing) and decoding (understanding) nonverbal messages. In terms of social interaction, this can be extraordinarily disabling.

There are many resources for improving our communication skills. There are courses, workshops, and reading material. It is worth your time and energy to find the resources that are best for you. As you know, good communication is at the very heart of good interpersonal interaction.

THE INFLUENCE OF CULTURE AND CONTEXT ON INTERACTION

Each person interprets actions, expressions, words, etc. based on their own cultural conditioning and experience. Cultures, or groups of people, have unique sets of rules and values. Organizations, families, and countries are examples of cultures. Each is different from the other, yet there may be important similarities.

Each of us has had multiple cultural influences, from our families, our religions, our communities, even our profession's culture. These have and do shape our beliefs and hence our interpretations. It is important that we recognize and respect the contributions of culture to communication. Some cultural influences on communication are listed in the chart below. As part of your self-exploration, you may wish to spend a few moments examining yourself and your biases and beliefs in each of these areas. Imagine how these could affect your interactions with others—negatively and positively. Through education and experience, you can increase your understanding of and appreciation of others' differences. You might read about people who are different than you, watch movies and television shows, and/or spend time with others from different cultures. Being open to diversity not only increases our enjoyment of others, it makes our caregiving more equitable, which is so important. Fill out Worksheet 15-1 to begin to examine this issue.

Context, or situation, is also very important to interaction and communication. Many of us are more comfortable in familiar environments, so we may be more open and welcoming if someone comes to our "turf," our home or office. Consider going to the office or home of your client or colleague in order to make them feel more comfortable, especially with difficult issues.

Think about how anxious new situations make most of us. Sometimes that anxiety is positive and exciting, other times, it is terrifying and immobilizing. Not only do we have emotional reactions to context, we also have physiological reactions, such as increased pulse and blood pressure experienced by many people, just from being in the doctor's office.

Context includes both animate and inanimate features of the environment, everything from furniture to acoustics. Personal interpretations of meaning vary from situation to situation. Again, respect for individual differences is critical here. For example, some therapists find case conferences highly intimidating. They may associate this context with their lack of confidence in their verbal abilities and they may experience a form of stage fright. Others may find case conferences a welcome opportunity to discuss important issues. Each person's ability to exchange important information is clearly influenced by the context of that communication.

THE IMPORTANCE OF LOOKING AND LISTENING

Remember when you were a child and your teachers and parents told you to stop, look, and listen? That was and continues to be very wise advice. As stated throughout this chapter, you are not alone in your work or in your life. Your interactions with others are key to the successful achievement of your goals. It is highly recommended that you spend the time to really see and really hear the perspectives of others. Hope that they will do the same for you. You have a lifetime of experience in interaction and communication behind you and ahead of you. Enjoy!

SUMMARY

This chapter reviewed important aspects of interaction, communication, and collaboration among OT professionals, clients, and colleagues. Formal and informal mechanisms for working with others, as well as influences on communication, were discussed. Not only will effective communication enhance the quality of care for your clients, it will also benefit you, the OTR or COTA. There are many ways to enhance your understanding of interpersonal communication, especially as it relates to work. You are encouraged to take advantage of the many opportunities available to learn more.

Worksheet 15-1

Cultural Influences	Who I Am	How I Feel About This
Ethnicity		
Race		
Gender		
Age		
Socioeconomic Status		
Health Condition		
Religion		
Sexual Preference		
Educational Background		
Political Orientation		

BIBLIOGRAPHY

Bird, A. (1990). *Early occupational therapy intervention.* Gaithersburg, MD: Aspen Publications.

Blechert, T., Christiansen, M., & Kari, N. (1987). Intraprofessional team building. *American Journal of Occupational Therapy, 41,* 580-581.

Case-Smith, J., & Wavrek, B. B. (1993). Models of service delivery and team interaction. In J. Case-Smith (Ed.), *Pediatric occupational therapy and early intervention* (pp. 127-159). Boston: Andover Medical.

Davis, C. (1994). *Patient practitioner interaction: An experiential manual for developing the art of health care* (2nd ed.). Thorofare, NJ: SLACK Inc.

Dunn, W. (1988). Models of occupational therapy service provision in the school system. *American Journal of Occupational Therapy, 42,* 718-723.

Dunn, W. (1991). *Pediatric service delivery: Facilitating effective service provision.* Thorofare, NJ: SLACK Inc.

Gardner, H. G. (1988). *Helping others through teamwork.* Washington, D.C.: Child Welfare League of America.

Gilfoyle, E. M. (1981). *Training: Occupational therapy educational management in schools.* Bethesda, MD: American Occupational Therapy Association.

Jaffe, E. G., & Epstein, C. F. (1992). *Occupational therapy consultation: Theory, principles, and practice.* St. Louis, MO: Mosby Year Book.

Maple, G. (1987). Early intervention: Some issues in cooperative teamwork. *Australian Journal of Occupational Therapy, 34,* 145-151.

Navarra, T., Lipkowitz, M. A., & Navarra, J. G. (1990). *Therapeutic communication: A guide to effective interpersonal skills for health care professionals.* Thorofare, NJ: SLACK Inc.

Purtillo, R., & Haddad, A. (1996). *Health professional and patient interaction* (5th ed.). Philadelphia: W.B. Saunders.

Schon, D. A. (1983). *The reflective practitioner.* New York: Basic Books.

Spencer, P. (1989). Team dynamics relative to exemplary early services. In B. Hanft (Ed.), *Family centered care* (pp. 4.43-4.49). Bethesda, MD: American Occupational Therapy Association.

Tickle-Degnan, L., & Rosenthal, R. (1992). Nonverbal aspects of therapeutic rapport. In R. S. Feldman (Ed.), *Applications of nonverbal behavioral theories and research.* Hillsdale, NJ: Lawrence Erlbaum.

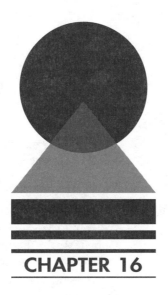

CHAPTER 16

MEDICAL TERMINOLOGY FOR THE OT STUDENT

Karen Sladyk, MS, OTR/L

INTRODUCTION

At some time in your career as an OT student, you will study medical terminology in great detail. It is likely that you will be required to buy a medical terminology textbook and will have to read it cover to cover. In this chapter, you will find ways to manage medical terminology and the most common medical terminology word roots. This chapter can be used as a tutorial of medical terminology or to test yourself in a different way than your textbook. There are several ways you can use this primer to help you master the large task of learning medical terminology. Check Table 16-1 to see what is the most appropriate way for you to use this chapter:

After you have determined the best way to use this chapter, develop an individual plan of study. Skim the section titles for the information you need. If medical terminology is new to you, begin here with the building blocks.

BUILDING BLOCKS OF MEDICAL TERMINOLOGY

Before you can begin to learn complicated medical words, it is useful to understand how the words are put together. Medical terminology generally follows some specific rules. Once you understand the rules, breaking down a very long word such as electroencephalogram (record of the electrical activity of the brain) becomes easy.

Most medical words are made up of **word parts**. These include:
- Word roots
- Prefixes (before a word root)

Table 16-1
How to Use This Chapter

Current Stage in Your Studies	How to Use the Chapter
Prior to medical terminology class	This chapter will give you a jump start and make your medical terminology class easier. Read the whole chapter, do all worksheets.
Currently taking medical terminology	This chapter will provide you with good review sheets in a style different from a medical terminology textbook. Read the whole chapter, do worksheets as a review for tests.
Ready for Level II fieldwork	You do not need to review the chapter but will find a review of the worksheets helpful. Focus on spelling, as documentation is an important aspect of fieldwork.
Finished fieldwork, studying for NBCOT exam	A review of the worksheets will provide a good start for studying for the NBCOT exam. Although terminology is not specifically tested on the exam, a solid foundation will make reading the questions easier and faster.
Passed the NBCOT exam, changing jobs, or re-entering the profession	Review the parts of the chapter that are most helpful.

- Suffixes (after a word root)
- Connecting vowels (between two word roots)

An example of how this works in the real world includes the words **player** and **replay**. In player, **play** is the word root, the foundation of the word. The suffix is **er**. In the word **replay**, **play** remains the word root and **re** is the prefix. This results in two different meaning words.

Now let us examine the word roots of some basic medical words. **Arthritis** and **hepatitis** are two medical words that most people have heard. **Arthr** means joints and **hepat** means liver. The suffix **itis** means inflammation. So arthritis is inflammation of the joints and hepatitis is inflammation of the liver. Generally speaking, the correct way to break down a word is to say the meaning of the suffix first. Arthritis becomes inflammation of the joints instead of joint inflammation.

Some of the most commonly used medical terminology suffixes include **logy** and **logist**. The suffix **logy** means **the study of** and **logist** means **one who studies**. So **terminology** breaks down as the study of terms and you are currently a medical **terminologist**, one who studies terms. Now that you know these common suffixes, you are likely to be able to break down the medical specialists in Exercise 16-1.

Connecting vowels are sometimes called combining vowels. Connecting vowels are almost always the letter **o**. A connecting vowel can go between two word roots or a word root and a suffix. **Arthropathy** is an example of the connecting vowel **o** between word root **arthr** meaning joint and suffix **pathy** meaning disease. Arthropathy would be broken down as disease of the joint. Once you have mastered word roots and combining vowels, spelling becomes an easy task. Check Table 16-2 for spelling hints.

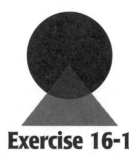

Exercise 16-1

Specialist	Definition
Cardiologist	
Neuropsychology	
Dermatologist	
Rheumatology	
Gastroenterology	

Table 16-2
Helpful Spelling Hints

- Medical words do not always have a prefix.
- Do not use a connecting vowel if the suffix begins with a vowel.
- Do not use a connecting vowel between a prefix and a word root.
- When unsure of which connecting vowel to use, use the letter o as it is the most common.

STUDY TECHNIQUES

Many OT educators believe that there are always several ways to learn particular skills. Teaching medical terminology is always a challenge to educators because it requires so much memorization. Before you can try out medical terminology in a practical way, such as note writing, you have to memorize the word roots. Memorizing is one of the more boring ways to learn something, but find comfort in the fact that thousands and thousands of OT students have memorized the same thing you are about to memorize.

Memorizing medical terminology is best done in short time sessions over a long period of time. Each time you master a group of terms, add in new terms to practice. Use both visual and auditory techniques to study. Organize your study environment to best meet your specific medical terminology learning needs. See Table 16-3 for suggestions.

A few words about the "all-night cram" for medical terminology. Educators generally agree that it is close to impossible to cram medical terminology into your head the night before a test. As mentioned above, medical terminology is best studied in short time sessions over a long time period. The reality of college life means some people prefer to do all-night cramming. If you are one of these types, do not oversaturate yourself with terms. Study only what you can manage.

Table 16-3
Study Techniques

Technique	How It Works Best
Study peer group	Form a group of peers to review medical terminology. Make sure that each member understands his or her responsibility to the group. Avoid asking only friends so that socializing does not inter-fere with studying. Share study techniques and resources, and quiz each other.
Flash cards	Put the word root on one side and the meaning on the other. Study the cards from both sides. Take the cards with you and review when you have 10 minutes before class, between studying for other topics, or while you wait for an appointment or ride.
Wall posters	Use large sheets of newsprint (craft store) or freezer paper (grocery store near tinfoil) to make large study sheets. Hang the posters in places you spend time, such as the kitchen while you clean up or bathroom while you brush you teeth.
Cassette tapes	Say the word root into a tape recorder, pause, and then say the meaning. While listening, try to say your answer before the tape gives you an answer. Make a second tape where you say the meaning into the tape recorder, pause, and say the word root. Share tapes with peers.
Worksheets	Before you write in this book or in the textbook that is required for class, make a photocopy of the exercises for practice or review later. Develop your own worksheets and share them with peers.
Game night	Invite your study peers over for medical terminology game night. Model your game after a favorite TV game show. Ask each partici-pant to come to game night with a category ready. Follow the rules of the game completely but substitute medical terminology ques-tions. Use snacks as prizes.

MOST COMMON WORD PARTS

The following section lists the most common word parts found in medical terminolo-gy. Medical terminology textbooks will cover a broader medical terminology base, but these most common word roots are a good start for mastering more advanced terms. Use this list for developing your study techniques outlined above or cover the columns with a bookmark and use the list to quiz yourself.

a	no, not, without	ar	pertaining to
ab	away from	arthro	joint
ac	pertaining to	audio	hearing
ad	toward	auto	self
adeno	gland	bi	two
aero	air	bio	life
al	pertaining to	brady	slow
albo	white	carcin	cancer
algia	pain	cardio	heart
an	pertaining to	cele	hernia
angio	vessel	cephal	head

chloro	green	kinesio	movement
chondro	cartilage	laryng	larynx
colic	large intestines	leuko	white
contra	against	lipo	fat
cranio	skull	litho	stone
cyan	blue	logy	study of
cyst	cyst, bladder	macro	large
cyto	cell	mal	bad
dento	teeth	malac	softening
derma	skin	mania	excessive preoccupation
di	two	megaly	large
dia	through	melano	black
dips	thirst	meso	middle
dynia	pain	meter	measure
dys	bad, difficult	micro	small
eal	pertaining to	mono	single
ecto	out, without, away	myel	spinal cord
ectomy	excision	myo	muscle
encephal	brain	necro	dead
endo	inside	nephro	kidney
epi	above	neuro	nerve and brain
erythro	red	oid	resembling
eu	good	oma	tumor
ex	out	orrhage	excessive bleeding
fibro	fiber	orrhagia	hemorrhage
gastro	stomach	orrhaphy	suture
genesis	beginning	orrhea	flow, discharge
glyco	sugar	orrhexis	rupture
gram	record	osis	condition of
graph	recording device	ostomy	new opening
hemi	half	oto	ear
hemo	blood	otomy	incision
hetero	different	ous	pertaining to
homo	same	patho	disease
hydro	water	penia	deficiency
hyper	high	peri	around
hypo	low	pexy	fixation
ia	condition of	phobia	fear
ic	pertaining to	phono	voice
in	not	plasty	surgical repair
inter	between	pnea	breathing
intra	within	pneumo	lung, air
ism	condition of	poly	many
ist	specialist	post	after
itis	inflammation	pre	before
ive	pertaining to	psych	mind

ptosis	prolapse	syn	joined, fused
pyo	pus	tachy	over
pyro	fire	thera	therapy
retro	behind, backwards	thermo	heat
rhino	nose	trans	across
sclero	hardening	trophy	nutrition, growth
semi	half, partly	uni	one
stasis	stopping, controlling	uro	urine
sub	under	xantho	yellow
supra	above, beyond		

The following are medical terminology practice exercises (Exercises 16-2 through 16-11). Although most of the exercises are based on the most common medical terminology, other word roots have been added. Use a medical dictionary if you are unfamiliar with a term or word. If you have a required medical terminology textbook, you should complete your class assigned activities first. If you have questions about medical terminology, you should seek the advise of your OT instructor.

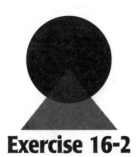

Exercise 16-2

WORD PARTS

Give the meaning of each word part.

kinesio	penia
rhino	megaly
tachy	gastro
litho	itis
pnea	algia
a	otomy
dys	trophy
myo	hypo
angio	patho
sclero	carcin
hemo	ostomy
neuro	cele
fibro	plasty
uro	inter
orrhagia	dento
colic	cyst
auto	phobia
homo	meter
mal	cranio
ad	pyo
derma	orrhea
cyto	oto
cardio	mono
mania	lipo
gram	brady

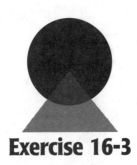

Exercise 16-3

MORE WORD PARTS

Give the meaning of each word part.

ectomy	hyper
oma	lipo
oid	dynia
osis	arthro
ab	ic
hydro	thera
phono	bio
graph	psych
thermo	micro
poly	aero
macro	eu
pyro	leuko
glyco	ecto
endo	meso
retro	mono
hetero	hemi
contra	semi
intra	peri
ology	post
trophy	ist
uni	trans
sub	audio
necro	xantho
meter	dys
sclero	ptosis

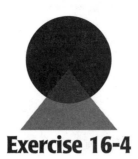

Exercise 16-4

LITTLE WORD PARTS

Small word parts can be confusing. Give the meaning of these.

a	ab
ac	al
an	ad
bi	di
dys	epi
eu	ex
hemi	ia
ic	in
ism	ist
itis	mal

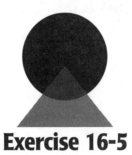

Exercise 16-5

MEDICAL SPECIALISTS

The following are specialists you may have contact with. Give the area that each specializes in.

Cardiologist	Neuropsychology
Dermatology	Endocrinology
Nephrology	Otolaryngology
Pediatrics	Oncology
Rheumatology	Gastroenterology

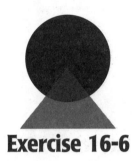

Exercise 16-6

COLORS

List all the word roots that mean a color.

_____

_____

_____

_____

_____

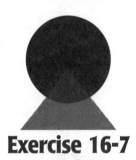

Exercise 16-7

COMBINED WORD ROOTS

Complete the following sentences.

Destruction or break up of nerve tissue is _____.

Surgical repair of the ear is _____.

The term for cancerous growth or malignant tumor is _____.

Dyskinesia is _____.

Pyrophobia is _____.

The term for paralysis of one side of the body is _____.

A chronic ailment that consists of recurrent attacks of sleep is _____.

Inflammation of the brain and spinal cord is _____.

A decreased heart rate is _____.

Cardiomegaly is _____.

A term for deficiency of oxygen is _____.

Condition of stiffness is _____.

Cystocele is _____.

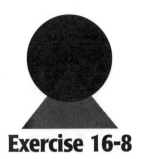

Exercise 16-8

BONES OF THE BODY

Label each bone.

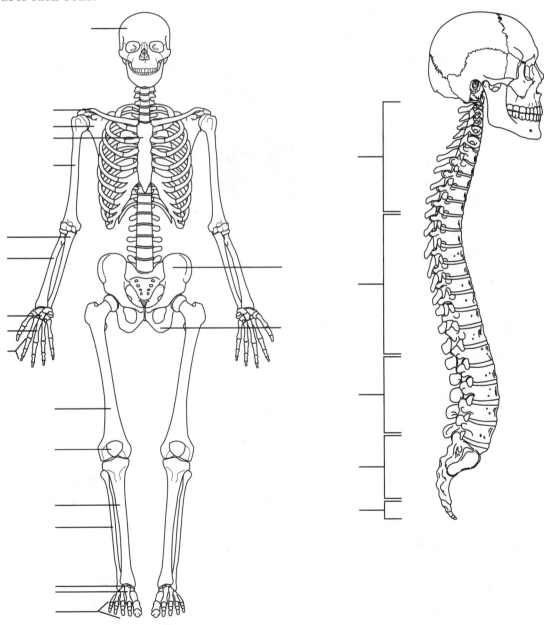

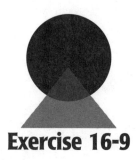

Exercise 16-9

CONFUSING WORD ROOTS

Give the meaning of the following often confused word roots.

orrhage, orrhagia, orrhaphy, orrhea, orrhexis _____

pyo, pyro, plasty, ptosis, pexy _____

myo, myel, mal, malac _____

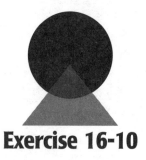

Exercise 16-10

PERTAINING TO

List the word parts that mean "pertaining to."

_____
_____
_____

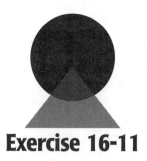

Exercise 16-11

DIRECTIONAL TERMS

Demonstrate on a peer the following directional terms.

Superior	Inferior	Extension	Flexion
Lateral	Medial	Abduction	Adduction
Proximal	Distal	Superficial	Deep
Posterior	Anterior	Unilateral	Bilateral
Prone	Supine		

BIBLIOGRAPHY

Kaplan, H. I., & Sadock, B. J. (1994). *Study guide and self-examination review for Kaplan and Sadock's synopsis of psychiatry.* Baltimore: Williams & Wilkins.

Leonard, P. C. (1990). *Quick and easy medical terminology.* Philadelphia: W. B. Saunders.

Smith, G. L., Davis, P. E., & Dennerll, J. T. (1995). *Medical terminology: A programmed text.* New York: Delmar.

Answers to Exercise 16-1

Specialist	Definition
Cardiologist	Cardio means heart, so a cardiologist is one who studies the heart.
Neuropsychology	Neuro means brain, psycho means mind, so neuropsychology is the study of the brain and mind.
Dermatologist	Derma means skin, so a dermatologist is one who studies skin. If the word was dermatitis, then it would mean inflammation of the skin.
Rheumatology	Rheuma means rheumatic disorders such as rheumatoid arthritis. Rheumatology is a specific specialty that studies rheumatic diseases.
Gastroenterology	Gastro means stomach, entero means small intestines, so gastroenterology means the study of the stomach and small intestines.

Answers to Exercise 16-2

kinesio	MOVEMENT	penia	DEFICIENCY
rhino	NOSE	megaly	LARGE
tachy	OVER	gastro	STOMACH
litho	STONE	itis	INFLAMMATION
pnea	BREATHING	algia	PAIN
a	NO, NOT, WITHOUT	otomy	INCISION
dys	BAD, DIFFICULT	trophy	NUTRITION, GROWTH
myo	MUSCLE	hypo	LOW
angio	VESSEL	patho	DISEASE
sclero	HARDENING	carcin	CANCER
hemo	BLOOD	ostomy	NEW OPENING
neuro	NERVE AND BRAIN	cele	HERNIA
fibro	FIBER	plasty	SURGICAL REPAIR
uro	URINE	inter	BETWEEN
orrhagia	HEMORRHAGE	dento	TEETH
colic	LARGE INTESTINES	cyst	CYST, BLADDER
auto	SELF	phobia	FEAR
homo	SAME	meter	MEASURE
mal	BAD	cranio	SKULL
ad	TOWARD	pyo	PUS
derma	SKIN	orrhea	FLOW, DISCHARGE
cyto	CELL	oto	EAR
cardio	HEART	mono	SINGLE
mania	EXCESSIVE PREOCCUPATION	lipo	FAT
gram	RECORD	brady	SLOW

Answers to Exercise 16-3

ectomy	EXCISION	hyper	HIGH
oma	TUMOR	lipo	FAT
oid	RESEMBLING	dynia	PAIN
osis	CONDITION OF	arthro	JOINT
ab	AWAY FROM	ic	PERTAINING TO
hydro	WATER	thera	THERAPY
phono	VOICE	bio	LIFE
graph	RECORDING DEVICE	psych	MIND
thermo	HEAT	micro	SMALL
poly	MANY	aero	AIR
macro	LARGE	eu	GOOD
pyro	FIRE	leuko	WHITE
glyco	SUGAR	ecto	OUT, WITHOUT, AWAY
endo	INSIDE	meso	MIDDLE
retro	BEHIND, BACKWARDS	mono	SINGLE
hetero	DIFFERENT	hemi	HALF
contra	AGAINST	semi	HALF, PARTLY
intra	WITHIN	peri	AROUND
ology	STUDY OF	post	AFTER
trophy	NUTRITION, GROWTH	ist	SPECIALIST
uni	ONE	trans	ACROSS
sub	UNDER	audio	HEARING
necro	DEAD	xantho	YELLOW
meter	MEASURE	dys	BAD, DIFFICULT
sclero	HARDENING	ptosis	PROLAPSE

Answers to Exercise 16-4

a	NO, NOT, WITHOUT	ab	AWAY FROM
ac	PERTAINING TO	al	PERTAINING TO
an	PERTAINING TO	ad	TOWARD
bi	TWO	di	TWO
dys	BAD, DIFFICULT	epi	ABOVE
eu	GOOD	ex	OUT
hemi	HALF	ia	CONDITION OF
ic	PERTAINING TO	in	NOT
ism	CONDITION OF	ist	SPECIALIST
itis	INFLAMMATION	mal	BAD

Answers to Exercise 16-5

Cardiologist	HEART	Neuropsychology	BRAIN AND MIND
Dermatology	SKIN	Endocrinology	GLANDS/EXCRETE IN
Nephrology	KIDNEYS	Otolaryngology	EAR AND THROAT
Pediatrics	CHILDREN	Oncology	TUMORS
Rheumatology	ARTHRITIS	Gastroenterology	STOMACH/SMALL INTESTINE

Answers to Exercise 16-6

ALBO	WHITE	LEUKO	WHITE
CHLORO	GREEN	MELANO	BLACK
CYAN	BLUE	XANTHO	YELLOW
ERYTHRO	RED		

Answers to Exercise 16-7

Destruction or break up of nerve tissue is NEUROLYSIS.

Surgical repair of the ear is OTOPLASTY.

The term for cancerous growth or malignant tumor is CARCINOMA.

Dyskinesia is DIFFICULT OR PAINFUL MOVEMENT.

Pyrophobia is ABNORMAL FEAR OF FIRE.

The term for paralysis of one side of the body is HEMIPLEGIA.

A chronic ailment that consists of recurrent attacks of sleep is NARCOLEPSY.

Inflammation of the brain and spinal cord is MYELOENCEPHALITIS.

A decreased heart rate is BRADYCARDIA.

Cardiomegaly is ENLARGED HEART.

A term for deficiency of oxygen is ANOXIA.

Condition of stiffness is ANKYLOSIS.

Cystocele is HERNIATION OF THE BLADDER.

Answers to Exercise 16-8

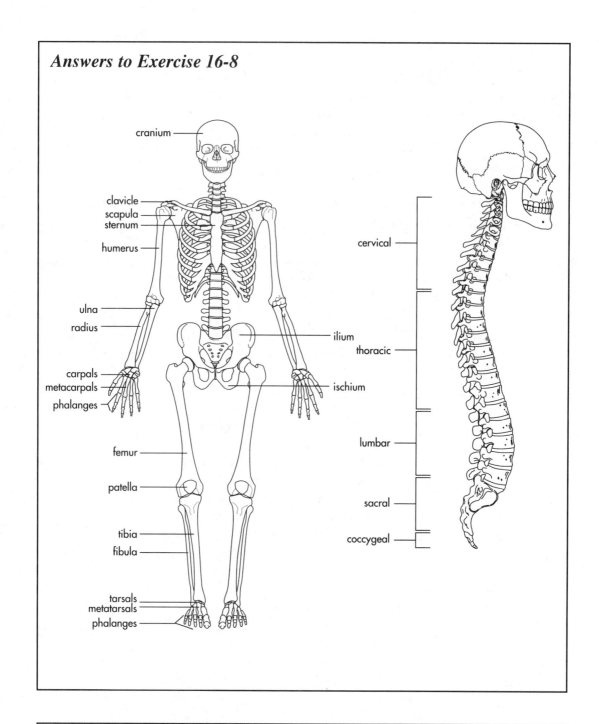

cranium

clavicle
scapula
sternum
humerus

ulna
radius

carpals
metacarpals
phalanges

femur

patella

tibia
fibula

tarsals
metatarsals
phalanges

ilium

ischium

cervical

thoracic

lumbar

sacral

coccygeal

Answers to Exercise 16-9

orrhage, orrhagia, orrhaphy, orrhea, orrhexis
EXCESSIVE BLEEDING, HEMORRHAGE, SUTURE, FLOW/DISCHARGE, RUPTURE
pyo, pyro, plasty, ptosis, pexy
PUS, FIRE, SURGICAL REPAIR, PROLAPSE, FIXATION
myo, myel, mal, malac
MUSCLE, SPINAL CORD, BAD, SOFTENING

Answers to Exercise 16-10

AC	EAL
AL	IC
AN	IVE
AR	OUS

Answers to Exercise 16-11

Superior	Inferior	TOP VS. BOTTOM HALF OF BODY
Lateral	Medial	OUTSIDE EDGE VS. CENTER OF BODY
Proximal	Distal	CLOSE TO CENTER VS. AWAY FROM CENTER
Posterior	Anterior	BACK VS. FRONT OF BODY
Prone	Supine	FACE DOWN VS. FACE UP OF BODY
Extension	Flexion	STRAIGHT VS. BENT, AS IN ELBOW
Abduction	Adduction	AWAY FROM VS. TOWARD BODY
Superficial	Deep	SURFACE VS. DEEP
Unilateral	Bilateral	ONE SIDE VS. TWO, AS IN USING ONE HAND OR TWO

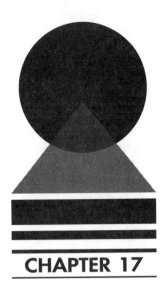

CHAPTER 17

DOCUMENTATION SKILLS

Karen Sladyk, MS, OTR/L

INTRODUCTION

Ask COTAs or OTRs what they dislike most about their job and the answer may be the documentation. Although often talked about in a negative manner, documentation is one of the most important skills an OT student can develop. Documentation is the means to which we communicate our treatment to other health professionals and third party payers. In addition, documentation is often used to demonstrate quality care of our consumers. Needless to say, documentation is an important aspect of our practice. It is important that OT students develop documentation skills early and continue to refine the skills throughout their careers. This chapter will address both the basic treatment plan and treatment notes. Tutorials and examples can be used to develop a foundation for more advanced skills.

THE TREATMENT PLAN

A treatment plan is likely to be the first formal piece of documentation an OT student is likely to write. Both the COTA and OTR participate in the treatment evaluation and the resulting treatment plan, but the OTR is ultimately responsible for the treatment plan. After the evaluations have been completed, a comprehensive treatment plan must be documented.

Each facility has established its own method for documenting a treatment plan. Some facilities have developed critical pathways that dictate the treatment plan, reducing the paperwork. Generally, a treatment plan includes problems, assets, goals/objectives, treatments, and outcomes/discharge criteria (Table 17-1).

This chapter is designed to help you write a basic OT treatment plan while you are in school. On fieldwork and in your career you will develop more advanced multidiscipli-

---

Table 17-1
Steps to Writing a Treatment Plan

1. Develop a list of problems and behavioral indicators, consider a frame of reference
2. Identify assets and prioritize the problem list
3. Develop goals and objectives that are clear and measurable
4. Design activities that are meaningful to the person
5. Identify expected outcomes and discharge criteria

---

nary treatment plan documentation skills. Before you can do that, you must have a working handle on the basic OT treatment plan. Case stories in this chapter will allow you to practice the skills you have learned.

Developing a Problem List and Behavioral Indicators

The first step in writing an OT treatment plan is to establish a list of problems the patient is facing and show behavioral evidence that these are problems. To do this, the OT student should review uniform terminology and make a written list of problems. If you are unfamiliar with uniform terminology, review Chapter 13 on activity analysis and uniform terminology in this primer before you continue with this chapter. To practice writing a problem list, consider the following case story.

Jim is a 40-year-old male who recently lost his management job due to downsizing of his workplace. Initially, he was happy to be laid off because he had the opportunity to look for a job he "really wanted" and catch up on reading. Lately, he has been disappointed because job offers are not coming in like he had thought. His unemployment support will be ending soon (6 weeks) and Jim has become depressed. He does not get out of bed until 10:30 a.m. and has not been showering or shaving. His wife has found him crying in his home office with the lights off. His wife further reports that he sits around all day doing nothing and does not even enjoy his hobby of fishing with his teenage son. Jim reports he is upset that he can no longer support his family and only wishes for a job. He says he is not suicidal but states he is an embarrassment to his family. His wife and son deny that he is an embarrassment and have been very supportive of him looking for a new job.

Jim is having problems in work, ADLs, and leisure. See Table 17-2 for an analysis of his problems and the behavioral indicators he shows.

Table 17-2
Analysis of Jim's Problems

Problem	Behavioral Indicator
Poor personal grooming	Does not shave, does not shower
Poor coping skills	Does not get out of bed until 10:30 a.m., cries
Provider role in family disrupted	Wants to work, feels embarrassed
Lack of enjoyment	Feels sad, does not like fishing, isolates self

---

Prioritize the List With Patient Assets

With many patients, the OT is likely to identify more problems than can be realistically addressed during treatment. Therefore, the therapist must set a priority list of problems to be addressed. To do this, one more list should be developed. Identifying patient assets can help prioritize treatment problems. In the case of Jim, he has several assets to draw on including:

- A good work history with management skills
- A supportive wife and son
- A history of good ADL and leisure skills
- Although ending soon, he currently has unemployment support

In developing a priority list of treatment problems, the issue of safety is always placed first. In this case, Jim is not suicidal and safety is not an issue. Looking at his problem list, the following prioritization might be successful:

1. Poor coping skills
2. Family role disturbance
3. Lack of enjoyment
4. Poor grooming

Poor coping skills is placed first because of its impact in all areas of work, ADLs, and leisure. Poor grooming is placed last because it is impacted by the other problems and Jim has a history of being successful in grooming prior to his recent depression. Looking at his list of assets also supports this priority list in that Jim appears to have support, but is not utilizing the support to help him cope.

Developing Goals and Objectives

The next step is to develop realistic goals and objectives for Jim to meet prior to his discharge. Considerations in developing goals and objectives include analyzing the type of facility the patient is being treated in, the expected discharge plans, and the limits of his third party payer. Most important is the patient's goals. In Jim's case, he is being treated in a day treatment program for professionals. He spends late afternoons and evenings in his home and will return home after his discharge. Jim's third party payer has agreed to cover 30 days of day treatment and because of the current financial strain, Jim is unable to pay for services beyond the initial 30 days. Jim states that his only goal is to return to work and be the breadwinner of the family.

To guide the development of the goals, objectives, and treatment techniques, the OT must consider a frame of reference. If you are unfamiliar with frames of reference, review Chapter 14 in this primer before you proceed with the treatment plan. In Jim's case, several frames of reference could be appropriate including model of human occupation, cognitive behavioral, or object relations. Choosing a frame of reference depends on your knowledge of the frames, the frames the facility uses, and the resources of the program. In Jim's case, the facility uses a cognitive behavioral approach because the program is for professionals with generally high levels of education and the stay is limited to 30 days. Several other frames of reference would be equally successful.

Writing goals and objectives for a treatment plan is a difficult task. Changes in laws and review organizations have led to the requirement that goals and objectives must be individualized and clearly measurable. Each goal and objective must be so clear that any professional reviewing the record would have an understanding of what is expected of the patient. Several methods have been developed to teach students how to write measurable goals. All of these methods lead to successful goal writing. It is not unusual to have different OT faculty teach you different methods. You should not get upset if each instructor asks you to write goals in a different way, just consider that each way adds to the flexibility of your thinking.

The goals and objectives are written in the same way, but the goal is the end product of several objectives. Think of goals and objectives as a staircase. The goal is written on the top step. Several objectives will lead to the final goal. Objectives may need to be adjusted as the patient moves through treatment, but the ultimate goal is the patient's highest functioning. Consider the diagram in Figure 17-1 on living a healthy lifestyle.

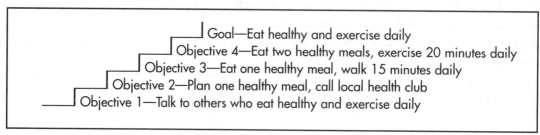

Goal—Eat healthy and exercise daily
Objective 4—Eat two healthy meals, exercise 20 minutes daily
Objective 3—Eat one healthy meal, walk 15 minutes daily
Objective 2—Plan one healthy meal, call local health club
Objective 1—Talk to others who eat healthy and exercise daily

Figure 17-1. Steps to a healthy lifestyle.

In this primer, we will use the ABCD method for writing goals and objectives. The ABCD method uses the following system for developing clear, measurable goals and objectives:
- Audience
- Behavior
- Condition
- Degree

The **audience** of the goal is the patient. The **behavior** is what is expected of the patient. The **condition** is the specific details, rules, or boundaries of the behavior. Lastly, the **degree** is when the behavior is completed. Each problem on the treatment plan must have a goal and set of objectives. In Jim's case (four problems), four sets of goals and matching objectives would be developed by the OT in the final treatment plan. First, consider the following goal for the problem of coping skills: *Within 30 days, Jim will verbally list three coping strategies for dealing with his depression using one strategy each day for the last 10 days.*
- Audience   Jim
- Behavior   Verbally list three coping strategies
- Condition   Use one strategy for the last 10 days
- Degree   Within 30 days

An appropriate first step to reaching this goal would be an objective that has Jim finding out what coping skills are. Consider the following objective: *Within 7 days, Jim will attend three coping skills groups, making a list of coping skills in a journal.*
- Audience   Jim
- Behavior   Attend three coping skills groups
- Condition   List skills in journal
- Degree   Within 7 days

Now try to develop your own problem list and goals. Consider the following case story.

Anna is a 65-year-old female who had a left CVA 3 weeks ago. She has rightsided weakness and some expressive aphasia. Prior to her stroke, she led an active retired life. She has three grown children and seven grandchildren all living in the area. Besides a large garden, two cats, and maintaining an older home, Anna tutors low income children after school. She is recognized as a community leader and this role is important to her. She is having problems dressing herself, maintaining her balance in the kitchen, and focusing her attention on tasks.

   Use Worksheet 17-1 to establish a problem list, an asset list, a priority problem list, and one possible goal and objective.

Anna shows several problem areas in ADLs, as well as in work and leisure. Until the motor and possible cognitive problems are addressed in the area of ADLs, returning to her prior lifestyle would be too difficult. The first priority problem that needs to be addressed is safety. Remember that safety is always addressed first no matter what the diagnosis is. Currently, Anna is having balance problems while working in the ADL kitchen in the OT clinic. In addition, she is not paying full attention, which may be either a cognitive problem or psychosocial adjustment to her illness. She might be prone to hurting herself in the kitchen. This area needs further evaluation. Anna has several assets including many family members, likely community support, and a prior active life. A possible goal might be: *Within 3 weeks of admission to the rehab unit, Anna will complete a hot meal in the ADL kitchen independently and free of safety issues.*

- Audience   Anna
- Behavior   Complete a hot meal
- Condition   In ADL kitchen independently and free of safety issues
- Degree   Within 3 weeks of admission to the rehab unit

Worksheet 17-1

Problems and Behavioral Indicators: _____

_____

_____

_____

Assets: _____

_____

_____

_____

Priority Problems: _____

_____

_____

_____

Goals and Objectives: _____

_____

_____

_____

Designing Activities

OT uses activities to improve function in patients. The next step in the treatment plan is to design specific activities to meet the individual goals and objectives of the patient. One problem that students often have when developing a treatment plan is to jump right into the treatment before laying the groundwork. When this happens, the results are an activity that the therapist wants to do, not an activity that has meaning or function to the patient. Before developing activities for your patient, review the individual problems, assets, goals, and objectives. Ask yourself, "Will this be meaningful to my patient?"

There are many resource books available for the student, COTA, or OTR to use to develop activities. With experience, practitioners are able to find activities off the top of their heads. Until you reach that point, consider having several OT activity books in your professional library. These OT resources can be supplemented by other activity books such as books from education, recreation, and community groups (i.e., scouting). See Appendix B at the end of this primer for a list of suggested activity books.

Let's return to the case story of Jim. His first problem involves coping skills and his goal is for him to identify and use coping skills. His family is trying to be supportive, but at this time Jim is not using them for support; he is trying to carry the burden of unemployment himself. Jim has been referred to a coping skills group where other people are dealing with the same issues. The nature of a group means that some of the members are dealing with coping better than Jim and some are not. OT practitioners can use these different levels to be therapeutic. For example, Jim's first objective is to identify coping skills. The therapist could simply read a list of coping skills to the group members but this would not be meaningful to Jim. Instead, the therapist asks Jim to develop a survey of coping skills and to survey both patients and staff on the use of coping skills. This allows Jim to use his management skills. After the survey is done, Jim begins to develop a journal where he can keep the results. Because Jim enjoyed reading, he may be interested in journaling. Even if he does not keep journaling after his discharge, he may find the written record of his survey helpful later.

Outcomes/Discharge Planning

The last step in developing and documenting a treatment plan is to set the criteria that the patient will need to be discharged and return to life outside of your program. This is a very difficult step for beginner treatment plan writers. Many students ask "How can I predict how my patient will look at discharge if I don't even know them yet?" This is a good question and true while you are just starting in your career. With experience, this task will become easier. The reality is that discharge planning should start the moment the patient is admitted. This allows for effective and efficient treatment to be started from the beginning. Discharge planning can always be adjusted along the way, but having an outcome vision from the beginning will allow the treatment to be focused from the start.

In Jim's case, the discharge plan was clear from the beginning. He would return home after the 30 days of day treatment. Community outpatient visits once a week or unemployment self-help groups might be appropriate referrals and are likely to be investigated by a social worker on the team with input from OT. The treatment team feels that Jim's outcome criteria include being able to maintain his ADLs independently, returning enjoyment of his leisure hobbies, and ability to return to actively seeking employment are attainable in 30 days. Besides OT and social work mentioned above, Jim has access to a medical doctor for medication, a clinical psychologist for insight therapy, a therapeutic recreation specialist for practicing his hobbies, and a nurse for medication education and case management. Together, the treatment team develops the outcome criteria and discharge plans using input from all team members, including OT.

SUMMARY OF TREATMENT PLANNING

This chapter has provided an outline for writing a basic OT treatment plan. Multidisciplinary treatment plans are routine in practice with OT contributing a part. Before you can write a multidisciplinary treatment plan, you must master a basic OT plan. The steps include identifying problems, identifying assets and prioritizing problems, setting goals and objectives, developing treatment activities, and setting outcome criteria and discharge plans. Two case stories will follow the end of this chapter to practice writing a treatment plan (Worksheets 17-2 and 17-3). The following section will address documentation after the initial treatment plan.

PROGRESS NOTE WRITING

After writing a treatment plan, the OT practitioner begins treatment and must document progress or lack of progress in the facility record. Just like treatment plans, each facility has developed policies on note writing that meets the needs of laws and review organizations. There are many different types or styles of note writing. In this section of the chapter you will learn the basics of a SOAP note and a narrative note.

SOAP Note

The SOAP format of note writing has been around for a long time and chances are that your fieldwork supervisors were trained in this format. SOAP is an acronym for:
- Subjective
- Objective
- Assessment
- Plan

The benefit of a SOAP note is that it provides a structure that all disciplines can use and understand. This consistency between disciplines allows for a quick review of the record for trends and patterns in patient behavior or treatment progress.

Writing a SOAP note is easy once you have the skill. The note begins with a **subjective** statement from the patient that is interesting because it shows current functioning. The **objective** data follow. This includes how many times the patient was seen, what type of activities were done, and any other measurable data. The **assessment** section includes the writer's interpretation of data and assessment of goals or objectives. Lastly, the **plan** section includes the next step.

Figure 17-2 shows how a SOAP note for Jim after the first week of his treatment may read.

Narrative Note

A narrative note allows for more flexibility than the SOAP note, but does not have the structure that some students like. In a narrative note, the writer is responsible for including all the data in a smooth, flowing, descriptive note. Generally, the writer begins with objective information, such as attendance and participation in treatment, then follows

Date

S: "I feel relief that I'm here in this coping skills group. I did not know there were other people that felt the same way I did."

O: Jim attended three coping skills groups this week and was treated in two individual sessions of 45 minutes each.

A: Jim was initially hesitant to join the coping skills group and needed an individual session to be convinced to try the group. He was encouraged to talk to his case manager about the group and agreed to try it once. Once in the group, he relaxed and began to actively participate. He was asked to develop a survey on coping skills used by others and is in the process of collecting his data. Jim has made friends in the group and has been seen socializing with them outside of group time. Although his affect remains depressed, he was seen smiling when talking about his projects. No evidence of suicidal ideation or psychomotor retardation was noted. First week objective was partially met.

P: Jim will continue to gather his data for his surveys. He will report the results to the group and document the results in his journal.

A. Nicenote, OTR/L

Figure 17-2. Sample SOAP note.

with interpretive information, such as patient reaction. Finally, a review of objectives met and plans for the next treatment sessions are included. The SOAP format can be easily converted to a narrative format (Figure 17-3) by switching the subjective and objective sections and leaving out the headings.

WRITING NOTES

The first step in writing any type of note is to gather the appropriate data. Be sure you have dates of attendance, information about participation, whether objectives were met, and future plans. The best way to get good at writing notes is to write a lot and to get feedback on your notes. Generally, this will happen during fieldwork. Class assignments might also include note writing. Like writing objectives, instructors teach note writing in many different ways. Although this may be frustrating as you try to master one style of note writing, remember that learning many different styles will improve the flexibility of your thinking.

Sometimes the best way to see how to write a note is to look at how not to write a note. Figure 17-4 is a narrative note full of problems.

Let us review the many errors in this note. First, grammar and spelling are serious issues. It is assumed that college-educated individuals will have notes free of grammar and spelling errors. Before you pass in a note or any other assignment in college, check for grammar and spelling errors. An occasional error is part of being human, but ask yourself, "What am I saying about my thinking when I pass in this assignment?" If you are happy with the answer, pass it in. If you get feedback that your writing is full of grammar and spelling mistakes, make sure your next assignment is perfect. A student once told me that she knew her paper

Date

Jim attended three coping skills groups this week and was treated in two individual sessions of 45 minutes each. He stated, "I feel relief that I'm here in this coping skills group. I did not know there were other people that felt the same way I did."

Jim was initially hesitant to join the coping skills group and needed an individual session to be convinced to try the group. He was encouraged to talk to his case manager about the group and agreed to try it once. Once in the group, he relaxed and began to actively participate. He was asked to develop a survey on coping skills used by others and is in the process of collecting his data. Jim has made friends in the group and has been seen socializing with them outside of group time. Although his affect remains depressed, he was seen smiling when talking about his projects. No evidence of suicidal ideation or psychomotor retardation was noted. First week objective was partially met.

The plan will have Jim continue to gather his data for his surveys, report the results to the group, and document the results in his journal.

A. Nicenote, OTR/L

Figure 17-3. Sample narrative note.

Date

Jim came too group all the time this week. He made a survey, a journal, a collage, a junk sculpture, and a god's eye for his wife. He didn't want to come to group at the start and had to be talked to and then saw his case manager and then came. He said he didn't want to do this stuff and wouldn't get anything out of it and didn't see the point anyway. When he came he was very depressed but did smile some. The plan is to encourage Jim to attend and to have Jim make an ashtray and a leather keychain.

I. M. Wayoff, OTR/L

Figure 17-4. Error-filled narrative note.

had spelling errors because her spellchecker was broken. I stood there amazed that she would freely admit this to her teacher. Remember, all your written work is a reflection of you. Project the image of a hard-working, competent student therapist.

One other major problem in this note is the endless list of tasks the patient completed. As you likely know, the profession of OT is not widely known or understood by many people, including other health professionals. When a note focuses on the things a patient made instead of how he or she responded to treatment, it appears that the OT department is nothing more than people who keep patients busy all day. As an OT practitioner, it is your responsibility to help other professionals understand how activity improves function. The focus of a note should be on function, not on what the patient created. See Table 17-3 for other helpful hints for treatment plan writing, note writing, and general college assignment writing.

Table 17-3
Helpful Writing Hints

- Check all data for correctness. Make sure everything from the date to the treatment results are accurately reported.
- Be spelling error free. Spelling errors project an image of an uneducated professional. Carry a dictionary with you at all times. If unsure of a spelling, consider a different word.
- Use professional language. Avoid street terms. "We had to stop her from talking" becomes "Patient was tangential and required maximum limit setting."
- Tell how the patient functioned. Avoid endless lists of projects the patient made.
- The plan must be the patient's. Many students make the mistake of writing what they plan to do in the plan section of a note. The plan must be the patient's not the therapist's. Bad example: The therapist will increase ROM 10 degrees. Good example: Patient will gain 10 degrees ROM.
- Stay in one tense. Do not jump tense, such as *is, was, are, were*. Past tense is preferred.
- Write in the third person. Do not use I. Call yourself the student therapist.
- No contractions. No *didn't, shouldn't, wouldn't*. In college-level work, write out both words.
- No run-on sentences. A sentence should have only one "and", with no more than two thoughts. If you have more than two thoughts, make a new sentence.
- No vague words. No *very, a lot, some, many*. These words have different meanings to different people. Tell exactly how much or do not use these words at all.
- Do not blacken out a mistake. If you make an error, put one line through the error and write "error" next to it. Blackened marks look like you are trying to hide something.
- Do not use correction liquid on a mistake. If you make an error, put one line through the error and write "error" next to it. Correction liquid looks like you are trying to hide something.
- Never use another patient's name in a record. This breaks confidentiality rules. Some facilities will allow you to use initials, but check before you write.
- Sign the note legibly. Review organizations will cite you if they cannot read your signature.

SUMMARY OF NOTE WRITING

Note writing can be a simple task after you have mastered the basic format and the specific facility rules. Use the treatment plan as a starting place to write a progress note. Comment on both subjective and objective data. Interpret the data and make a plan for the future. Make sure your notes are free of grammar and spelling errors. Follow the helpful hints outlined above for problem-free progress notes.

EXERCISES FOR TREATMENT PLANNING AND PROGRESS NOTE WRITING

The best way to master treatment plan writing and progress note writing is to practice. Use the following case stories to practice writing a basic OT treatment plan and progress note (Worksheets 17-2 through 17-5). For a more realistic case story, use a patient that you have observed in fieldwork or a more detailed case story provided to you by your teacher. The worksheet outline that follows the case stories can be helpful in organizing an assignment for OT school. Remember to use uniform terminology when identifying problems.

Worksheet 17-2

Kathy Smith: Depression

Kathy Smith is a 44-year-old female who began to suffer from major depression 3 weeks ago on the anniversary of her best friend's accidental death. She lives in a two-story house with her husband and 15-year-old son. She is currently on medical leave from her job as a deli clerk at a local supermarket. Although Mrs. Smith worked outside the home, she felt it was important to see her son off to school each morning and was home just after her son returned from school. Prior to her depression, Mrs. Smith led an active social life. She and her husband played tennis with other couples and she enjoyed going out for coffee and chatting with girlfriends.

Mrs. Smith was hospitalized for 15 days for depression at a local hospital and received OT services twice daily during her stay. Since her discharge from the hospital, she has been living at home with her husband and son. Mrs. Smith has been receiving therapy services at a local outpatient mental health center where you are a student. During the day, Mrs. Smith has her sister with her until it is time for therapy, however, her sister is from out of state and will be returning home in 2 weeks. Mrs. Smith's OT is your fieldwork supervisor and you have been assigned to her treatment.

Current status:

- Chief complaint: "I have no energy to do anything."
- Motor activity: Slow and lethargic, ambulatory.
- Speech: Slow, low volume, no hearing impairment.
- Mood and affect: Mood is sad, affect is sometimes sad, sometimes flat, or sometimes agitated. Endurance for activity depends on other therapy scheduled.
- Thought: Content of thought is around friend's death, and what death was like for friend. Denies suicidal thoughts or plans. Is easily distracted from conversations or tasks and is easily confused in situations outside of her home.
- Perception: During inpatient hospitalization, she did hear her friend's voice calling to her, however, this stopped with medication and she is not experiencing this currently.
- Appearance: Neat and clean.
- Intellectual functioning:
     *Orientation: Oriented X3, however, slow and needs time to process questions.
     *Fund of knowledge: Bright woman with 2 years of college.
     *Abstract: Can abstract if given time, however, needs to be refocused to thought.
- ADLs: Sister sets everything out and helps her get ready for her appointments. Appetite is poor.
- Insight and judgment: Aware of her depression and has expressed an interest in getting well, however, has had a difficult time making changes in her behavior.

The recreational therapist has just brought Mrs. Smith into your waiting area after her RT evaluation. The therapist tells you to look out because "Kathy is a little cranky today." You greet Mrs. Smith and begin to explain what you were thinking about working on in treatment. Mrs. Smith looks at you and says "Whatever" in a monotone voice.

Treatment Plan Practice Worksheet

Treatment Problems, Behavioral Indicators, Possible Frame of Reference. What are the problems
and what evidence do you have to indicate these are problems?

Assets.

Prioritized Problems. Safety is always considered first.

Goals and Objectives. Audience, Behavior, Condition, Degree.

Treatment Activities. Separate groups from individual activities.

Outcomes/Discharge Plans.

Worksheet 17-3

Bill Jones: CVA

Bill Jones is a 44-year-old male who suffered a CVA 4 weeks ago. He lives in a two-story house with his wife and 16-year-old daughter. He is currently on medical leave from his job as a department store manager. Although his job requires him to work long hours, Mr. Jones is a devoted father and makes breakfast for his daughter each morning before she goes to school. Prior to his CVA, Mr. Jones led an active social life. He and his wife bowled with other couples and he enjoyed drinking coffee while ice fishing with his "guy friends."

Mr. Jones was hospitalized for 15 days following his CVA at a local hospital and he received OT services twice daily during his stay. Since his discharge from the hospital, he has been living at home with his wife and daughter. His wife works full-time to maintain the family's health insurance. Mr. Jones has been receiving therapy services at a local outpatient rehabilitation center where you are a student. During the day, Mr. Jones has a home health aide with him until it is time for therapy, however, he is only eligible for a home health aide for 6 more weeks. Mr. Jones's OT is your fieldwork supervisor and you have been assigned to his treatment.

Current status:

- ROM: Right is normal for AROM. Left is normal for PROM.
- Strength: Right is normal. Left is flaccid, however, MMT last treatment showed trace movement.
- Endurance: Fluctuates between 20 to 35 minutes depending on PT/OT schedule.
- Sensation:
    - *Proprioception: Right is normal. Left is impaired. However, left has improved since beginning outpatient therapy.
    - *Hot/cold: Both left and right are normal.
    - *Localization of tactile stimuli: Right is normal. Left is diminished on both anterior and posterior sides as well as diminished on left side of face.
    - *Perception: Displays hemianopsia and constructional apraxia, normal receptive understanding.
    - *Gross and fine motor: Right is normal but unable to assess left upper extremity due to flaccidity. He walks with a quad cane (a stable, four-legged cane).
- Affect: Sad or flat at times. Progressively becoming less cooperative during treatment. Sad when family visits or when he talks about his daughter.
- Oral functioning: Tends to choke on liquids, especially coffee, mouth droops, mild tongue lateralization from midline to right, he is able to speak.
- Daily living skills: Mild dressing apraxia, aide sets up meals and assists grooming and hygiene.

The PT has just brought Mr. Jones into your waiting area after his PT evaluation. The therapist tells you to look out because "Bill is a little cranky today." You greet Mr. Jones and begin to explain what you were thinking about working on in treatment. Mr. Jones looks at you and says "Whatever" in a monotone voice.

Treatment Plan Practice Worksheet

Treatment Problems, Behavioral Indicators, Possible Frame of Reference. What are the problems and what evidence do you have to indicate these are problems?

_____

_____

_____

_____

_____

Assets.

_____

_____

_____

Prioritized Problems. Safety is always considered first.

_____

_____

_____

Goals and Objectives. Audience, Behavior, Condition, Degree.

_____

_____

_____

Treatment Activities. Separate groups from individual activities.

_____

_____

_____

Outcomes/Discharge Plans.

_____

_____

_____

_____

NOTE WRITING CASE STORIES

The people in the case stories presented in the treatment planning section of this chapter have now completed 1 week of treatment under your care. Use the following information to practice writing both a SOAP progress note and a narrative progress note. Be sure to check the first week information against what you know in the treatment plan. Include the date and sign the note with your name and your credentials (Worksheets 17-4 and 17-5).

Worksheet 17-4

Kathy Smith: First Week of Treatment

Data Collected:

Attendance: Three socialization groups, five relaxation groups, two evening family groups, and was seen for five short (15 minute) individual sessions.

Affect: Varied between depressed (tearful) to sad but appropriate to the discussion. Expressed embarrassment to not being able to control crying during family group.

Attention to task: Fine with some verbal redirecting. In relaxation she said, "I really like these exercises because I can remember the good times with my friend without crying."

Motor activity and speech: Improved but still slow.

ADLs: No changes in home life.

Progress Note Writing Practice Worksheet

Use a SOAP note format to document progress made in the first week of treatment.

_____

_____

_____

_____

_____

_____

Convert the SOAP note above to a narrative note.

_____

_____

_____

_____

_____

_____

Self-evaluation:

[] Data accurate	[] Spelling correct	[] Grammar correct
[] Used professional language	[] Focus on functioning	[] No contractions
[] Written in past tense	[] No run-on sentences	[] No vague words
[] Plan is patient focused	[] No blackened words or correction liquid	[] Signed legibly

Worksheet 17-5

Bill Jones: First Week of Treatment

Data Collected:

Attendance: 1 hour of individual OT treatment daily and four self-range of motion groups.

Perception: Continues to display hemianopsia and constructional apraxia, normal receptive understanding.

Gross and fine motor: Right is normal. Left upper extremity showing beginnings of tone. He walks with a quad cane (a stable, four-legged cane).

Affect: Sad or flat at times. Progressively becoming less cooperative during treatment. Started to cry when he talked about his daughter. Counseling techniques were used and patient reported relief.

ADLs: Choked on liquids when he rushed but was able to drink 2 oz. of coffee. Stated he "was very proud and that was the best coffee he ever had."

Progress Note Writing Practice Worksheet

Use a SOAP note format to document progress made in the first week of treatment.

_____

_____

_____

_____

_____

_____

Convert the SOAP note above to a narrative note.

_____

_____

_____

_____

_____

_____

Self-evaluation:

[] Data accurate	[] Spelling correct	[] Grammar correct
[] Used professional language	[] Focus on functioning	[] No contractions
[] Written in past tense	[] No run-on sentences	[] No vague words
[] Plan is patient focused	[] No blackened words or correction liquid	[] Signed legibly

BIBLIOGRAPHY

Acquaviva, J. D. (Ed.). (1992). *Effective documentation for occupational therapy.* Bethesda, MD:

American Occupational Therapy Association.

Hemphill, B. J. (1988). *Mental health assessment in occupational therapy: An integrative approach to the evaluation process.* Thorofare, NJ: SLACK Inc.

Hemphill, B. J., Peterson, C. Q., & Werner, P. C. (1991). *Rehabilitation in mental health: Goals and objectives for independent living.* Thorofare, NJ: SLACK Inc.

Joe, B. E. (Ed.). (1991). *Quality assurance in occupational therapy.* Bethesda, MD: American Occupational Therapy Association.

Reed, K. L. (1991). *Quick reference to occupational therapy.* Gaithersburg, MD: Aspen Publications.

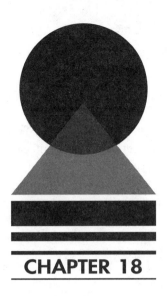

CHAPTER 18

GONIOMETRY

Signian McGeary, MS, OTR/L

INTRODUCTION

The measurement of joint motion is a technique that therapists employ to evaluate a patient's extremities and spine. In order to assess dysfunction, set goals, and measure progress in treatment, the technique of goniometry is necessary. Educators in allied health programs teach this skill. Students have different levels of integration of the subject matter based on the multifaceted nature of the topic. This chapter is written to assist the novice, the rusty, and the bewildered. It is assumed that a complete resource is or will be available for you (see Bibliography at end of chapter).

Since all COTAs and OTRs must exhibit thorough mastery of goniometry, this chapter is a tutorial to help you gain skills by providing Exercises (Answers are at the end of the chapter) from arthrokinematics, visualization, and practice suggestions. The term *arthrokinematics* refers to movement of joint surfaces. Goniometry is the measuring of motion that occurs at a joint as a result of movement of one joint surface in relation to another.

Goniometry is fundamental to the biomechanical model of OT practice. This model is used in most, if not all, settings for the treatment of physical dysfunction. The biomechanical frame of reference assumes that motion is essential for success in performance of occupation. The study of motion involves kinetics and kinematics. Kinetics looks at forces that produce motion. Kinematics is the description of motion without force factors. The three components that underlie the capacity for motion are joint range of motion (ROM), strength, and endurance. Dysfunction is noted when one of these components impedes occupational function. For example, a client who has arthritis may have loss of ROM. A therapist therefore needs the skill of goniometry to evaluate the extent of loss of motion in order to plan treatment.

Goniometry generally comes first in the progression of a therapist's skill development education. Only when you have mastered goniometry can you learn more advanced testing and treatment techniques such as mobilization. You should review the bones of the human skeletal system and the bone landmarks before beginning this chapter. Once the student understands how the supporting structure of the body and the skeleton functions, then the consideration of muscles can be added to the picture. Finally, the application of the mechanics of movement, anatomy, and kinesiology or kinematics comprise the next domain for further student development.

JOINT CLASSIFICATION

From a biomechanical standpoint, the body is simply a system of levers. Muscles act to move the bony endpoints of these levers. The joints form the fulcrum or pivot points of the lever systems in the body. For example, when the biceps muscle flexes the forearm, the elbow acts as the pivot point in this lever system. To appreciate movement of the human skeleton, one must first closely examine the features of disarticulated bones. Only then can one properly envision the three-dimensional relationship of one bone to another as they form a joint.

Nearly every bone in the human body connects to another bone. There are three main classifications of articulations or connections of bone to bone:
- Amphiarthrodial (Cartilaginous)
- Synarthrodial (Fibrous)
- Diarthrodial (Synovial)

It is important to consider that form dictates function. Thus, the type of joint articulation or connection allows us to understand or predict the type of motion that will occur at that joint. A review of the joint types and their subclassifications will permit a greater appreciation of the relationship of form to function.

Amphiarthrodial and Synarthrodial Joints

The amphiarthrodial and synarthrodial joint types can be grouped together as nonsynovial. Since the joints are fixed and non-movable, we cannot measure movement at such nonsynovial joints. An amphiarthrodial joint, which is the direct union of one bony surface to another, can be subdivided into two types. According to Norkin and Levangie (1992) the symphysis (e.g., pubis symphysis uniting the os coxae) and the synchondrosis (e.g., where the ribs connect to the sternum via hyaline cartilage) are amphiarthiodial joints.

Synarthrodial joints employ a fibrous tissue to connect bony components. Norkin and Levangie's (1992) subdivision of synarthrodial joints include: sutures as seen in the skull, gomphosis as seen in teeth, and syndesmosis as found between the shafts of bones connected by interosseous membranes (e.g., the radius and ulna).

Diarthrodial Joint

The diarthrodial joint is a joint that indirectly connects one bone to another via a joint capsule. All joint capsules enclose a joint cavity lined by a slippery, synovial membrane. A layer of cartilage covers the ends of the two articulating bones. The cavity itself is filled with synovial fluid.

The joint capsule is composed of fibrous connective tissue and acts like a sleeve that holds the bones securely but permits their movement. The articular cartilage covering the ends of the bones acts like a rubber heel on a shoe and absorbs jolts. The synovial membrane secretes a lubricating fluid called synovial fluid that facilitates movement by decreasing friction (Exercise 18-1).

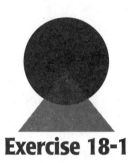

Exercise 18-1

Label the drawing below with the five main qualities of a synovial joint.
1. Joint capsule
2. Joint cavity
3. Synovial membrane
4. Synovial fluid
5. Articular cartilage

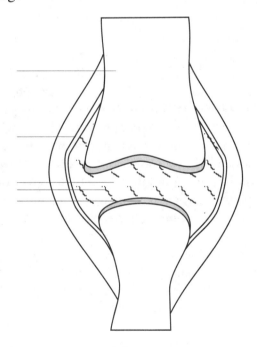

Motion at Diarthrodial Joints

Subclassifications of the synovial diarthrodial joint are based on the extent of motion possible at such joints. The true subclassifications are uniaxial, biaxial, and triaxial. Uniaxial indicates one degree of freedom which means motion occurs in one plane with one axis. The elbow is a good example of a uniaxial joint. The biaxial joint has two degrees of freedom indicating motion occurs in two planes along two axes. A good example of a biaxial joint is the metacarpal phalangeal joint of the index finger which can easily be demonstrated as showing two degrees of freedom. The third type of synovial joint is the triaxial with three degrees of freedom. It permits movement in three planes along three axes. The shoulder or hip are good examples since ball and socket joints allow motion in three directions. Of the synovial joints, try to list all the joints in the body that have:

- Three degrees of freedom
- Two degrees of freedom
- One degree of freedom

ROM

The amount of motion available at any particular joint is called the range of motion, or ROM. In order to expand this concept of joint motion, new terms must be explained. Physiological motion, called voluntary motion and/or osteokinematics, is the movement of the bones. Physiological motion is that motion that we observe visually and which is measured in goniometry. Another type of joint motion is considered nonvoluntary and not easily measured or observed. Nonvoluntary refers to the movement of joint surfaces. Arthrokinematics and accessory motion refer to the joint articular surface movement. In order to appreciate accessory motion, a closer look at bone ends is necessary.

Bone ends (epiphyses) have many different configurations. For our present purposes assume there are just two types: concave and convex (Figure 18-1).

Let's now consider motion at these bone ends. When a convex surface moves on a stable concave surface, the sliding of the convex articulating surface occurs in the opposite direction to the motion of the distal end of the bone or bony lever. This is what we mean when we use the expression "accessory motion" of the joint. Put your right hand in the shape of a fist. This is a convex bone end. Fit the right hand into the hollow shape you make in the left hand. As the convex fist moves down in the concave palm of the left hand the right forearm acts as a bony lever moving up in the opposite direction. This simulates the way in which the head of the humerus moves in the glenoid fossa. The convex humerus head surface is moving in the opposite direction than the distal aspect of the humerus in voluntary shoulder flexion. Practice this simulated movement to clarify your understanding of the concept. Consider working with a disarticulated scapula and humerus to enhance the image of a convex surface moving on a stable concave surface.

When a concave surface is moving on a stable convex surface, the sliding occurs in the same direction as the motion of the distal end or bony lever. An example would be the concave surface of the proximal phalanx moving on the fixed convex surface of the metacarpal. Simulate this motion as the right fisted hand is the fixed convex metacarpal and the cupped concave left hand moves as the phalanx. Note that both ends of the phalanx are moving in the same direction.

The bony part that is moving is described or named first. Thus, the convex on con-

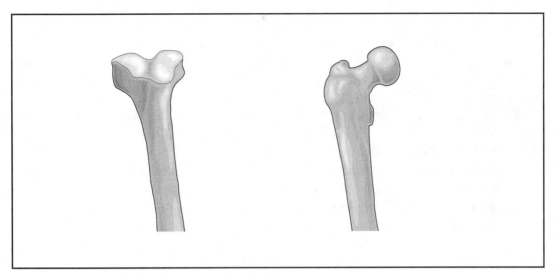

Figure 18-1. Examples of concave and convex.

cave rule indicates the convex surface is moving; conversely, the concave on convex rule indicates that the concave surface is moving.

Remember, it is the accessory motion in the joint that occurs during the physiological motion. The most important point to keep in mind is when movement of the bones in the body are occurring, both ends of the bone are moving. The design of the bone end dictates what type of motion occurs.

PLANES AND AXES

There are three planes (cardinal) of the body. Motion at a joint takes place in these planes. The planes are transverse, frontal, and sagittal. The transverse plane is a cut made to divide the body in half at the midsection, resulting in a top and bottom half. The transverse plane is also called the horizontal plane. The frontal plane cuts the body from front to back, and the sagittal plane divides the body into right and left sections that are mirror images of one another. Review the planes until you have them mastered.

Movement occurs in planes and the body segments are being rotated or moved about an axis. The axis is always perpendicular to its corresponding plane. Rotary motion occurs around a vertical axis in a transverse or horizontal plane. Examples of rotary motion include pronation and supination of the forearm, rotation of the head and trunk, as well as internal and external rotation at the shoulder.

Motion that occurs in the frontal plane occurs around the anterior-posterior axis. To visualize the anterior-posterior axis, consider the motion of a pinwheel, the center pin is the axis around which motion of the wheel occurs in the frontal plane. Another example would be the hands of a clock moving in the frontal plane and the axis is the center point where they originate. Abduction of the shoulder and leg occurs in the frontal plane around an anterior-posterior axis.

The sagittal plane divides the body into right and left halves. Motion in this plane occurs around a coronal axis. Note the term *frontal* axis is also used to denote the coronal axis. Consider a wooden toy soldier or a teddy bear with movable arms that only move forward in a sagittal plane around a coronal axis. Flexion of the elbow, shoulder, and knee also occur in this plane.

TERMS AND REVIEW OF MOVEMENT

The terms used to describe movement or action of the joints must be learned just like a new language. There should be immediate recall of the meaning of the terms, as well as the action in the body. This is a minimum basic requirement on which to build skills.

Movement is described from the anatomical position. Remember, the anatomical position is one in which the subject stands facing you with palms toward you, the examiner. Movement occurs at fixed points throughout the human body. The fixed point is the joint. Terms to understand in relation to movement are:

- Flexion   Extension
- ABduction   ADduction
- External Rotation Internal Rotation
- Supination   Pronation
- Ulnar Deviation   Radial Deviation
- Inversion   Eversion

Such classic definition of movement within planes assumes the body is in the anatomical position. Exercise 18-2 allows for additional practice and visualization of the concept of planes and axes.

The terms of motion listed can be applied to uniaxial, biaxial, and triaxial joints. If the joint is uniaxial, only one choice is possible (i.e., flexion and extension). If the joint is biaxial, the choice is two of the above. If the joint is triaxial, the choice is three of the above.

Flexion occurs in the sagittal plane around a coronal axis. This is also true of elbow flexion, as well as shoulder, hip, knee, wrist, and finger flexion. Extension is the return from flexion back to the anatomical position. Practice flexion in the sagittal plane on yourself, in front of a mirror. Ask a friend or family member to demonstrate his or her flexion of the elbow, shoulder, wrist, fingers, neck, hip, knee, or toes.

Abduction is the next movement to consider. This motion occurs in the frontal plane around the anterior-posterior axis. The shoulder, specifically the triaxial glenohumeral joint, flexes and also abducts. Consider abduction as making angels in the snow, except you're standing in the anatomical position. The arm will get closer to the ear. Adduction would be the return from abduction in the frontal plane. What other joints in the body can abduct? Because abduction and adduction sound similar, it is a good idea to start the practice of stating "A B duction" and "A D duction" when referring to the motion. This ensures that faulty hearing or diction will not cause confusion.

Rotation is sometimes more of a challenge to consider. This motion can occur at the neck, trunk, shoulder, forearm, hip, and foot. The transverse plane is the direction of motion around a vertical axis. The neck rotates from right to left to allow an expansion of the visual field. Imagine a pin at the top of the head around which the neck rotates on a vertical axis. This is similar to how a spinning top moves.

Consider the rotation of the palm in the anatomical position. The palm faces out or is supinated. When the palm faces inward or rotates into the pronated position, it does so in the transverse plane around a vertical axis.

Rotation of the glenohumeral joint can be palpated at the superior aspect of the shoulder. With the palm of your left hand cupped on the top of your right shoulder, feel for the movement of the humerus while the right hand supinates. You can palpate the greater tubercule moving as the head of the humerus rotates externally or outwardly. This same

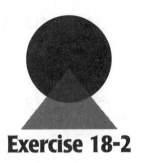

Exercise 18-2

One can visualize an axis by using a pencil. Place a pencil pointing at the shoulder of a partner so that if it went through the shoulder joint, your could imagine the humerus turning on it (e.g., the pencil acting as a pivot point for the head of the humerus). Now with the shoulder starting in the anatomical position, for each movement below, place the pencil so the humerus turns on it to produce (Perry, Rohe, & Garcia, 1996):

1. Flexion and Extension

2. ABduction and ADduction

3. Internal and External Rotation

Name the plane and axis for each motion above.

1. _____

2. _____

3. _____

motion can also be called lateral rotation of the shoulder. Thus, three terms—*outward, external,* and *lateral rotation*—describe the change of position or rotation of the shoulder in the transverse or horizontal plane with a vertical axis. *Internal rotation, inward rotation,* and *medial rotation* all describe the same motion in the transverse plane around a vertical axis.

Inversion and eversion define movement of the lower extremity as the sole of the foot changes position. Inversion, the foot turns inward, and eversion, the foot turns outward.

SUGGESTIONS FOR PRACTICE

Practice the motions presented with another student. Quiz each other and ask for demonstration of specific upper extremity and lower extremity movements. Create a list of flexion, abduction, and rotation of specific joints throughout the body.

Cut out pictures of your favorite movie star, athlete, television personality, or model and identify the position of his or her limbs and trunk. Create your own study guide reference of specific limb positions and label the plane and axis of motion. Now complete Exercise 18-3.

ACTIVE AND PASSIVE ROM

Now that specific motions are mastered, the review of the differences between active and passive ROM is our next objective to address. Remember that ROM, both passive and active, will vary among individuals according to age and gender, as well as other factors. A review of medical records and patient history usually precede a ROM evaluation. Medical status will impact how you approach the patient and overall therapeutic clinical reasoning issues.

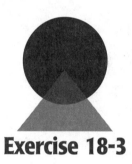

Exercise 18-3

What do you call the movement when you are standing erect in the anatomical position and you (Perry et al., 1996):

1. Bend your elbow from a fully straight to a bent position?_____
2. Maintain the elbow bent position, but turn your palm up? _____
3. Maintain the elbow bent position, but turn your palm down? _____
4. Maintain the elbow bent position, keep your elbow touching your side and turn your arm out so your fingers are pointing directly away from your side? _____
5. Straighten your elbow? _____
6. Move your arm away from your side so it sticks straight out to the side away from your shoulder? _____

Give the planes in which the following motions take place.

1. Stepping up a step _____
2. Abduction of the femur at the hip _____
3. Shaking head "no" _____
4. Straight sit-up _____

Active range of motion (AROM) is just that—the individual activates the motion and completes it. The muscles are used by the individual to whatever degree the individual is capable of controlling.

Passive range of motion (PROM) is just that, passive—the individual's joint ROM is evaluated in a passive condition. The individual does not participate in any movement at the joint. The therapist is manipulating the individual's limbs for therapeutic factors that are evaluated or treated.

Prior to evaluating the patient's PROM, a patient demonstration of his or her AROM is necessary. By initially observing patient AROM, the limits of the voluntary range are observed and potential problems noted. Likely to be issues are joint stiffness and decreased muscle strength, which impede the patient's ability to have complete AROM. Thus, the display of the patient's AROM allows the therapist to make a hypothesis of the general muscle strength in a particular muscle group. For example, if a client is unable to actively reach full range in shoulder flexion, a fair grade of the deltoid muscle group is suspected. Observing the patient results is a valuable evaluation opportunity for the skilled therapist. Observation skills are a fundamental key in the evaluation process and therapist's clinical reasoning.

AROM is the joint range attained by the individual voluntarily moving the joint. Take time to observe AROM of fellow students, friends, and family members. Consider the variety in AROM you will observe based on age or gender differences. Prior to considering the actual degrees of ROM, the issue of end feel will be reviewed.

What is learned about a patient when ROM is assessed? PROM provides the therapist with information about the integrity of the articular surfaces, extensibility of the joint capsule, and associated ligament and muscle (Norkin & Levangie, 1992). PROM allows us to evaluate the end feel of a joint—how the movement feels and responds at the endpoint of the range. PROM is generally slightly greater than AROM. As the therapist moves the limb, an observation of the patient's response should be noted. Is the patient's facial expression changing secondary to discomfort? Pain during the passive movement of the limb can be due to moving, stretching, or pinching of noncontractile structure (Norkin & Levangie, 1992). Pain at the end of PROM may be due to stretching of contractile tissue, as well as noncontractile tissue (Norkin & Levangie, 1992). PROM allows us to anticipate areas of difficulty for the client.

END FEEL

When performing PROM on an individual, all physiological movement has a point where movement stops. Depending upon the type of joint and where it is located in the body, predictable normal end feel can be anticipated. Abnormal end feel is also a factor to be considered in evaluation and treatment; however, that is beyond the scope of this text. Refer to Norkin and Levangie (1992) to explore this topic in detail.

The hands of the examiner are used to palpate the end feel. Sensitivity to the end feel is learned with practice. The examiner learns to feel the resistance to further motion at the end of PROM. The feeling is palpated through the examiner's hands. There are three normal end feels. The first is a soft end feel. Soft is when one muscle belly is hitting another and will stop movement that otherwise might continue. An example of a soft end feel is noted in elbow flexion. The forearm hits the biceps muscle and movement is stopped by this contact. Depending upon the size of the biceps, such as in weightlifters or bodybuilders, PROM could be stopped well before any actual joint restriction would play a role.

The second type of end feel is called firm. In this type, the examiner feels a taut resistance to further movement. Like a rope that will not give, or an elastic with no give remaining, the firm end feel is a muscular, capsular, or ligamentous stretch. A motion of shoulder flexion in the glenohumeral joint results in a firm end feel during PROM.

The last normal end feel to review is labeled hard. In this situation, it is bone coming in contact with bone. It feels hard, the movement is clearly stopped. The example here is at the elbow in extension. The olecranon fitting into the fossa stops any further PROM in extension. Once again, practice on yourself and on a person who is willing to be your patient. Take care to respect the limits of range and to anticipate that deviation from the norm will occur. Always remember to listen to the verbal response or feedback your patient provides. Adjust your approach or methods accordingly.

GONIOMETRY TECHNIQUES AND PROCEDURES

Goniometry provides data about ROM. When this data are used in conjunction with observation, palpation, and medical history, a plan of therapeutic intervention can be made. The tool itself employed in goniometry will be described and general procedures as to its usage. *Gonia* is a term meaning angle. *Metron* is a term for measure. The goniometer is a type of ruler that measures ROM.

The goniometer is usually made from plastic or metal and has two arms (Figure 18-2). One arm is called the stationary arm and the other is the movable arm. The movable arm is attached to the goniometer body via a screw or rivet that permits rotation of the arm. There are many different sizes of goniometers. For example, small versions are used for joints in the fingers, and large types for the hip or shoulder joint. A medium-sized goniometer might be used for wrist or ankle evaluation.

Just as the hands of a clock or a gauge on a dial move, so too can the movable arm of

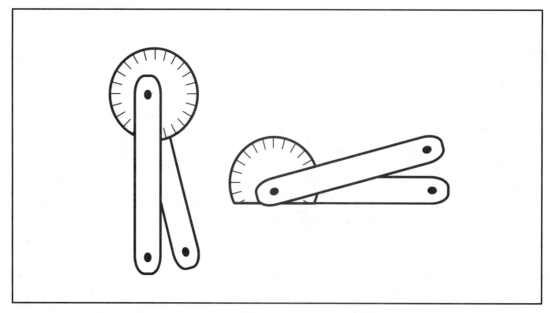

Figure 18-2. Goniometers.

the goniometer. The axis of the goniometer is placed over the joint during measurement assessment. The increments on the scale usually go from 1 to 10 degrees. The scale can be a full circle of 360 degrees, or a half scale or circle of 1 to 180 degrees. Review Figure 18-2 and then review the goniometer you will be using. Can you identify the movable vs. the stable arm? Find the axis of your goniometer.

Practice reading the goniometer. Set the movable arm at 45 degrees, 64 degrees, 90 degrees, and 145 degrees. Try another experiment with your goniometer. Take a plain white piece of paper and trace the goniometer while it has been set at 10 degrees, 25 degrees, 45 degrees, 75 degrees, 90 degrees, and 175 degrees.

With those same degrees listed above, try to position those angles on your partner's elbow. Ask your partner to hold a designated angle at the elbow. Eyeball the angle. It is a good practice to visually assess the angle at a joint prior to the use of the goniometric measurement. In this way you have an idea as to the approximate range. Visual estimation before measurement is taken to prevent gross errors caused by reading the goniometer incorrectly. Practice reading the goniometer. Practice the concept of eyeballing the range of the joint under examination.

Another idea to practice is visualizing the bones and their articulation while first eyeballing the range at the joint. The next area to incorporate in measurement technique is the ability to locate anatomical landmarks. By imagining the bones under the flesh, the relationship of body part and landmark will be facilitated.

Take time now to review the landmarks on a skeleton or textbook model. We use landmarks to provide a reference point to help ensure that alignment of the goniometer is correct.

Formal evaluation of joint ROM requires an understanding of preferential test positions. In order to achieve optimal range in your patient, particular positions of body segments are required. Positioning of the goniometer for assessment is also specific for each joint to be evaluated. The body should be stabilized so that the specific motion can be isolated to the joint being measured. The therapist may be doing a complete evaluation or just one or two joints in the upper extremity.

Alignment and positioning of the goniometer and patient require an absolutely clear understanding and familiarity with the list of terms provided (Table 18-1). It is the reader's responsibility to check the required reference text for definition of terms.

Alignment of the goniometer requires understanding that the mobile arm is the distal arm. The stable arm is the proximal arm. The fulcrum of the goniometer is the axis of the tool. The axis or fulcrum is positioned over the axis of the joint being measured. The proximal arm of the goniometer will be positioned on the part of the bone that is stable and does not move. The distal arm of the goniometer is placed adjacent to the part that does move.

The consistent use of the same test position for successive measurement increases the reliability and validity of test procedures. Consistent methods of evaluation will result in increased accuracy and credible data. (Norkin & Levangie, 1992). Furthermore, if all therapists in a clinical setting have consistency of approach, intertester reliability will result. Once again, I recommend the review of resources in joint measurement techniques.

Formal test procedures are not standardized, but there are approaches that have been adopted by many clinicians. The aim of this section is to review the basic considerations in positioning the limbs for assessment of ROM. The knowledge of joint structure, under-

Table 18-1
Important Terms

• Acromion	• Anterior superior iliac spine
• Olecranon process	• Patella
• Lateral epicondyle	• Lateral malleolus
• Radial head	• Fibular head
• Styloid process	• Tibial tuberosity
• Capitate	• Calcaneous
• Greater trochanter	• Prone
• Medial	• Dorsal
• Lateral	• Dorsum
• Proximal	• Volar
• Distal	• Anterior
• Plantar flexion	• Posterior
• Dorsi flexion	• Supine

standing of end feel, understanding of the skeletal system's important landmarks, in combination with alignment skill of the goniometer, and the ability to read the goniometer result in the ability to record data that then impact on treatment. The next section will review the exact procedure for the measurement of one joint in the upper extremity.

PROCEDURE

The sample review of ROM will be restricted in this primer to elbow flexion with the expectation that the reader can integrate the material and will refer to other references for the procedures of total body assessment.

Elbow flexion occurs in the sagittal plane around a coronal axis. The patient should be comfortably positioned in a supine position. The arm should be positioned close to the body in shoulder adduction with the elbow extended. As previously noted, the patient will be asked to exhibit his or her AROM first. Next you will assess PROM and eyeball a visual estimate of range. Lastly, the stationary arm of the goniometer will be aligned with the midline of the humerus and the mobile (distal) arm will be aligned with the lateral midline of the forearm. The patient's hand is supinated. The mobile (distal) arm of the goniometer will move with the distal aspect of the limb. The axis of the goniometer will line up with the lateral epicondyle of the humerus. Your hands will support the client's forearm and the arms of the goniometer. You will passively move the client's limb into elbow flexion. The shoulder should be stabilized to prevent flexion. As you read the scale on the goniometer at the end of range, recheck your alignment of the tool. The end feel of the motion is soft. Review the end feel section if needed. Elbow flexion range is 0 to 150 degrees as a general norm. Record data on the evaluation sheet.

Review the tables found in Norkin and White (1995) of the average ROM available per joint in the body and review the evaluation forms included in Appendix C. Review the reading of the goniometer and continue to practice on willing subjects. Always note the limb orientation of your patient on your evaluation sheet. Right vs. the left limb, the date of the evaluation, and the type of range (i.e., passive or active) that was assessed should be recorded. Data collection is only as valuable as the precise nature of the recording of information.

As you acquire confidence with elbow range assessment, move on to the joints in the hand. Remember that the size of the goniometer you will use changes depending on the joint being tested. Note that the position of the patient will change depending on the joint being evaluated. Alternative positioning is also an issue when a patient cannot accommodate to standard procedures. The concern for stabilization of joints is necessary to avoid substitution or movement in another part of the body invalidating the goniometer reading. This is noted, for example, in the evaluation of shoulder flexion; a patient might laterally flex his or her trunk in order to achieve increased shoulder flexion.

The larger or more complex the joint under evaluation, the more detailed the procedure to complete that evaluation. The shoulder girdle complex is an area that has multiple joints, all of which need to be considered when assessing range. Review of the Norkin and White (1995), Pedretti and Zoltan (1990), and Trombly (1995) texts are required in order to continue your practice work in goniometry.

EXPLAINING GONIOMETRY TO YOUR PATIENT AND YOUR PATIENT'S FAMILY

The ability to introduce yourself to a patient and explain the evaluation procedure must be practiced. You must develop your own style and professional demeanor that allow you to competently describe what you do to others. Patients need to be treated with respect and valued given the cultural and environmental context of their lives. Consider then how you will explain goniometry to the patient. How will you introduce yourself to the patient? Can you demonstrate in a clear, concise, competent fashion how the goniometer works to the patient? How will you explain to the patient what he or she will be doing during the evaluation? How will you know if the patient is comfortable and understands what you will be doing? Practice first with a mental image of your professional role during a goniometry evaluation. Next, once again ask a friend or family member to be your patient and role play the process of introduction and explanation of goniometry. Practice moving your patient from supine to sidelying to sitting, and handling the patient. Ask your patient for feedback as to whether your touch is reassuring. Do you have a firm, secure touch? Ask your friendly role-playing patient to give you his or her impression of your professional style.

Laboratory practice is essential for the successful completion of any course in goniometry. Providing ROM without this skill competency can result in injury to the patient. Even family members assisting and providing ROM to a patient must be trained by a rehabilitation expert before it is safe for him or her to provide this procedure to the patient.

SUMMARY

The foundations for good skill development in measuring joint ROM have been reviewed. Specifically, planes, end feel, joint classification systems, and accessory vs. physiologic motion were presented. The exercises you have completed will anchor your knowledge base and increase your confidence in the acquisition of skill and knowledge. A final exercise practice of the elbow was presented to further your mastery of goniometry.

It will take practice to know how you actually support the limb you are moving during PROM of the patient. You must consider this a skill development. No one should perform

PROM without an understanding of the skeletal system and must have supervision. Supervision from a skilled professional will confirm your competency.

Respect what you do as a therapist. Respect the skill required to provide your services to a patient. Lastly, respect your patient and listen to his or her response to the service you provide. Listen both with your ears and with your hands as you manipulate and palpate the body during the goniometric evaluation.

BIBLIOGRAPHY

Daniel, M. S., & Strickland, L. R. (1992). *Occupational therapy protocol management in adult physical dysfunction.* Gaithersburg, MD: Aspen Publications.

Norkin, C. C., & Levangie, P. K. (1992). *Joint structure & function: A comprehensive analysis.* Philadelphia: F. A. Davis.

Norkin, C. C., & White, D. J. (1995). *Measurement of joint motion: A guide to goniometry.* Philadelphia: F. A. Davis.

Pedretti, L. W., & Zoltan, B. (1990). *Occupational therapy: Practice skills for physical dysfunction.* Philadelphia: C. V. Mosby.

Perry, J. F., Rohe, D. A., & Garcia, A. O. (1996). *The kinesiology workbook.* Philadelphia: F. A. Davis.

Trombly, C. (1995). *Occupational therapy for physical dysfunction.* Baltimore: Williams & Wilkins.

Answers to Exercise 18-1

1. Joint capsule
2. Joint cavity
3. Synovial membrane
4. Synovial fluid
5. Articular cartilage

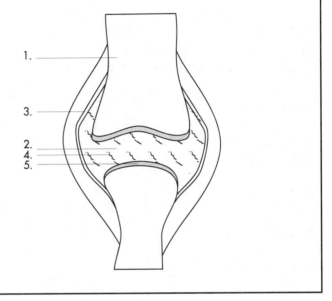

Answers to Exercise 18-2

1. Sagittal plane/Coronal axis
2. Frontal plane/Anterior-posterior axis
3. Transverse plane/Vertical axis

Answers to Exercise 18-3

1. Flexion
2. Supination
3. Pronation
4. External rotation
5. Extension
6. Abduction

1. Sagittal
2. Frontal
3. Sagittal
4. Sagittal

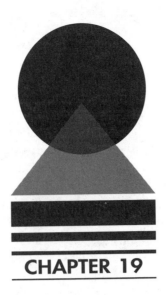

CHAPTER 19

THERAPEUTIC COMMUNICATION

Roseanna Tufano, MFT, OTR/L

INTRODUCTION

There are many different forms and styles of communication in our world. Each of us has a native language, which is part of our self-identity. Each generation also has its own subcultural street language and/or dialect which identifies a certain period in time and place. For example, a typical way American teenagers greet each other in the 1990s is to say, "What's up?" Along with the various ways we verbally communicate, there exists another level of nonverbal interaction. Most American teenagers will initiate a multistepped handshake (nonverbal) as they say, "What's up?" (verbal).

A unique form of communicating includes the verbal and nonverbal interactions between a therapist and client. Therapeutic communication refers to the ways that therapists and clients exchange information, thoughts, and ideas. This chapter will introduce you to a philosophy called humanism and discuss Carl Roger's work on the therapeutic relationship. You will also learn specific communication tools and skills based on this humanistic philosophy needed for effective communication when conducting initial interviews and sessions. These tools will allow you to establish rapport and to build trust between therapist and client. Tutorials will allow you to practice basic skills.

A PERSON-CENTERED APPROACH TO THERAPY

Carl Rogers (1902-1987) was a psychologist who focused much of his work on the therapeutic relationship. His approach is known as the person-centered theory of personality. The basic aspects of this theory include two major concepts: self-actualization and self-direction. Rogers believed that each person has an innate or inherent tendency to develop oneself to his or her fullest potential. This level of personal completeness is called self-actualization. He also believed that each person is capable of directing oneself in the healthiest way, a concept he referred to as self-direction. Rogers viewed the personality as everchanging and influenced by communications, relationships, and self-concept. The relationship between a therapist and client is used to guide the treatment plan.

The humanistic philosophy highlights the characteristics unique to people vs. animals. The basic premise states that humans are rational beings who possess the capacity for truth and goodness. This belief emphasizes the dignity and worthiness of each person. People are viewed as equally valuable regardless of their ethnicity, race, religion, gender, socioeconomic status, health, and intellectual capacity.

Carl Rogers is a prominent example of a humanistic philosopher. He has emphasized the need to regard clients with a positive and open attitude that remains nonjudgmental at all times. He has defined this attitude as unconditional positive regard. Within this treatment approach, Rogers encouraged his clients to select their own goals for treatment. He believed that clients could discover their own solutions to their problems trusting that they knew best what was healthiest for themselves. By regarding the client in this unconditional way, Rogers believed that one's innermost feelings and behaviors will be revealed to the therapist because the client no longer fears rejection. Rogers concluded from his research studies that the more clients felt accepted, prized, and valued by their therapists, the more likely they were to identify therapy as successful.

In OT practice, we incorporate both the humanistic beliefs and Rogerian approach within our treatment modalities. We emphasize the potential of all our clients and include them as part of their own treatment plan, trusting their own ability for self-direction. We offer services to anyone in need regardless of their ethnicity, race, religion, gender, socioeconomic status, health, and intellectual capacity.

OT personnel should remain nonjudgmental and supportive of the positive attributes of every person. We structure activities to allow for problem solving and desired change in behaviors. We listen and regard each of our clients for his or her individual and unique concerns, even when we do not agree with his or her perceptions.

The therapeutic relationship is the backbone of all our OT interventions. The therapist's spirit and behavior are conveyed to clients through both verbal and nonverbal communication. Without effective communication, we could not develop the trusting bond that is needed to ensure successful treatment outcomes nor support the clients through their many struggles and advances.

THE HELPING PROCESS

Within the framework of using a humanistic and Rogerian approach, COTAs and OTRs integrate values. Values are qualities and standards considered worthwhile and/or desirable. The values inherent within the humanistic philosophy include regarding each person as a unique individual and prizing his or her humaneness. A therapist using the Rogerian approach to treatment believes that every person can make choices about his or her life and come up with personalized solutions to problems. OT personnel are concerned about what the client identifies as a problem and what the client values about the change process.

At times, therapists and clients differ on what the therapeutic problems are for treatment. This difference of opinion may be reflective of each person's own set of values. It is important to remember that each client has the right to treatment and should be included in the process of determining goals and solutions whenever possible. Sometimes clients choose to refuse treatment. Although this decision may differ from the therapist's judgment, the client should still be valued as a human being making a personal choice. COTAs and OTRs do not always agree with their client's actions, but should always value them as people.

Among the various values that therapists possess, respect and genuineness are significantly important to establishing a trusting rapport with clients. We communicate these values through both verbal and nonverbal means. Each of these qualities will be discussed separately in the next two sections.

Respect

Another word for respect is honor. Therapists show respect for their clients by showing consideration and unconditional regard. There are various ways to communicate respect to our clients. Consider the following points.

Prize each client for his or her individuality. OT personnel should consider the unique lifestyles and nature of problems as part of our job. Remember to respect your client's feelings regardless of whether or not you agree with him or her. Many clients feel that they do not have much control in their lives except for their own feelings. Avoid making statements like: "Don't cry!" or "Don't worry!" While your intentions may be good, you are actually telling the client how to feel or not feel. It is the client's behavioral response to feelings that may need to be changed, not the emotion itself. Encourage your client to identify his or her personal needs and wants and incorporate them into the treatment plan. Be sure to always ask the client what he or she considers to be the problem. Do not assume that you know what is best for the client without including him or her in the treatment process.

Be nonjudgmental. Roger's term *unconditional positive regard* means that the client should be respected consistently and without bias and/or prejudice. This also means accepting the person who may refuse your treatment approach today and still inviting him or her to participate tomorrow. In our professional roles, we must learn to regard and find something positive in everyone. In order to become truly nonjudgmental, we must be aware of our own prejudices, own up to them, and consciously put these personal feelings aside when we are working as therapists. This process is part of our own professional development and takes great time and personal effort. Consider the following.

> *Therapist:* I could see that you are having a hard time during your therapy session today. I will stop by to see you this afternoon and perhaps we could try the exercises again. It is not unusual for clients to feel unmotivated at times. I am here to support you all the way.

Be present in mind and body. It is important to convey through our body language and psychological presence that we are committed to being available to our clients. It takes discipline to learn how to put aside one's own concerns and to fully attend to another. We could probably all remember an experience when someone was staring at us but not really seeing us as a person because he or she was preoccupied with self-concerns.

Clients feel respected when the therapist devotes full attention, in body and attitude, for the whole treatment time. Whenever possible, do not allow disruptions and/or personal distractions to interfere with your sessions.

Incorporate the client's own resources. OT personnel make every effort to include the client in the treatment process. It is important to ask and/or guide our clients to solve their own problems even if their approach does not match our ideas. There are many ways to convey to a client that you value his or her input and ideas even if the actual treatment approach has to be adapted in some way. Consider the following.

> *Therapist:* That's an interesting way to approach your problem, Mr. Williams. I see how hard you are trying to correct the problem. Let's also try one of my ideas and see how it works for you. Let's try and find the best solution to this problem.

Notice how Mr. Williams is respected for the act of trying to correct the problem regardless of whether or not the approach is appropriate. This is an example of how to regard the person even when the therapist does not agree with the client's actual behavior. Try to reinforce people's intentions and goodwill even when the manner in which they tried to implement a behavior may not be appropriate. Many times a client may need the help of the COTA and OTR to assess his or her way of doing things. Clients are more likely to ask for help or admit their unsuredness if they believe that the therapist will remain accepting and nonjudgmental.

Genuineness

Another word for genuineness is sincerity. COTAs and OTRs show genuineness through their honest attitude and real behaviors. Consider the following points.

Be open. Many clients will have alternate lifestyles and habits from your own. Be prepared to hear about their stories. Avoid pretending that you understand or agree unless it is true. Clients could sense from your nonverbal mannerisms whether or not you are being honest. Consider the following.

> *Therapist:* You are right. I don't know how to survive on the streets. However, I am very interested in understanding what it is like for you. Tell me about it.

The therapist is admitting to not experiencing the same lifestyle as the client. However, that does not mean that the therapist is incapable of understanding. Remember that you will not always agree with your client's decisions and actions but could still be genuinely interested in their well-being.

Be real. Your clients will trust you more readily if you appear as a person and not as an actor playing the role of a therapist. Find the balance to being friendly yet not being a friend, to showing caring yet not getting overly involved in the client's problems. Learn how to express your feelings while being sensitive to your client's feelings. Do not hide behind your professional role nor pretend that you have power over the client. Admit that you do not have all the answers but will attempt to find solutions with the client's help and resources. Incorporate your personal qualities such as use of humor, spontaneity, energy level, sense of timeliness, and commitment to the profession. Remember the saying: "It's not what you say but how you say it that counts." OT is an active and direct profession, one that affords us the opportunity to relate person to person.

Be non-defensive. At times, clients may express negative attitudes toward staff. It is important to listen and to entertain the client's feelings, thoughts, and behaviors about a particular person or situation. As a general guide, allow the client to tell you about his or her feelings. Consider the problem from the client's point of view. Support the client's direct and appropriate disclosure of the issue. Clearly respond to the issue raised by the client, leaving your personal feelings aside. Expert therapists recognize their own strengths and weaknesses and admit to learning from their clients and experiences. Be willing to explore your role in contributing to the problem, remembering that in a healthy relationship, each partner contributes 50% and is partially responsible for the outcome of the relationship. Consider the following.

> *Therapist:* I can see how disappointed you are about our session. I'm interested in discussing the problems and figuring out together how we could better manage your care in this department.

Sometimes the act of acknowledging a person's feelings and allowing them to vent will diffuse some of one's anger. At other times, you might need to table the discussion until the client is calmer and clearer about the situation. Consider the following.

> *Therapist:* Mrs. Miller, I am going to suggest that we talk about what is making you angry when we both have had a chance to think more clearly and calmly about the situation. I will check back with you this afternoon.

In either situation, it will be beneficial for the therapist to remain non-defensive in the presence of the client. OT personnel should have their own support network, which may include a supervisor, colleague, friend, or mentor to work through their own personal feelings about clients.

Be consistent. A good indication of whether someone is truly genuine is to listen to one's statements and then to observe one's behavior. Genuine people are consistent in their words and actions or at least could account for any discrepancy. If you tell a client that you will go by his or her room to talk with him or her later, it is important to follow through on your word. Inconsistent behavior on the therapist's part will lead to a non-trusting and superficial relationship. Clients will be likely to show dedication and commitment when the therapist is consistent in supporting them and the treatment process.

INTEGRATING COMMUNICATION SKILLS

Communication skills are useful tools to forming an effective therapeutic relationship. They are also helpful in our everyday interactions with family and friends. Knowlege of how to use these skills, however, is only one part of the therapeutic process. Students who are beginning to practice and learn the skills often comment that they sound mechanical. This is an excellent point to remember. At some time in our learning, we must integrate the mechanics of these skills into the helping process. The art of therapy is knowing when and how to use certain therapeutic techniques while always valuing the human condition. With increased experience and practice of these skills, therapists will begin to sound more natural as they integrate their own unique styles of interacting. It is the combination of a humanistic view of people, incorporating respect and genuineness, and actual knowledge of communication skills that will allow each of us to therapeutically establish relationships with our clients.

To help you understand and grasp the concepts of these various communication tools, each skill will be discussed separately in the following sections. The goal is that you will eventually be able to integrate all of them into a style that represents your therapeutic self and that will suit the needs of your clients.

We will begin by examining the skills of attending and listening. Both have a significant nonverbal component to their application.

Attending

When we attend to another person, we are present with them. As therapists, we must convey to our clients that we are both physically and psychologically "with them." Therapists show their respect and genuineness in their attending styles. As effective helpers, we must give of ourselves in hopes that our clients will give of themselves in return. The therapeutic relationship is an everchanging and interactive process.

One of the first things that clients will notice about you is your attending style. This skill transcends any words you may speak and will communicate to the client how interested and available you are to them on a nonverbal level. Consider the following example.

> *Therapist:* Hello, Mr. Sanchez. I am going to be working with you in occupational therapy so I wanted to just come by to introduce myself and to see how you are doing.

We could all agree that the words spoken sound appropriate as an introduction. Now consider this same therapist with the following conditions.

> The COTA or OTR knocks on the client's door but does not wait for the client to say "Come in." He or she has the client's chart in hand and is flipping through pages while making the above statement.

How does this therapist's attending style influence the words spoken? There are two different messages being conveyed to the client. The verbal message sounds like the therapist is interested in getting to know the person. However, the nonverbal message shows inattention for the person and perhaps more interest in the condition to be treated. Which message would impact you the most as a first time meeting?

Our nonverbal behaviors have significant impact on our clients. It is highly important to attend wholly to our clients, especially when we first meet them and are trying to establish some rapport and trust.

Egan (1990) has developed an acronym, SOLER, describing important microskills in the attending process. They are summarized as follows.

- **S=Squarely.** When meeting with a client, position your body so that you are facing the person directly. This posture will convey a message of involvement and interest.
- **O=Open.** Keep your posture open. Notice your tendency to cross your arms and legs

or to hug your own body while communicating. By keeping your posture open, you will convey that you are both physically and psychologically available to the client and also feel confident about yourself.

- **L=Lean.** Adjust your upper body posture to enhance communication. By leaning toward a client, you are suggesting concern and interest in what he or she is saying. It is important to respect your client's personal space, so be aware of how your posture is affecting him or her. If a client leans back as you are leaning forward, he or she may be uncomfortable with the level of closeness at this time. Leaning toward a client at significant periods of interaction could be assuring and comforting.
- **E=Eye contact.** Keep an even and direct flow of eye contact. While one does not want to stare at the client, it is important to look at him or her with a comfortable amount of contact. An occasional shift of one's eyes is natural but a deliberate looking away may convey reluctance, unsuredness, or discomfort. Many of us associate a level of confidence by how one maintains eye contact.
- **R=Relaxed.** Attempt to appear as relaxed and natural as possible. Your body is a powerful tool for communicating with your clients. Avoid fidgeting behaviors and signs of nervousness. It is a good idea to watch yourself on a videotape to better understand how you convey relaxed or nervous behaviors. We all have habits that we may be unaware of such as playing with our hair or rocking our legs. Learn how to adjust your body to portray a comfortable and confident therapeutic style.

Consider the above microskills as guidelines for yourself. Try to learn about your natural tendencies in these areas and decide how you may want to enhance or decrease their intensity.

Along with monitoring your own attending style, develop your therapeutic observation skills of your clients using these same parameters. You will become more proficient at recognizing your client's nonverbal messages and be able to provide him or her with feedback about his or her attending to you as the therapist.

Listening

Attending skills allow the therapist to become an available listener. There is a difference between hearing the sounds that someone makes as he or she talks to you, and actually listening to the person. Recall a time in your life when you told someone, "You are not listening to me!" Chances are that you did not feel understood or attended to in your conversation.

The skill of therapeutic listening involves various levels. One level is to accurately perceive a client's nonverbal messages, as introduced in the section on attending. Another level is to understand the spoken messages. In order to truly listen and grasp what another person is communicating, the therapist must also consider the context of the conversation and how the messages relate to the client's life.

In OT, we use purposeful activities as our treatment modality. A client's participation in these activities allows us to see many forms of expression and communication on both the verbal and nonverbal levels. We must become effective listeners and learn how to interpret various types of responses. Consider the following behaviors and characteristics.

- Body movements: posture, coordination, motor control, gestures
- Facial expressions: smiles, frowns, tics, movement of eyebrows and lips, eye movements, appearance

- Voice quality: pitch, tone, level, intensity, inflection
- Autonomic nervous system responses: breathing rate, blushing, paleness, pupil dilation, perspiration, trembling

You have probably heard the expression "Listen to your body." There is a great deal of truth to this statement because the body will reflect one's thoughts and feelings honestly. Part of our socialization process is to learn how to choose words and to talk in ways that will be socially accepted by others. At times, we may say what we think others may want to hear or accept, rather than how we truthfully feel about a situation. Clients may tell you that they are "feeling better" because they think that you want to hear this from them. However, by observing their nonverbal behaviors, including the responses stated above, you will know the genuineness of this statement. If your client appears pale and trembling, looks away from you as he or she softly tells you that he or she is feeling better, an observant therapist will note the discrepancy between words and appearance. It is necessary to check out your concerns with the client at that time.

Chances are high that you have been told already that you are a good listener. Many prospective therapists have natural, inherent qualities of caretaking and concern for others. Listening to a client's verbal messages is different from listening casually to a friend. It is our job to actively pay attention and to listen even when we feel disinterested, bored, or preoccupied. Before we can formulate any feedback, we must first listen and grasp the content of conversation. Therapists ask themselves about the core messages and themes that are part of our clients' stories. We wonder why the client is telling us about a particular topic, asking ourselves what does he or she want me to know about him or her at this time? We wonder how this conversation reflects his or her life.

There are a variety of obstacles that could interfere with our therapeutic listening skills. The following is a list for your consideration. Could you think of other obstacles to add to this list?

- Prejudgment of a client before knowing him or her
- Prejudice regarding his or her gender, race, religion, status, etc.
- Over- or underidentifying with the client
- Treating the client as a diagnosis rather than a person
- Rehearsing answers to the client while he or she is talking to you
- Time restraints
- Preoccupation with personal problems
- Non-therapeutic interrupting of the client
- Illness and physical discomfort
- Physical and emotional reactions to the client's content

Rogers talked about how therapists need to put aside their *self* in order to enter the world of another. Therapists must make a conscious decision to bracket off their personal needs, wants, and feelings for a designated amount of time to successfully listen and attend to their clients. This ability, to give of oneself unconditionally, takes maturity and experience. There are many intrinsic rewards for therapists who can give of themselves regardless of whether or not the client succeeds in therapy. OT gives us an opportunity to touch lives in a warm and active way.

GATHERING INFORMATION

As necessary as it is for therapists to listen and attend to their clients, it is also important to know how to ask and clarify information from the client. Various OT interviews contain preset questions that a therapist will ask during an initial assessment. During sessions, it will be necessary for you to question the client about his or her response to the treatment process. In this next section, the skill of probing and clarifying information will be discussed.

Open Vs. Closed Questions

Whenever therapists want to know about the client's thinking and feeling process, they will ask an open question. Open questions will require the person to explain rather than to answer yes or no. An example is: "How did you manage with your exercises this weekend?" Whenever therapists want a specific response to a concern, they will ask a closed question. An example is: "Did it hurt you when I pressed down on this muscle?"

In OT, you will need to be able to utilize both open and closed questions and to select the best time for their usage. The ability to prompt and probe a client is particularly important when he or she needs encouragement or guidance to explore problem situations. The goal of the therapist is to gather pertinent information from the client to further define and organize treatment. You will need to seek information about experiences, behaviors, and feelings by asking questions in a variety of ways.

There are some general guidelines for using questions effectively and efficiently. Consider the following list of suggestions.

- **Do** ask open questions to attain specific experiences, behaviors, and feelings. *Example:* How did you fall in your house that caused this injury? What do you want to focus on in our session today? What are you feeling about being in the hospital?
- **Do** ask open questions to encourage a quiet or withdrawn client. *Example:* I am not so sure how you are feeling about being in the hospital. What has it been like for you to come here?
- **Do** be specific and clear in your manner of questioning. *Example:* I want to clarify a point that you just made. What will motivate you to get better?
- **Do** ask the client to fill in missing information. *Example:* I am unclear about a certain piece of information. Where exactly will you be living upon discharge?
- **Do** keep the focus on the client. *Example:* I know that you are worried about your husband but I am wondering how you are feeling since you broke up with him?
- **Do** select the best tense (past, present, future) to obtain needed and current information. *Example:* When did you actually fall down in your apartment? How are you feeling now that you finished your therapy session? What would you like to be able to do when you go home next week?
- **Do not** ask too many questions in a row or ask multiple questions in one sentence. *Example:* What did you say and what did you do?
- **Do not** ask random questions to fill space and time. *Example:* So did you hear about the rumor that is going around the OT department?
- **Do not** lead the client to an answer by giving him or her the information in the question. *Example:* Did you feel hurt when he hit you?
- **Do not** ask questions that will take the focus off the client. *Example:* What is your boyfriend going to do about his living situation?

- **Do not** sound like you are conducting an interrogation. *Example:* Where were you on Thursday when you were supposed to come for your therapy session?

Now that you understand the possible uses and misuses of asking questions, let's review some general guidelines for asking open vs. closed questions.

To ask open questions, begin your sentence with the following words:

- What
- How
- When
- Where
- Why
- Describe
- Tell

Use "Why" sparingly because most people will associate this as a judgmental question.

To ask closed questions, begin your sentence with the following words:

- Are
- Did
- Have
- Will
- Can
- Could

Use closed questions sparingly and only when you need to know a yes or no answer.

In OT, it is particularly useful to ask questions when the client is being vague in his or her conversation. Consider the following example.

> *Client:* Life stinks!
>
> *Therapist:* What do you mean exactly?
>
> *Client:* Don't you know? It's too hard to explain.
>
> *Therapist:* I understand that you are frustrated but I do not know what is causing you to feel this way. How about telling me what has happened to you?

Clients may not disclose about their life issues or feelings for various reasons. It is difficult for some people to identify clearly and specifically what they are feeling. For those clients, it is helpful to gently probe their vagueness. You will find that the more respectful and genuine you sound, the more likely your client will tolerate your questions. Learning how to ask open questions takes practice and retraining from our usual ways of social interaction. Once you have become accustomed to asking open questions, you will find that the content of your conversation will become more diverse and interesting. Practice during your everyday conversations and notice for yourself how much more you will learn about the other person.

Vague Statements

Practice asking open questions that will give you concrete information about content and feelings. Read the following examples; use Exercise 19-1 to practice open-ended questions.

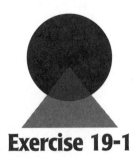

Exercise 19-1

Write an open question to obtain information and seek clarification from the client.

1. I can't do this!

2. My life is one big flop.

3. This therapy stuff is not working.

4. You don't really expect me to do all this.

5. I never had to depend on anyone before this accident.

6. You know what I mean, don't you?

7. Everything is fine.

8. I don't have any control in my life.

9. I'm feeling okay.

10. I just don't want to come to therapy anymore.

Client: I can't figure this out.

Therapist: What exactly are you confused about? (or) How are you feeling about your situation?

Client: This hurts!

Therapist: Where exactly are you feeling pain? (or) What specifically is causing you pain?

Client: Go away! You just don't get it, do you?

Therapist: What is making you angry right now? (or) Tell me about what is upsetting you.

EMPATHY

The various communication tools and skills that have been identified in this chapter are all used interchangeably. There is no certain order, no predictable sequence to determine when and how the therapist should use them. The art of therapy includes one's therapeutic sense of when and how to intervene with communication skills. When you attend to your clients closely and accurately, you will learn how to follow the lead of your clients. Most clients will identify that "feeling understood" by their therapists is critical to the therapeutic relationship. In this next section, you will learn how to communicate your understanding of a client's content using a form of primary accurate empathy.

Empathy may be defined as communicating to another that you understand his or her experiences, behaviors, and feelings. By conveying the therapist's understanding to clients in OT, you can move the person forward in the problem solving and healing process of treatment. The exchange of empathy is a powerful and supportive way to make emotional contact with clients.

In order to respond empathically, the therapist must listen and attend closely to the client. The therapist then tries to recognize the core messages being discussed by asking him- or herself "What is this person trying to tell me regarding feelings, behaviors, and experiences? What is the main feeling and importance of this conversation?" As the therapist recognizes the core messages, he or she will check out this perception with the client.

When communicating an empathic statement, the therapist will convey two levels of understanding to clients. One level is the feeling or affective component. For example, the therapist may say: "So you are feeling happy in our session today." This statement identifies the possible feeling of the client but does not convey the behavioral context of this reaction. In order to fully understand the basis for feelings, therapists listen to the client's experiences and the behavioral context during which these feelings emerged. It is useful to consider the formula "You feel_____because_____." In initial practice, you are advised to use this formula. As you become more familiar and accustomed to communicating both the feeling and behavioral levels, you may want to deviate and use your own natural style.

Primary Accurate Empathy

A primary accurate empathy statement is a first-level empathic statement that begins to acknowledge the patient's feeling. Table 19-1 lists guidelines to use when formulating a primary accurate empathy response and Table 19-2 lists guidelines to avoid.

Consider the following examples of empathy.

Client (a 50-year-old man who recently experienced a right CVA who is to be discharged next week): My life will never be the same again. I can't walk. I can't work. How am I going to spend the hours of my day? I don't think that I can remember all you taught me in here.

Therapist: So you are feeling scared because you are not sure how you will manage on your own at home. Is that true?

Client: Yeah. I've never been the type to depend on anyone.

Client (a 20-year-old female who is about to finish college): I have always been a perfectionist. I get upset with myself if I get anything lower than an "A" on my tests. Yesterday, as I was beginning to take my psychology test, I began to get shaky. Then I felt like I couldn't breathe. My heart was racing. My mind went blank! That has never happened to me before!

Therapist: So you are feeling surprised because you experienced such a strong reaction to stress unlike other times in the past. Does that sound right?

Client: You bet. I'm shocked! I've always been able to handle stress before. Now I'm afraid that these symptoms will come back again!

Empathy is an important skill to integrate into your OT practice. You can convey your warmth and understanding to a client who is struggling to problem solve and adapt his or her life in some way. This is a skill that takes a lot of practice and experience since it is made up of so many parts. Take some time to review Exercise 19-2. You will discover that empathy is a useful and powerful skill to be used with clients and personal acquaintances as well.

TERMINATION OF SESSIONS

In this next section, you will learn about various ways to end a session with a client. It is important to remember that time is a form of a therapeutic boundary. COTAs and OTRs should maintain schedules and punctuality because time represents an important aspect of the treatment session known as closure.

In this chapter, we discussed various ways to establish a trusting relationship with clients. Each session has a beginning and an ending. As OT practitioners, you provide your clients with an opportunity to start and to end a therapeutic relationship with you during every session. Depending on your own personal experiences with beginnings and endings, you may find that you are more or less comfortable with this process. This same

Table 19-1
Guidelines to Help Form a Primary Accurate Empathy Response

- Attend fully to the client, especially to nonverbal clues. (Refer back to the section on attending and listening skills.)
- Identify the feelings expressed by the client in the present. Do not become distracted by focusing on the past. Even when your client is telling a story in the past tense, he or she is experiencing feelings in the present.
- Select the most dominant feeling expressed. Clients may experience more than one emotion at a time. Choose the one that is most evident.
- Match the correct intensity of feeling expressed. Think of feelings as having three levels— mild, moderate, and severe. For example, a mild form of the feeling word anger is upset, a moderate form is mad, and a severe form is rage. Practice identifying the levels of intensity on your own.
- Paraphrase the main idea associated with the client's experiences and behaviors. Stay close to the client's words but deviate enough to let him or her know that you are listening.
- Formulate a verbal response consisting of "You feel____ because_____."
- Check your empathic response for accuracy. After formulating your verbal response, ask the client what he or she thinks about your statement. Does he or she agree or disagree?

Table 19-2
Guidelines of What to Avoid When Formulating an Emphatic Response

- Avoid not responding at all. Sometimes therapists lack a response because they are not sure how to phrase their statement. The client may interpret this lack of response as not caring or disinterest.
- Avoid asking a question when you should be conveying understanding. The client may interpret your question as a sign of inattentiveness and may think that his or her statement was not worth responding to.
- Avoid using clichés (e.g., Don't worry, be happy). You want to individualize your responses and support the uniqueness of each person.
- Avoid giving advice. During the early stages of developing a therapeutic relationship, it is not timely to jump into action. Take the time to listen and understand your client thoroughly. Many people want to be heard and are not interested in your solutions.
- Avoid pretending to understand when you genuinely do not. If you are genuinely confused, the appropriate skill to use is open questioning. Clients can tell whether you are trying to understand or just placating them.
- Avoid parroting the client's exact words. You want to avoid sounding mechanical or incapable of understanding.
- Avoid giving sympathy in place of empathy. Sympathy connotes identification with the client's feelings such as pity, condolence, compassion, and commiseration. It also suggests that you agree with your client's feelings. When you use empathy effectively, it does not matter whether you agree with the client or not. One does not have to agree to understand where the client is coming from.

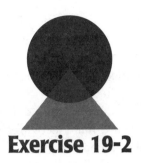

Exercise 19-2

Practice writing an empathic statement based on the following client's statements. Use the formula "You feel ___ because ___." Be sure the first blank is filled with a true feeling word.

1. *(a 65-year-old male with early signs of dementia)* This woman is in my room and she says that she is my neighbor. I don't know who she is. She knows my name and everything, but I can't figure this out. What am I supposed to do?

2. *(a 15-year-old male diagnosed with attention deficit hyperactivity disorder)* Hey man! Don't you have anything more interesting to do in group today? This will take me 5 minutes to put together.

3. *(a 40-year-old female in recovery from heart surgery)* I've started to realize that I am getting older but I never thought that I could die so young. This whole hospitalization seems like a nightmare. When I get out of here, I'm going to take the time to enjoy my life and to spend quality time with my children.

4. *(a 55-year-old male with left hemiplegia)* I have never had to depend on anyone before. I don't know if I want to live like this. I used to take care of myself. Now look at how pathetic I am.

5. *(a 17-year-old female with anorexia)* You keep saying that I am thin but I know that I am fat. I'm tired of everyone in my family trying to shove food down my throat. How would you feel if I tried to force feed you?

6. *(a 25-year-old male with a brain injury)* There is no excitement in this place! Every day is the same old routine. I can't wait to go out on pass so that I could live it up for a few hours. It's too quiet around here for me.

statement is true about your clients. For example, if you are working with a client who was abandoned in childhood, he or she may have difficulty starting a relationship with you because it will be difficult for him or her to trust and to get close to someone. This client may also have difficulty ending sessions because saying "good-bye" may represent leaving and abandonement to him or her.

Inherent in our work, we aim to establish and role model a healthy relationship with our clients. Therefore, as OT personnel, we must recognize the importance of beginnings and endings in the therapy process as they come to represent life and death on a deeper level. Our role is to be consistent and clear with our clients during all phases of the session and the therapeutic relationship. We begin by connecting initially and attending both physically and psychologically to our clients. We end by recognizing the closing and separation process, which means letting go and reinstating a boundary between the client and therapist.

In this section, you will learn guidelines to ending a session. It is important to understand that ending a session is just as significant as establishing a rapport with our clients.

One of our functions as therapists is to be the timekeeper. OT practitioners are responsible for starting a session and ending on the designated time allotted per treatment session. There are certain points to consider about terminating a session. Consider the following guidelines.

- Remind the client that you are approaching the end of a session. *Example:* We have a few minutes left of our session today. Let's wrap up our discussion.
- Summarize the significant events of the session by either asking the client to review the session or doing this yourself. *Example:* Tell me what you learned from our treatment session today and how you plan to practice these techniques at home this week. *Example:* Today you learned specific strategies for coping with your anger that include doing physical exercise, writing in a journal, talking with someone you trust, and using assertive techniques.
- Give homework when appropriate. *Example:* I want you to do all the exercises that we performed today in your own home. Here is an exercise sheet as a reminder. You are to try and repeat each exercise 10 times every day. Do you have any questions about this?
- Refer any new topics, introduced by the client or yourself, to be discussed at the next session. Refrain from starting anything new at the end of a session. *Example:* You are asking me a very good question about strengthening your left arm. We will talk about this in more depth at our next session since we are out of time for today. I will show you some ways to exercise and strengthen the left side of your body next week.
- Evaluate the client's degree of both emotional and physical safety before terminating the session. Do not allow a client to leave your session without notifying staff or family members of your concerns for his or her safety. If a client is unsafe with you, or if you suspect that he or she may harm him- or herself when leaving your session, you must treat this situation as an emergency and notify your next appointment that you will be delayed to take care of an urgent situation.

Example: Mrs. Pratt, I am very concerned about your ability to drive home safely. I am going to notify your doctor that you are feeling extremely tired and dizzy from our treatment session today. I am also going to call your husband to see if he can pick you up since it is not a good idea to have you drive home alone. Susan, our aide, will wait here with you while I make these phone calls.

Example: I am very concerned that you have thoughts of harming yourself. If you were to hurt yourself, how would you do it ? Do you have a suicidal plan? Let's go and talk with your primary nurse on the unit and tell her how you are feeling. She can reach your doctor for you.

In summary, remember to end your sessions on time, unless your client is feeling unsafe. Model an appropriate way to say "good-bye." This will signify to the client that the session is ending and coming to a close. Whenever appropriate, you may disclose your own feelings about ending the session. For example, you may say, "This was a great session. I enjoyed working with you today," or " I am sorry that you did not progress as far as you hoped to in our session today." Remember that whenever you disclose your own feelings in sessions, you are selecting information that will be useful to your client. Admitting your own sadness about ending a therapeutic relationship is modeling appropriate feelings around leaving and separation. Crying and clinging to the client is detrimental because it suggests that you are unable to handle ending the relationship yourself. Denying that the session is actually ending is also inappropriate. Since endings are often difficult for most of us, do not hesitate to talk more subjectively about your feelings with fellow colleagues, your supervisor, or a mentor. Even when our clients have progressed and are getting better at the time of their discharge, we are often left with mixed feelings about their leaving. Take the time to work through your own feelings around termination and you will in turn be more effective with your clients

ADVANCED COMMUNICATION SKILLS

In this chapter, you have learned about communication tools and skills to establish rapport, to use during interviews, and to terminate a therapy session. There are other more advanced skills that could be used by COTAs and OTRs once a trusting relationship has been established with the client. Here is a brief summary of some of these skills.

- **Advanced Accurate Empathy.** This is a more in-depth form of basic empathy. Based on various forms of client data, OT practitioners could make an interpretation of underlying themes, hidden meanings, patterns of behaviors, and feelings.
- **Confrontation.** This skill is a form of an invitation to the client to investigate discrepancies in feelings and behaviors. It is used to allow the client to discover ambivalence and mixed messages that he or she may be giving during treatment. When used correctly, it is presented in a nonjudgmental fashion and does not create a power struggle with the therapist.
- **Immediacy.** This skill invites the client to explore the therapeutic relationship between the client and OT practitioners. It is used to explore issues around transference and countertransference that include anger, dependency, personal attractiveness, and inappropriate boundaries (i.e., ethical and moral behaviors).
- **Self-Disclosure.** This skill is used by OT practitioners who are willing to share a personal story that relates to their client's treatment issue. The purpose of self-disclosure is to give an example of new alternatives for problem solving regarding a therapeutic issue. It is important that the therapist has resolved this problem in a productive manner so that he or she may serve as a role model. Therapeutic self-disclosure is always used to benefit the client and should not be used as a way of venting one's own frustrations.

These skills are useful in the actual problem-solving process for the patient. They require further understanding and experience by OT practitioners. These skills could be found in texts included in the Bibliography.

SUMMARY

This chapter described various communication tools and skills that can be utilized by OT practitioners. These specific skills included attending and listening, respect and genuineness, open vs. closed questions, basic or primary accurate empathy, and termination. While it is necessary to understand the mechanics of using these skills, they are most effective when combined with a humanistic approach to working with the client. Establishing person-to-person contact in therapy is the key to developing a therapeutic relationship. Together, OT personnel and clients can identify and resolve problems in the helping process that are based on the inherent needs and values of the client.

BIBLIOGRAPHY

Bruce, M., & Borg, M. (1987). *Frames of reference in psychosocial occupational therapy.* Thorofare, NJ: SLACK Inc.

Cole, M. B. (1993). *Group dynamics in occupational therapy.* Thorofare, NJ: SLACK Inc.

Corey, G. (1996). *Theory and practice of counseling and psychotherapy* (5th ed.). Pacific Grove, CA: Brooks/Cole.

Davis, C. (1994). *Patient practitioner interaction: An experiential manual for developing the art of health care* (2nd ed.). Thorofare, NJ: SLACK Inc.

Egan, G. (1990). *The skilled helper* (4th ed.). Pacific Grove, CA: Brooks/Cole.

Hemphill, B. (1988). *Mental health assessment in occupational therapy.* Thorofare, NJ: SLACK Inc.

Kaplan, H., Sadock, B., & Grebb, J. (1994). *Kaplan and Sadock's synopsis of psychiatry* (7th ed.). Baltimore: Williams & Wilkins.

Yalom, I. (1985). *The theory and practice of group psychotherapy* (3rd ed.). New York: Basic Books.

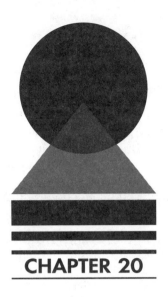

CHAPTER 20

UNIVERSAL PRECAUTIONS

Catherine Meriano, MHS, OTR/L

INTRODUCTION

Universal precautions are not only mandated by law, but more importantly, they are vital to your health and safety while working as an OT practitioner. These precautions are easily followed, but because of their simple nature, are easily forgotten as well. Unfortunately, injury or infection can occur with even one exposure to a contaminant. It is your professional responsibility to protect yourself and your patients.

TERMS TO KNOW

Before understanding the use of universal precautions, there is a set of definitions that must be reviewed. Understanding the definitions will make universal precautions easier to follow correctly. The following are basic definitions of organizations and disease processes related to universal precautions.

Occupational Safety and Health Administration (OSHA). A federal agency that was developed in 1970 with the primary objective of providing a safe work environment. Originally, OSHA was concerned with workplace injury and workplace-acquired illnesses such as chemical or environmentally induced illnesses. OSHA established voluntary guidelines for reduction of hepatitis B in 1983, and then the Bloodborne Pathogens Standard in 1991 (Gershon, Karkashian, & Felknor, 1994).

Centers for Disease Control and Prevention (CDC). A federal agency developed to record disease epidemics, assist in research, and eliminate diseases through education and the development of vaccinations. The CDC established universal precautions in 1987 for use with all blood products (Gershon et al., 1994). This became a federal law as part of the Bloodborne Pathogens Standards in 1991 (Muraskin, 1995).

Tuberculosis (TB). A life-threatening illness caused by the *Mycobacterium tubercu-*

losis, of which there are several strains. The most important of the *Mycobacterium tuberculosis* strains is the human variety. The most common location of TB infection is in the lungs, and infection is airborne or spread by coughing. Once infected, the cells become inflamed and scar tissue called nodules or tubercles are formed. The cells adjacent to these nodules begin to die leaving a fibrotic or hardened area which causes decreased lung capacity. This is a chronic disease in which phases of spread alternate with phases of healing and fibrosis. Symptoms include persistent cough and low grade fever (Walter, 1992).

Hepatitis B. An illness caused by the hepatitis B virus (HBV) which destroys cells primarily in the liver. The virus is spread through blood and body fluid exchange. Once infected, this is considered a chronic disease and the symptoms include fatigue, nausea, vomiting, low grade fever, or, in acute cases, jaundice (Walter, 1992).

Acquired Immunodeficiency Syndrome (AIDS). A life-threatening illness caused by the human immunodeficiency virus (HIV) which destroys the immune system. The virus is spread through blood and body fluid exchange. Once infected, a person is diagnosed as HIV-positive. An individual is not diagnosed with AIDS until the symptoms of AIDS are evident. The symptoms of AIDS include chronic digestive problems, pneumonia, and a skin rash called Kaposi's sarcoma. The amount of time an individual is HIV-positive before being diagnosed with AIDS is varied (Walter, 1992).

Methicillin Resistant Staphylococcus Aureus (MRSA). An illness caused by the *Staphylococcus aureus* bacteria. Commonly found in all humans, particularly in crowded areas such as hospitals (Walter, 1992), it typically infects mucous areas such as the nose or open wounds. This particular strain is most dangerous because it is resistant to traditional antibiotics and is easily spread.

Universal Precautions. A term used to describe the handling of blood products and body secretions, and the use of protective barriers. This is also called body substance precautions. Protective barriers include gloves, masks, gowns, goggles, and the ambu bags for use during CPR. It is important to be trained in the use of the ambu bag for CPR.

As a general rule, gloves should always be worn during any type of ADL treatment. If working in an acute care setting, many therapists will wear gloves with every patient treatment. Review Table 20-1 on contaminated items that OT practitioners may use. Understanding the proper disposal of items after contamination is important for safe OT treatment.

Now that the terminology is clear, the next sections will discuss responsibility of the federal government, the employer, and the employee.

FEDERAL GOVERNMENT RESPONSIBILITY

The regulations for universal precautions were established by OSHA in 1991 as stated earlier. The CDC and OSHA monitor different aspects of the regulations. OSHA monitors employer compliance and will enact penalties if regulations are not followed. OSHA has also developed a list of high risk positions based on a 1 in 1,000 chance of becoming infected at the workplace (Gershon et al., 1994). The CDC monitors exposure to any diseases while in the workplace. One such study in 1993 showed that 120 health care workers had documented or possible occupationally acquired HIV infection. The majority of the workers were nursing staff and laboratory staff, which is not surprising as the primary cause of transmission is by needlestick (Muraskin, 1995). No cases involving OT prac-

Table 20-1
Contaminated Items That OTs May Use

Contaminated Items	Possible Causes of Contamination	Universal Precautions General Guidelines
Needles	May be used with certain modalities such as iontophoresis	Do **not** recap needles. Both needle and cap are placed into a sharps container.
Safety pins	Used for sharp/dull sensory testing	Do **not** re-use. Safety pins should be put into a sharps container.
Scissors, tweezers, and scalpel	May be used during wound debridement	All items should be placed into a sharps container.
Bandages, soiled linens, or personal protective equipment	May result from wound debridement or dressing	If lightly soiled, these may be placed in a linen hamper or regular trash. If soaked with blood or contaminated body fluids, the material needs to be placed in a medical waste container. Waste containers are red or have a red label.
Blood or body fluid spill	May result from injury (cut) or incontinence/illness	Some facilities have a "spill team." Other facilities have trained the environmental services staff in proper clean-up procedures.

Note: It is important to become educated by your specific facility regarding universal precaution policies and procedures.

titioners were reported.

The actual standards set forth by OSHA can vary slightly depending on the type of facility and if more stringent state guidelines exist. For example, in the hospital setting there are containers in each room for medical waste and sharps, but dirty linen is carried through the halls to dirty linen carts or dirty linen rooms. In the nursing home setting there are fewer receptacles for medical waste and sharps because the volume is low, but dirty linen cannot be carried through the hallways. Dirty linen carts must be brought outside the resident's room and this can only be done when meal trays are not in the residents' rooms. It is best to learn the particular standards for whatever setting you are working, and for the state you are working in, but always remember the basic practices of universal precautions as stated earlier.

EMPLOYER RESPONSIBILITY

The employer's responsibility is defined by the OSHA standards. The first aspect of this responsibility is education. Employees must be provided with information regarding the use of universal precautions, personal protective equipment, and facility policies regarding disposal and cleaning of contaminated blood products and body secretions. This education is to be provided at an orientation and yearly after hire.

The second aspect is the employer's responsibility to provide the necessary personal

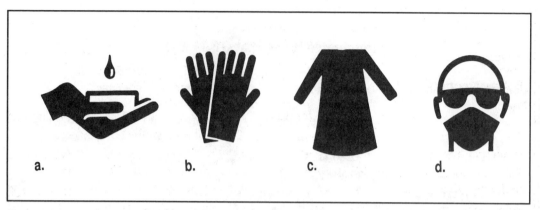

Figure 20-1. Common health care symbols. a) Wash hands. b) Gloves. c) Gown. d) Mask and eye protection.

protective equipment. These include, but are not limited to, the following: gloves, lab coats, gowns, face shields, masks, eye protection, mouth pieces, resuscitation bags, pocket masks, and other ventilation devices. The employer may also need to supply protective clothing in appropriate sizes. If an employee is allergic to latex, the employer must supply hypoallergenic gloves, glove liners, or powderless gloves in appropriate sizes. All personal protective equipment needs to be readily available for all appropriate staff. Some employers will also provide signs with symbols that can be posted outside a patient's room if extra attention toward universal precautions is warranted. This sign is universal and therefore does not breach patient confidentiality in any way. Examples of these symbols are shown in Figure 20-1. Keep in mind that if you are working in the home care setting you need to plan ahead for your needs.

The third aspect of the employer's responsibility is the availability of "employee health services." This includes a mandatory annual TB test, an optional HBV vaccine, and maintaining employee records of these shots, as well as exposures to any infectious disease. The employee health service must also offer or be able to refer a health care worker for counseling and treatment if an exposure does occur.

There are federal penalties that OSHA can use to enforce compliance by employers. These are usually monetary. Because of the risk of employee illness and lawsuits, most employers follow the regulations without the need of these penalties.

EMPLOYEE RESPONSIBILITY

The employee's responsibility is also defined by the OSHA standards. The employee must attend the educational programs offered regarding universal precautions and adhere to the infectious control/universal precaution policies.

An important area of infectious control that is vital but often overlooked is handwashing. Employees should wash their hands between each treatment and any time hands are obviously soiled. Even though gloves are worn, hand washing is still essential. The instructions in Table 20-2 will describe the proper techniques to use during handwashing.

The employee must also report any exposures to the employee health department and complete any follow-up care recommended. The employee is required to have a TB test annually. There is no vaccine for TB; this is only a test to determine if a health care work-

Table 20-2
Proper Handwashing

Steps	Rationale
Pull out a paper towel before washing.	This allows a clean paper towel to be available for drying without touching contaminated cranks.
Turn on the water and adjust the temperature to warm.	Cold water does not allow for proper cleansing.
Rub your hands and wrists vigorously under the water.	Your hands and wrists need to be thoroughly moistened.
Apply soap, and work up a good lather, making sure you cover the entire hands, wrists, fingernails and between fingers. Clean around your rings also.	Microorganisms like close spaces.
Briskly rub your entire hands together under the running water for at least 15 seconds.	You do not want the soap to become dry. You also want to scrub enough to eliminate any microorganisms on the hand and wrist surfaces.
Rinse your hands and wrists well while keeping your hands facing down.	You do not want water to run down your forearms.
Dry your hands thoroughly with the paper towel and then use the paper to turn off the water.	The faucet is contaminated and you do not want to touch it.
Throw the paper towel away without touching the wastebasket.	The wastebasket is also considered contaminated.

er has been exposed and infected with TB. Once a health care worker tests positive, there is no further need for testing as the result will always be positive. In most cases, with proper treatment of medications, an exposure will not result in TB symptoms.

The employee will have the option of a three-part series of the HBV vaccine or will need to sign a waiver to deny the vaccine. Unless contraindicated by a physician, the HBV vaccine is highly recommended. The likelihood of contracting HBV as a health care worker is far greater than the likelihood of contracting HIV. For this reason, all OT practitioners should receive the vaccination. Fieldwork sites and new employers may request verification of the HBV vaccine. Once you have completed the set of shots for the vaccine, be sure to keep a record of the vaccinations for verification.

There are no federal penalties for an individual who does not follow the universal precautions, however, most employers will terminate employment if the employee is putting him- or herself at risk. Not only is the individual taking a chance with his or her own health, but with that of the patients and co-workers. Universal precautions are taken very seriously in the health care setting and lack of compliance will not be tolerated. The majority of health care workers comply without complaint as they are aware that these regulations are in place for their safety. The areas with the lowest compliance are emergency medical service workers and emergency room personnel (Gershon et al., 1994). Unfortunately, the emergent needs of the patient cause these workers to occasionally forget their own protection.

SUMMARY

This chapter has reviewed the history, implementations, and areas of responsibilities in relation to universal precautions. These precautions have been established for the safety of both the patient population and the health care workers, and should become a "second nature" part of the therapy routine.

BIBLIOGRAPHY

Gershon, R., Karkashian, C., & Felknor, S. (1994). Universal precautions: An update. *Heart-Lung, 23,* 352-358.

Muraskin, W. (1995). The role of organized labor in combating the hepatitis B and AIDS epidemics: The fight for an OSHA bloodborne pathogens standards. *International Journal of Health Services, 25,* 129-152.

Walter, J. (1992). *An introduction to the principles of disease.* Philadelphia: W. B. Saunders.

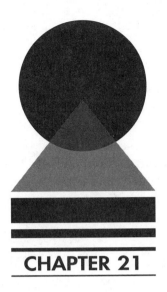

CHAPTER 21

ETHICS FOR STUDENTS

S. Maggie Reitz, MS, OTR/L

INTRODUCTION

As an OT student, it is very important to be aware of the values and the Code of Ethics of your chosen profession. This knowledge will assist you in resolving dilemmas you will encounter in both your academic and clinical experiences. This chapter will briefly describe the core values of the profession, ethical language, and the OT Code of Ethics. Following this foundation, potential ethical dilemmas commonly faced by students will be identified. A process that can be used to resolve these dilemmas will also be described.

CORE VALUES AND ATTITUDES OF OT

The AOTA has identified seven core values and attitudes of the profession (1993): altruism, equality, freedom, justice, dignity, truth, and prudence. These values and attitudes are centered on the belief that OT students and practitioners should be giving, caring, practical, honest individuals who uphold the rights and dignity of all humans. The Code of Ethics (AOTA, 1994) provides a guide which mandates how these values and attitudes are to be enacted through professional behavior.

OT CODE OF ETHICS

The Code of Ethics (AOTA, 1994) is an important reference for OT students and practitioners alike. This code stresses the professional responsibilities of OT students and practitioners and provides guidance to ensure ethical behavior. The ethical rules and principles espoused include: beneficence, autonomy, confidentiality, duty, competence, justice, veracity, and fidelity (AOTA, 1994). These principles provide guidelines for professional behavior and interactions with patients, peers, students, supervisors, supervisees, other health professionals, and faculty.

AOTA's Code of Ethics may not be the only code available to students for guidance. Frequently, OT academic departments utilize an additional separate code of ethics or there may be a college- or university-wide code of ethics. In addition, states, territories, and the District of Columbia may have regulatory boards which often have a code of ethics for practitioners in their jurisdictions. Academic OT departments and regulatory boards have often adopted AOTA's Code of Ethics or one that is very similar. It is important that students be aware of the specific ethical principles that are included in the codes which apply to them.

ETHICAL TERMINOLOGY

Terminology in a discussion of ethics can be confusing and intimidating at first. However, after learning a few basic terms, the richness and importance of ethics to the profession's ability to enact its values becomes readily apparent. During discussions of ethics in medicine and health, the terms *nonmaleficence* and *beneficence* are used. Nonmaleficence means "above all [or first] do no harm" (Beauchamp & Childress, 1989, p. 120). On the other hand, beneficence means besides not harming the patient, health care providers have a duty to remove or prevent harm, to provide a benefit or beneficial service to the patient, and to balance "benefits and harms" (Beauchamp & Childress, 1989, pp. 194-195).

The words veracity, fidelity, and duty also appear frequently in writings on ethics. These terms are similar but not identical. Veracity simply means being truthful, while fidelity means keeping your word (Beauchamp & Childress, 1989). Duty is a broad term which includes the important behaviors of meeting one's responsibilities and performing one's work competently. Specifically, for OT students this means completing the tasks required by your role as an OT student in a safe, ethical, and skilled manner.

STEPS IN RESOLVING AN ETHICAL DILEMMA

Sometimes the ethical dilemmas that students find themselves in may have been prevented by foresight, problem solving, and an awareness of the profession's core values and Code of Ethics. Here is a hypothetical example of a dilemma students can face. Two friends, Sally and Joe, are both OT students but are in different sections of an anatomy class. Sally asks Joe, who has already taken the midterm exam, what was on the exam. Trying to be a good friend, Joe describes some of the questions without thinking through the ethical issues involved or the possible ramifications of his action. Can you identify the core OT values that would be in conflict with this behavior? Are there competing values, such as friendship vs. honesty? What are the possible ramifications of these students' behaviors? Could other people, such as other students or faculty members, be impacted by Joe's and Sally's behavior? Jot down your initial thoughts (Worksheet 21-1). You will be expanding on your ideas later.

There is a process of ethical reasoning that can help organize and guide the student through problem solving ethical issues such as the one described. This process poses some of the same questions you were just asked. There are different descriptions of the steps that can be taken in the process to resolve an ethical dilemma. However, most versions are similar to the one presented in Table 21-1, which was adapted from Aroskar (1980) and used previously by me and my colleagues (Hansen, Kamp, & Reitz, 1988; Reitz, 1992).

Worksheet 21-1

Thoughts on Joe's and Sally's Behaviors

Table 21-1
Five Steps to Resolving an Ethical Dilemma

1. Gather relevant information. Possible examples: identify all individuals affected by the issue, prior history of the issue, dynamics and culture of the setting(s).
2. Determine conflicting values and areas of agreement. Possible example: commitment to patient autonomy vs. the principles of beneficence and nonmaleficence.
3. Identify as many relevant actions as possible. This process is often referred to in writings on ethics as seeking alternative courses of action.
4. Determine all possible positive and negative outcomes for each possible action. This should include outcomes for all participants in the dilemma. An ethical dilemma never involves just one person. Sometimes it takes time and thought to identify all those who may possibly have a "stake" or will be touched by a specific decision.
5. Weigh, with care, the consequences of each outcome. This step includes the process of reordering or rearranging parts of different decisions to arrive at a new alternative which may be the best possible course of action.

Adapted from Aroskar, M. (1980). Anatomy of an ethical dilemma: The practice (Part II). American Journal of Nursing, 80, 661-663.

Worksheet 21-2

Ethical Analysis Worksheet

Using either the dilemma of Sally and Joe described in the text or another dilemma, diagram your thought process as you unravel the dilemma. You may find it helpful to review two references that use this type of reasoning process before you proceed. This process is applied to clinical issues in the Hansen, Kamp, and Reitz (1988) article and to documentation issues in a chapter (Reitz, 1992) in AOTA's *Effective Documentation for Occupational Therapy* publication.

Steps to Resolve Ethical Dilemma	Notes
Gather relevant information.	
Determine conflicting values and areas of agreement.	
Identify as many relevant actions as possible.	
Determine all possible positive and negative outcomes for each possible action.	
Weigh, with care, the consequences of each outcome.	

The choice of a course of action should be based on which alternative is most consistent with the codes of ethics which apply to you, while not conflicting with your beliefs. Sometimes individuals may have difficulty weighing their personal beliefs and the OT Codes of Ethics. There are experts available to OT students and practitioners alike who can help in resolving these dilemmas in a professional and ethical manner. These resources are identified at the end of this chapter. Worksheet 21-2 is also provided for you to formally analyze the dilemma of the two students described above or another dilemma of your choosing.

COMMON ISSUES THAT OT STUDENTS FACE

It is not uncommon for OT students to face a variety of ethical dilemmas during the course of their academic careers. Table 21-2 includes a list of the more common issues which will be discussed.

Additional issues can arise during the course of the clinical portion of your education. Your fieldwork supervisors will be available to educate and assist you with ethical issues faced in fieldwork. The issues faced in fieldwork tend to be more complex and serious than those faced in academia. However, the practice and thought given to ethical issues in academia is good experience for resolving ethical issues you will face later in clinical settings.

Table 21-2
List of Common Ethical Issues in Academic Education

- Collaborating vs. Cheating
- Late Assignments and Absences
- Confidentiality
- Plagiarism
- Copyright
- Seeking Assistance From Other Faculty Members
- Use of Work Supplies for School Assignments
- Library Materials

It is also good to consider the relative seriousness of an ethical dilemma. For example, failure to return a book on time is unethical in that it impedes other students' abilities to learn and complete assignments. However, witnessing an episode of cheating and failing to report the incident is more serious. The seriousness of the issue should be taken into consideration when deciding on the amount of energy and attention to focus on the dilemma.

Collaboration Vs. Cheating

Sometimes class assignments are designed to foster collaborative teamwork where ideas are shared. This type of assignment models one type of possible future practice. Other assignments, however, are designed to provide the instructor with information regarding your current level of competence independent of others. You will not have a study group or "study buddy" present with you during your Level II fieldwork when you are evaluating and treating patients. You must be able to demonstrate independent clinical reasoning. Both types of assignments are beneficial and enhance skills to ensure that you become a competent practitioner.

It is very important for students to recognize when an assignment is a collaborative learning experience and when the assignment must be completed independently. If at any time you do not believe you understand the parameters of an assignment then you need to take the responsibility of seeking clarification from the instructor. Once you understand the parameters you must abide by them.

Late Assignments and Absences

The life of an OT student can be very busy and stressful. Most students fulfill multiple roles and have many responsibilities. Outside responsibilities can at times interfere with a student's ability to complete an assignment on time. When this happens, students are sometimes tempted to provide false information regarding the reasons for a late submission. Other times, students fail to provide any information to the faculty member, including the fact that they are not turning in an assignment that is due. This behavior is not ethical.

There are different types of reasons for missing class or failing to hand in an assignment on time. Two of these types will be discussed here:

- Lateness/absence due to lack of time and conflicting demands on one's time
- Lateness/absence due to personal illness or the death of a family member or close friend

In the first case, if you are unable to hand in a paper on time, you should let your instructor know as soon as possible. This allows you and the instructor to examine the issue together. If you do not contact the instructor early, it is imperative you communicate with the instructor at the time the paper is due. If you fail to do this, then the instructor may waste time looking for a paper to grade, fearing that the paper was inadvertently lost when, in fact, you never turned it in. There are several ways to avoid this situation. The most professional way is to see the faculty member during office hours. If this is not possible, a message should be left for the faculty member as soon as possible. In addition, you can turn in a piece of paper with your name and the fact that you are not handing in the paper when the other papers are collected. This acts as a reminder to the faculty member. You do not need to tell the instructor personal details of your life, but do not fabricate excuses and do not expect that points will not be deducted. All students should be familiar with course requirements and grading policies regarding submittal of late assignments. If you find that you are at increasing risk of not keeping up with your assignments, you need to contact your advisor regarding options early, before failure is imminent. Specific issues can be discussed and options considered.

This scenario is further complicated if other students are involved. As an OT student, you have responsibilities to your fellow students. This especially includes students with whom you are working on a group project. You have a duty to keep appointments with your group for planning and preparing the assignment as well as contributing your share of outside research.

As an OT student, you have certain duties to your peers and your instructors. For example, when you are late to class you disrupt the other students' learning. In addition, you interrupt the instructor's flow of thought. If you are unavoidably late to class, it is your responsibility to get the information already reviewed at some other time from either the instructor or your classmates. Do not expect the whole class to sit through a rehash of what has already occurred. It is also unreasonable to expect the instructor to stay after class to review what you missed, that is one of the purposes of office hours. You should not inconvenience others due to your tardiness, whether it was under your control or not.

Most OT programs and the institutions in which they are taught have policies regarding serious illness or death of a family member or significant other. Be aware of these policies. If you are aware of these policies ahead of time, it is easier to manage the situation if it should, unfortunately, arise. Sometimes documentation of an illness or death may be required.

Confidentiality

Students have frequently volunteered or worked at some type of health care setting before entering OT programs and are familiar with the need to protect the confidentiality of patient information. Its importance cannot be overly stressed. In addition, sometimes students do not think to apply this same idea to personal information that is shared in class. Due to the nature of OT education, sometimes students and instructors have personal examples that are relevant to class discussions. This information should be respected and not be used for gossip.

Plagiarism

One of the most frequently misunderstood writing skills is when and how to credit sources of information. If you did not come up with the idea you are writing about, then a citation of where the idea came from is required. Most OT schools require students to develop skills at citing sources using the format described in the 1994 edition of the *Publication Manual of the American Psychological Association* (4th ed.) by the APA. If, for example, you are writing a paper on adaptations for a patient who has had a hip fracture and you found ideas in a textbook, you must cite the chapter in the textbook. An example of this type of citation can be found on page 204 of the APA *Publication Manual* (1994). If you used a description of the type of fracture from another textbook, you also need to cite that chapter. If you referred to the incidence rate of hip fractures in older adults from a journal article in the introduction of your paper you need to reference this article as well. Examples of this type of citation can be found on pages 194 through 196 in the *Publication Manual of the American Psychological Association* (APA, 1994). Chapter 8 of this primer reviews writing papers using APA format.

It is best to paraphrase or reword material into your own words. When you do this you still must cite the source (i.e., the author and year). If you do not paraphrase, you must place the author's words in quotation marks and cite the page number along with the author and the publication date (APA, 1994). Students often think it is acceptable to avoid using quotations marks or even citing the original author if they reorder the wording of the sentence or just change one word in the middle of a sentence. This is not paraphrasing, it is plagiarism! If you have questions, seek the assistance of the instructor.

Copyright

Students should respect copyrighted material. If materials are used in a paper for a class or for a presentation, they must be appropriately referenced. If copies are going to be distributed or the materials submitted as part of a publication, permission must be obtained from the copyright holder. A brief article by Kornblau (1995) summarizes this issue.

Seeking Assistance From Other Faculty Members

Students occasionally place faculty in awkward positions by seeking assistance from one faculty member on an assignment given by another faculty member. This approach is particularly unethical if the student does not make it clear that his or her questions are part of an assignment. Open-ended questions such as, "What do you think about using a resting hand splint for a patient with arthritis?" can be perceived by a faculty member as a general quest for knowledge and the faculty member may answer the student's question in detail. If the faculty member's perceptions are accurate the student should be encouraged and applauded. However, if the student has been given this question on a take home exam or on an assignment where the directions specify that the assignment is to be done independently, then there is a significant problem. In this case, the instructor has structured the assignment in this manner to assess the student's independent clinical reasoning abilities. Asking for assistance from others in this example is unethical behavior. More directly put, it is cheating.

Students should ensure they know the parameters of an assignment. For example, is the assignment to be completed independently or are they to seek additional expert opinions and collaborate? Students should clearly present these parameters to any faculty members they seek assistance from. For example, "Our take home exam includes a question on splinting for people with arthritis. We were told that we can and should seek opinions from professors and clinicians regarding this issue. What do you think?"

Use of Work Supplies for School Assignments

The typical OT college student now works at least one part-time job. Frequently, this job provides access to a copying machine and other office supplies. Is it ethical to use this equipment and supplies for your schoolwork? It is ethical only if you have direct permission from your employer and if you do not abuse this privilege. It is unethical and illegal to use these materials without permission. Businesses and employers are increasingly policing this type of theft.

Library Materials

While performing library research, there are few things as frustrating as finding what appears to be an excellent article on your topic and then realizing that some individual has ripped out the article. It is especially frustrating when whole issues of OT journals are missing from the library. Ripping out articles or "borrowing" journals are forms of theft. Theft is illegal and unethical.

Returning library materials in a timely manner allows others to access the material and is professional behavior. This is especially true if you have a book and receive a note that it is being "recalled." A book is recalled because someone else has requested it, and needs it soon. Fines for failing to return books that have been recalled are significant. Paying these fines is your responsibility. Make sure that the library has your current address on file. Libraries send notices to you via the filed address in order to notify you that a book is being recalled. Keeping your current local address on file at the library, therefore, can save you from having to pay a costly library fine.

RESOURCES TO RESOLVE ETHICAL DILEMMAS

It is important to realize that regardless of the ethical issue there are resources, both printed materials as well as experts, to assist and support you through the process of resolving an ethical dilemma. As a student it is important that you are aware of these resources. Reviewing professional periodicals is a way of keeping abreast of ethical issues. Articles from a variety of OT publications have recently appeared that discuss ethical issues involving student recruitment (Kyler-Hutchison, 1996), behavior at professional meetings (Stancliff, 1996), and making a career change (Reitz, Melvin, & Winkler, 1996). Resource persons include your faculty advisor; your fieldwork supervisors, both at the academic and clinical sites; the president of your state or local OT association; members of your state regulatory board; AOTA's ethics program manager at the national AOTA office; the chairperson of AOTA's Standards and Ethics Committee; and the National Board for Certification in Occupational Therapy. Most issues that students face can be resolved independently or with the assistance of faculty. However, if the ethical dilemma is of a very complex or highly serious nature (e.g., student observed fraud or patient neglect), then faculty can assist the student in determining which resources would be most appropriate to contact for additional assistance.

SUMMARY

This chapter has focused on introducing you to the language of ethics and alerted you to possible dilemmas you may face in your student role, primarily involving academic issues. Related ethical issues can arise during your fieldwork experiences. Remember that ethical dilemmas are part of everyday life and are best addressed early, directly, and honestly.

As an OT student and future OT practitioner, you have the responsibility to embrace AOTA's seven core values and attitudes, and to uphold the OT Code of Ethics. The profession's values and ethics are important tools that facilitate competent role performance as a student and a future clinician. Use them well.

BIBLIOGRAPHY

American Psychological Association. (1994). *Publication Manual of the American Psychological Association* (4th ed.). Washington, DC: Author.

American Occupational Therapy Association. (1993). Core values and attitudes of occupational therapy practice. *American Journal of Occupational Therapy, 47,* 1086.

American Occupational Therapy Association. (1994). Occupational therapy code of ethics. *American Journal of Occupational Therapy, 48,* 1037-1038.

Aroskar, M. (1980). Anatomy of an ethical dilemma: The practice (Part II). *American Journal of Nursing, 80,* 661-663.

Bailey, D. M., & Schwartzberg, S. L. (1995). *Ethical and legal dilemmas in occupational therapy.* Philadelphia: F. A. Davis.

Beauchamp, T. L., & Childress, J. F. (1989). *Principles of biomedical ethics* (3rd ed.). New York: Oxford University Press.

Hansen, R. A., Kamp, L., & Reitz, S. (1988). Two practitioners' analyses of occupational therapy practice dilemmas. *American Journal of Occupational Therapy, 42,* 312-319.

Kornblau, B. (1995, June 26). Who has the legal rights to written materials? [Legal Line]. *ADVANCE for OTs,* 4.

Kyler-Hutchison, P. (1996, February 22). The role of the educator: Ethical implications in recruiting. *OT Week,* 11.

Purtillo, R. (1993). *Ethical dimensions in the health professions* (2nd ed.). Philadelphia: W. B. Saunders.

Reitz, S. (1992). Ethical issues in documentation. In J. D. Acquaviva (Ed.), *Effective documentation for occupational therapy* (pp. 219-229). Rockville, MD: American Occupational Therapy Association.

Reitz, S. M., Melvin, J. A., & Winkler, L. (1996, May). Ethical guidelines for making a change. *OT Practice,* 32-37.

Stancliff, B. L. (1996, April). Conference ethics etiquette. *OT Practice,* 32-37.

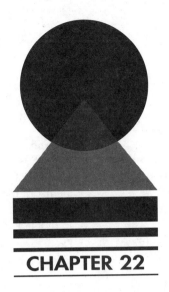

CHAPTER 22

CLINICAL SKILLS: PRECAUTIONS AND TECHNIQUES

Catherine Meriano, MHS, OTR/L

INTRODUCTION

This chapter will address multiple miscellaneous areas related to the treatment of persons with disabilities or injuries. At first glance, it may seem relevant only to those therapists working in a physical disabilities setting, but even if a therapist is working in a mental health setting this information will be useful. There are more and more individuals treated in mental health settings who also have physical limitations. Ethically, you cannot have tunnel vision in any specialty area, as we are all treating people, not a diagnosis.

GENERAL PRECAUTIONS

When certain behaviors or special conditions are dangerous to your patient, the patient is put on "precautions." Table 22-1 is a listing of precautions that are necessary to know despite what specialty area you choose to work in. These are only the most basic precautions. It is important that you establish the needs and precautions of each individual client through discussions with the physician and the treatment team. Understanding patient precautions will keep patients safe.

Table 22-1
Precautions

Precaution	Definition
• Cardiac: Used for individuals who have high blood pressure, or any history of cardiac illness or surgeries.	• Do not use isometric or heavy resistive exercises. Do not exercise above the level of the heart. Monitor blood pressure, heart rate, and fatigue. (See text below regarding how to monitor blood pressure and heart rate.)
• Fatigue: Used for individuals who have been diagnosed with any type of progressive neuromuscular disease such as multiple sclerosis (MS), amyotrophic lateral sclerosis (ALS), and post-polio syndrome.	• Do not use heavy resistive exercises because fatigue can cause progression of these illnesses rather than improvement. Avoid treatment in extreme heat or cold.
• Total Hip: Used for individuals who have had a total hip replacement.	• Do not bend the hip past 90 degrees of flexion, adduct hip (cross legs), or internally rotate hip. These can cause the new hip to dislocate.
• Weightbearing: Used with individuals who have had surgery or an injury to a leg.	• These are fully described in this chapter.
• Universal: Used with every individual.	• Please see Chapter 20 on universal precautions.

CARDIAC PRECAUTIONS

In order to complete the cardiac precautions listed in Table 22-1, you must be able to check your client's heart rate and blood pressure. The heart rate of an individual is usually taken at the radial pulse for adults and the brachial pulse for infants. If a radial pulse is difficult to find, the carotid pulse can be used. The radial pulse is located on the radial, palmer surface of the wrist. The brachial pulse is located on the anterior surface of the elbow. The carotid pulse is located on either side of the neck. All heart rate checks are completed with only the index and middle fingers placed gently over the areas described above. If too much pressure is applied, the circulation is stopped. It is best to check a heart rate for 60 seconds rather than 15 or 30 seconds and multiplying the number. A normal heart rate in the adult is 80 to 120 beats per minute. There are a variety of formulas to establish the exercise "target heart rate," but each individual will have his or her own "normal" and it is important to establish a baseline and exercise parameters prior to any treatment sessions.

A normal blood pressure of an individual under the age of 40 is considered to be 140/90 or under. A normal blood pressure of an individual over the age of 40 is considered to be 160/90 or under. Remember that the top number is called *systolic*, and is defined as the reading of the pressure that results from the heart contracting to pump blood into the arteries. The bottom number is called *diastolic*, and is defined as the reading of the pressure as the heart relaxes between contractions. There are individuals who complete their daily activities with high blood pressure, or hypertension, and those who function well despite having low blood pressure, or hypotension. For this reason, it is

Table 22-2
Taking a Blood Pressure Reading

Position the client	Either sitting or lying is acceptable as long as the client is comfortable.
Position the arm	Roll up the sleeve past the elbow. Support the arm on a surface or your hip with the palm facing upward.
Prepare the blood pressure cuff	Open the cuff and loosen the thumbscrew. Press the cuff to release all the air. Wrap the cuff around the arm so it is tight, but comfortable.
Place the stethoscope	Find the brachial pulse at the anterior elbow with your fingers. Place the stethoscope over the brachial pulse and hold it in place with your hand. Place the earpieces in your ears.
Inflate the cuff	Tighten the thumbscrew and pump the bulb to inflate the cuff. Stop when the pulse sound stops. Loosen the thumb screw slowly.
Systolic pressure	Read the number when you hear the first noise. It will sound like a heartbeat.
Diastolic pressure	Read the number when the noise stops.

vital that the proper exercise parameters are established on an individual basis with the client's physician. If abnormal blood pressure is noted during a therapy session, it is always best to stop the session and notify the physician immediately.

When taking a blood pressure, you will need a blood pressure cuff, or sphygmomanometer, and a stethoscope. Table 22-2 provides a set of directions which will define the proper method of taking a blood pressure reading.

WEIGHTBEARING PRECAUTIONS

Whether using an ambulation device, a wheelchair, or no equipment for mobility, you must know each individual's weightbearing precautions. These precautions must be followed during transfers and ambulation. It is the responsibility of the physician to establish these precautions, and the responsibility of the therapist and the nursing staff to reinforce these precautions. The following is a list of the most common weightbearing precautions and their corresponding abbreviations.

- **Non-weightbearing (NWB).** No weight can be applied to the affected leg.
- **Toe touch weightbearing (TTWB).** Weight should not be applied to the affected leg, but the toe can touch the floor for balance purposes only.
- **Partial weightbearing (PWB).** A small portion of weight can be applied to the affected leg.
- **Weightbearing as tolerated (WBAT).** Weight can be applied as the individual's pain tolerance will allow.
- **Full weightbearing (FWB).** There are no restrictions for applying weight to the affected leg.

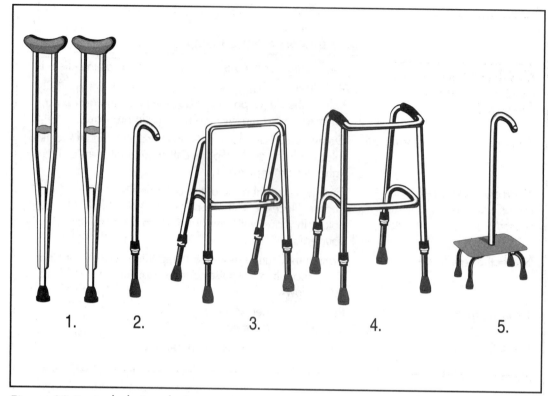

1.   2.   3.   4.   5.

Figure 22-1. Ambulation devices.

MOBILITY

Most new graduates of OT programs are surprised at how much mobility is required during OT sessions. Walking or wheelchair use is required during ADLs training, homemaking training, work hardening, and many types of functional activities. Before you begin any type of activity that requires walking or wheelchair mobility, there is basic information that you must know. The following sections cover these topics, which include ambulation devices and use, wheelchair parts, and wheelchair use. Figure 22-1 and Table 22-3 will describe ambulation devices and the use of these devices.

WHEELCHAIR

There are a multitude of possible configurations for wheelchair parts. Many of these possibilities are custom made for a particular individual and are usually costly. When ordering a custom wheelchair for a person, it is best to consult a rehabilitation specialist who has the experience and the training to provide the best possible solutions for the individual's seating deficits. This specialist may be located at a rehabilitation facility or may be a vendor of wheelchairs. It is your responsibility as the referring therapist to investigate the qualifications of this specialist before spending your client's time and money on a wheelchair. It is also essential that you and all the treatment team members participate in the design of the wheelchair. Each discipline within the team will be able to offer a different viewpoint of the client's needs to the specialist.

When a standard chair is required, there are also several options that need considera-

---

Table 22-3
Ambulation Devices and Uses

Ambulation Device Name	Proper Use
Number 1: Crutches. A person can use one or two.	Three point (two crutches and one leg) use is for a person who cannot use one leg (e.g., broken leg). The crutches are brought forward and the person swings the strong leg through, never allowing the injured leg to bear weight.
Number 2: Standard cane. A person can use one or two. Typically one cane only is used.	The cane is used opposite the injury. If the left leg is injured, than the cane is usually held in the right hand. The proper sequence for ambulation is cane, weak leg, strong leg.
Number 3: Hemiwalker.	The hemiwalker is used opposite the injury. This provides greater support than canes, but less than a walker. These are typically used when a person cannot hold a walker with both hands due to weakness. The proper sequence for ambulation is hemiwalker, weak leg, strong leg.
Number 4: Walker.	The walker is placed directly in front of the person and is held with both hands. The person's body should always be inside the walker when an ambulation sequence has been completed. The proper sequence for ambulation is walker, weak leg, strong leg.
Number 5: Quad cane. This variation of the cane allows greater stability than a standard cane because it has four small feet protruding off the base of the cane. There are two varieties named small-based quad cane (SBQC) and large-based quad cane (LBQC).	The quad cane is used in the same manner as a standard cane. This is held in the hand opposite the injured leg and has a sequence of cane, weak leg, strong leg.

---

tion. In most cases, an OT practitioner can order a standard chair without difficulty. Examine Figure 22-2, which shows a wheelchair labeled with the most common wheelchair parts. Table 22-4 describes the parts shown in Figure 22-2, and some options available on a standard wheelchair.

Lastly, examine Table 22-5, which describes the proper technique to measure a client for a wheelchair.

ADLS

As an OT practitioner, you may be involved in ADLs, or activities of daily living, training. The following sections will instruct you in the proper sequencing of bathing and dressing. It is vital that the client's modesty and safety are considered constantly throughout each ADL session. It is also important to realize that bathing and dressing can and will cause fatigue to the client. Most of us take for granted the ease with which we get

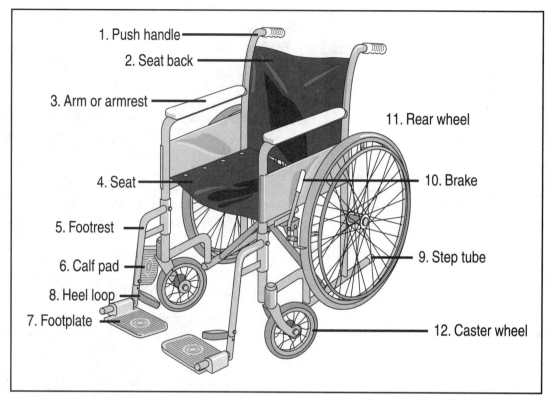

Figure 22-2. Parts of a wheelchair.

ready every morning to start the day. Cardiac and fatigue precautions all need to be incorporated into the ADL training session.

These instructions are primarily focused on ADL training in a chair. Bathing and/or dressing in bed is possible, but not ideal. Getting washed and dressed in a chair or wheelchair is much more functional in most cases and usually preferred by the clients. For this reason it is important to be aware of the weightbearing precautions discussed earlier as you transfer a client out of bed and into a chair.

Bathing

The following list of directions describes a recommended sequence for bathing in a chair. Bathing in bed would be the same, except when washing the buttocks the client will need to roll to the side.

1. Uncover the upper one-half of the body and allow the patient to wash the face, chest, arms, and stomach.
2. Cover the upper one-half of the body and uncover the lower extremities. Allow the patient to wash the lower extremities.
3. If the client has good standing balance, he or she stands to wash the genitals and buttocks. If your client appears uncomfortable with the terms genitals or buttocks, you can use terms such as private parts or backside, but remember that you are the professional and should not use derogatory terminology even if the client uses this terminology. If the client has poor standing balance, it is best to wash these areas in bed before getting into the chair.

Table 22-4	
Wheelchair Parts and Options	
Number 1: Push handle	This is the handle that is held by someone pushing the wheelchair.
Number 2: Seat back	The back of the chair can be custom made for different widths, heights, and textures.
Number 3: Arm or armrest	Choices include desk length, which are short or full length, fixed or removable, pull off or swing away, and can be custom fit for height.
Number 4: Seat	The seat of the chair can be custom made for depth, width, and length. Cushions can be added for skin protection, comfort, or positioning.
Number 5: Footrest	Choices include elevating or fixed, removable or fixed, and the length is adjustable.
Number 6: Calf pad	These are optional and serve the purpose of keeping the leg on the footrest. Heel loops serve the same purpose.
Number 7: Footplate	Provides a footrest and properly positions the ankle when used correctly.
Number 8: Heel loop	These are optional and serve the purpose of keeping the leg on the footrest. Calf pads serve the same purpose.
Number 9: Step tube	This is where a "helper" should step while pulling back on the pull handle to get a wheelchair up onto a curb. With pressure placed on the step tube the caster wheels should come off the ground.
Number 10: Brake	Located on each rear wheel to stabilize the wheelchair during transfers. Brake extenders are also available to allow the person with a hemiplegia to reach both brakes with one hand.
Number 11: Rear wheel	The larger wheels on a standard wheelchair. If the client propels him- or herself, there is an inner ring to propel with. If the client has a hemiplegia and propels him- or herself, there will be two inner rings: one for turning right and one for turning left.
Number 12: Caster wheel	The smaller wheels on a standard wheelchair.

4. Cover the lower one-half of the body.
5. Complete grooming in the chair (hair, teeth/denture care, etc.).

Dressing

The following list of directions describes a recommended sequence for dressing in a chair. Dressing in bed would be the same, except when hiking the pants the client will need to roll from side to side or "bridge" his or her hips. The first set of directions is for a client who has a hemiplegia.

Table 22-5 **How to Measure for a Standard Wheelchair**	
Wheelchair seat and back width	Measure across the hips and thighs at the widest part and add 2 inches. If using a seat cushion, add the width of the cushion.
Seat depth	Measure from the most posterior aspect of the buttocks, along the thigh, to the posterior, proximal knee bend. Subtract 2 to 3 inches so that the knee does not touch the front of the seat. If using a back (lumbar) cushion, add the width of the cushion.
Seat height	Measure from the posterior, proximal knee bend to the heel and add 2 inches so that the knee does not touch the front of the seat. If using a seat cushion, add half the height of the cushion.
Back height	Measure from the wheelchair seat to the axilla and subtract 4 inches to allow movement of the upper extremities. If using a seat cushion, add half the height of the cushion.
Armrest height	Measure from the wheelchair seat to the elbow while flexed at 90 degrees. If using a seat cushion, add half the height of the cushion.
Footrest height	Measure from the posterior, proximal knee bend to the heel and add 1 inch. If using a seat cushion, subtract half the height of the cushion.

Donning a Shirt: "Pullover" Method

This can be used with pullover or button-down shirts.

1. Position the shirt on the lap with the collar on the lap and the tag facing upward.
2. Create a "well" within the affected arm shirt sleeve to put the affected arm into.
3. Place the affected hand into the "well" using the unaffected arm.
4. Pull the sleeve up over the affected elbow.
5. Put the unaffected arm into its sleeve.
6. Gather into the unaffected hand and raise the shirt over the head.
7. Straighten the shirt.
8. Fasten the buttons.

Donning a Shirt: "Wrap Around" Method

This can be used with button-down shirts only.

1. Position the shirt and don the affected arm sleeve as in steps 1 through 4 above.
2. With the unaffected arm, grab the tag or the collar on the unaffected side of the shirt.
3. Bring the unaffected arm over and behind the head to pull the shirt around to the unaffected arm.
4. Place the unaffected arm into the shirt sleeve.
5. Straighten the shirt.
6. Fasten the buttons.

Donning Pants

1. Cross the affected leg over the unaffected leg at the knee.
2. Place the pants over the affected foot.
3. Allow the foot to return to the floor and pull up the pants past the affected foot.
4. Place the unaffected leg into the pants and pull up the pants as far as possible while sitting.
5. If there is any function in the affected hand, hook a belt loop or hold the pocket to keep the pants from falling when standing.
6. Stand and hike the pants. If the client has good standing balance, he or she should remain standing to zip and button/snap the pants. If the client has poor standing balance, he or she should sit in the chair to zip and button/snap the pants.

Donning Shoes and Socks

1. Socks can be put on following the same sequence of crossing the legs as described for donning pants.
2. Shoes can also be put on by crossing the legs, or can be placed on the floor. When placed on the floor, the affected foot is lifted by the unaffected arm and placed into the shoe. The unaffected foot steps into the shoe. Elastic laces or closures are commonly used to avoid tying laces.

Donning a Brassiere: "Pullover" Method

1. Hook the brassiere and place it on the lap facing down.
2. Place the affected arm into the strap.
3. Place the unaffected arm into the strap.
4. Pull the hooked area up and over the head.
5. Straighten.

Donning a Brassiere: "Wrap Around" Method

1. Tuck the brassiere into the unaffected side waistband.
2. Reach behind the body with the unaffected arm and bring the brassiere around the back.
3. Hook the brassiere in front and slide it around to the back.
4. Place the affected arm into the strap.
5. Place the unaffected arm into the strap.
6. Straighten.

Donning Ankle Foot Orthosis (AFO)

An AFO is used to compensate for a foot drop.

1. Place the AFO into the shoe.
2. Lift the affected leg with the unaffected arm and place it into the shoe. Make sure the heel is lined up with the back of the AFO.
3. Pull on the AFO like a shoehorn and push on the affected knee with the unaffected arm. Repeat this until the foot is completely inside the shoe.
4. Fasten the AFO calf strap.
5. Fasten the shoe.

The next set of directions is specifically for the client who has had a total hip replacement. Upper extremity dressing is usually not an issue as the upper extremities are unaffected by the surgery. Before reading these, it may be beneficial to review the total hip replacement precautions listed in Table 22-1.

Donning Pants

1. Using a reacher, hook a belt loop or clamp the top of the pants.
2. Lower the pants to the affected foot being careful not to bend the hip past 90 degrees.
3. Place the affected foot into the pant leg and pull the pants up with the reacher until within arm's reach. Remember not to bend the hip past 90 degrees.
4. Place the unaffected leg into the pant leg.
5. Pull the pants up as far as possible while sitting.
6. Stand and hike the pants.
7. If the client has good standing balance, he or she should remain standing to zip and button/snap the pants. If the client has poor standing balance, sit in the chair to zip and button/snap the pants.

Donning Shoes and Socks

1. Place the sock on a sock aid.
2. Lower the sock aid to the affected foot by holding onto the ropes.
3. Place the affected foot into the sock aid and pull the sock on by pulling the ropes.
4. Place the unaffected foot into the sock by bending the unaffected leg. Do not bend forward because this will also bend the affected hip.
5. Place the shoes on the floor and step into them by bending the knees. A long shoehorn may be useful.
6. Elastic laces or closures can be useful temporarily for shoe tying until hip flexion is allowed.

All of the hemiplegic and total hip replacement dressing techniques will work correctly in reverse for undressing.

BIBLIOGRAPHY

Christiansen, C., & Baum, C. (Eds.). (1991). *Occupational therapy: Overcoming human performance deficits.* Thorofare, NJ: SLACK Inc.

Foti, D., Pedretti, L., & Pedretti, L. (1996). Activites of daily living. In L. P. Pedretti (Ed.), *Occupational therapy practice skills for physical dysfunction.* St. Louis, MO: Mosby.

U.S. Department of Health and Human Services. (1995). *Post-stroke rehabilitation clinical practice guidelines.* Rockville, MD: Agency for Health Care Policy and Research.

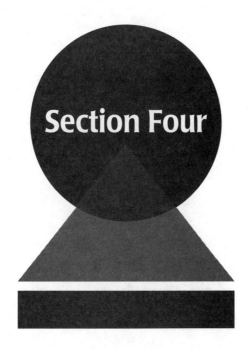

Section Four

Transition Skills

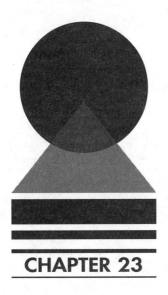

CHAPTER 23

FIELDWORK CHALLENGES

Mary Alicia Barnes, OTR/L
Mary E. Evenson, MPH, OTR/L

INTRODUCTION

Your fieldwork experience is a vital part of your professional education. It is viewed as a "critical link," bridging classroom learning to the realities of service delivery. This is often referred to as the application of theory to practice (Cohn & Crist, 1995). Fieldwork provides you the opportunity to interact with professionals and clients from diverse backgrounds. You are exposed to a variety of concepts, approaches to practice, and treatment settings. It is a unique opportunity to learn about professional cultures, therapeutic relationships, and the art and science of practice. Your fieldwork experience helps to shape your knowledge, attitudes, and skills in OT as one of the first steps in your path of career development and lifelong learning. This process involves pulling together self-awareness, life experience, and academic information while engaging in practical applications of these bodies of knowledge. A key component of this process is developing "a set of attitudes and feelings" (Fidler, 1966, p. 2) which will enhance your ability to think critically and creatively, and to function collaboratively. These capacities are considered by many to be the foundation for professional development (Cohn & Crist, 1995; Crist, 1995; Fidler & Gerney, 1994; Hughes & Opacich, 1990; Kasar, 1994).

The following information aims to help prepare you to meet the challenges of fieldwork. This chapter addresses the shift from classroom to clinic, supervision, domains of learning and practice, coping with student role transitions, and dealing with fieldwork-related problems. Thoughtful reflection and completion of the learning exercises and activities in the areas of the therapeutic use of self, professional development, and the affective domain of learning can guide you in gaining a greater sense of self-awareness. Engaging in this process can help you to anticipate and monitor your personal and professional preparation for effectively engaging in your fieldwork education. Information discussed in previous chapters is referred to as it is integral to the fieldwork experience.

CLASSROOM TO CLINIC: KNOW WHERE YOU ARE GOING

It is important to realize and recognize that there are distinct differences between academic and clinical environments. Academic settings see their main purpose as conveying knowledge and facilitating creative thinking, whereas clinical settings focus on providing services to clients and families. In that the academic program sees its mission as serving the students' needs, the clinic directs its attention to the business of service delivery. While in school, a student is accountable to him- or herself. However, once in the clinic, expectations are that you be accountable to clients, their families/caregivers, your supervisor, and others in that setting.

Academic settings may be adaptable to student and/or faculty needs and have some control over the amount of work and work pace. For example, in an academic setting, workloads may be timed in regard to midterms and finals, as well as other assignments and break periods. This structure and your syllabi can assist you with planning and time management. In the clinic, workload and pace fluctuate for a number of reasons, such as census or caseload, clients' needs, site regulations, and resources to manage the demands. Since serving clients is the primary focus, students may perceive the clinic as less adaptable or flexible in comparison to their academic program.

Depending upon the students' personal obligations and simultaneous role demands, there can be benefits and trade-offs for the schedule requirements of either the academic or clinical environment. For example, for students used to a set schedule, learning to adjust to the schedule changes of classes may be difficult. However, for students used to free time between classes, adjusting to a full-time work schedule in the clinic may take some effort. In terms of understanding a system's culture or dynamics, in settings where the medical model prevails, the health care professionals may be seen as support services and students may be quite removed from the chain of command. For students with previous professional experience, this status change may be confusing and/or frustrating.

Another significant difference between the academic and clinical environments is in the student to instructor ratio. There are generally many students per instructor in a classroom setting, which may limit opportunities for direct interaction. In the clinic, this ratio may be as small as 1:1, which can result in increased opportunities for direct interaction with the clinical educator/supervisor and a sense of closer scrutiny. In addition, in school, students primarily receive grades as a source of feedback. In a clinical environment, feedback may be provided verbally (and/or nonverbally) on an ongoing basis from clients, families, and other staff. It also is provided with varying degrees of frequency, both verbally and/or nonverbally, as well as in writing from your supervisor. Furthermore, a student's performance is publicly observed. It may be observed by the entire health care team, especially at team meetings. Most notably, your performance has a direct impact on the client, who may potentially offer the most immediate, as well as meaningful and relevant, feedback.

Primary learning tools in the academic setting include books, readings, lectures, audiovisual materials, case studies, small group projects, labs, observations, and simulations. Clinically, learning is situation based and, at times, self-directed. It is provided through interacting and problem solving with clients, families, and other professionals. In general, classroom learning tends to be more passive, set up by the structure of the syllabus, course objectives, and assignments, whereas clinic learning is more active. It is part of a dynamic process of engaging with others, gathering data, and problem solving while providing treatment. This is commonly referred to as "thinking on your feet" (Crist, 1995, p. 5). Typically, the learning process shifts from teacher-directed to self-directed. Therefore, as a student, you have increasing responsibility to assess your existing knowledge and, if necessary, utilize resources to enhance your knowledge base.

Part of this shift involves understanding more subtle, qualitative differences in learning and self-management. In doing so, it is important to consider your skills in self-management (see Chapter 10). In school, knowledge may be demonstrated through recall of facts or theoretical information. The need or opportunity to ask questions or formulate opinions may not always arise. Clinically, it is expected that you ask questions, seek needed information, problem solve, and collaborate. Academically, you may demonstrate understanding through written assignments without having to verbally present your opinion or information. Time may be given for analysis of information and in-depth explanation about what you think and why. In a clinical setting, being able to assert and express yourself clearly and succinctly, verbally and in writing, is crucial.

One of the most difficult variables to ascertain is your tolerance for ambiguity or uncertainty. In academic settings, instructors may have a high threshold for tolerating ambiguity, whereas for students seeking the "right" answer, this lack of certainty may be difficult to accept. In the clinic, the client may become anxious when faced with uncertainty about his or her future, whereas the professional's tolerance may vary greatly, depending upon the setting or situation. Learning to bear this ambiguity may take time.

The transition from the classroom to the clinic is clearly a major change that involves moving from the student role to that of an entry-level practitioner. It is a time to examine your understanding of OT philosophy, as well as theories, ideas, and techniques learned in school. It is also a period of continued self-reflection and learning about yourself as an individual, an adult learner, and an aspiring OT practitioner.

Crist (1995) states that the primary skills of the successful practitioner in today's rapidly changing health care environment include the ability to "...take responsibility, act dependably, be accountable, adaptable, resourceful, and ethical in decision-making" (p. 5). Crist feels that these skills, in conjunction with a strong academic knowledge base, will empower and enable you as a therapist to adapt your clinical skills to the demands or needs of a specific work environment.

Fieldwork is an opportunity to practice these skills, most notably, communication, self-direction, time management, and active problem solving, within the context of the treatment relationship and session (Crist, 1995). It is also a crucial time to begin the vital process of preparing, refining, and communicating your conceptualization and definition of OT which can be adapted to any environment in which you are working. The characteristics of the successful fieldwork student include themes of flexibility, adaptability, doing, risk taking/active experimentation, teamwork, communication, and delay of gratification (Crist, 1995; Herzberg, 1994). Depending upon your personality, experience, and learning style, these qualities may come easily to some and require significant effort and attention on the part of others.

KNOW THE EXPECTATIONS

Level I Fieldwork

The Accreditation Council for Occupational Therapy Education's (ACOTE) *Essentials and Guidelines for Accredited Educational Programs* (1995a, 1995b) for both OT and OTA describes Level I fieldwork as experiences intended to enhance coursework through guided observation and selected participation in various aspects of the OT process.

Generally, Level I fieldwork offers students practice-related experiences which are usually integrated throughout the academic program. The overall purpose of the Level I fieldwork experience is to provide students with exposure to the values and traditions of OT practice through observation of and interaction with a variety of populations and personnel. This may occur with "incapacitated or well populations; age-specific or diagnosis specific clients" (Commission on Education [COE], 1992a, p. 1). Supervision can be provided by academic or clinical OT personnel. Supervision may also be provided by other professionals such as teachers, nurses, social workers, physical therapists, etc. (ACOTE, 1995a, 1995b). Through these experiences, you have the opportunity to examine your reactions to clients, systems, related personnel, and potential role(s) within the profession.

Level I fieldwork can be an opportunity for building skills in observation, activity/occupation analysis (Nelson, 1996), and clinical reasoning. It may be seen as a beginning phase in your professional growth and development. Mission, program philosophy, performance expectations, and specific objectives of the Level I fieldwork experience vary throughout each academic program. Therefore, the timing, length, requirements, and specific foci of the Level I fieldwork experience are negotiated with each academic program on an individual basis (COE, 1992a).

Level II Fieldwork: Guidelines for the OTA

The purpose of Level II fieldwork is "to provide in-depth experiences in delivering OT services and to develop and expand a repertoire of OT practice" (ACOTE, 1995b, p. 10). Students are required to complete the equivalent of 12 weeks or 440 total hours of Level II fieldwork on a full-time basis "with various groups across the life span, persons with various psychosocial and physical performance deficits, and various service delivery models reflective of current practice" (ACOTE, 1995b, p. 10). Within the 12-week period, there should be opportunities for practice of entry-level roles which are "supervised by an OTR or COTA with a minimum of 1 year of experience" (ACOTE, 1995b, p.10). The student's schedule should align with that of the on-site supervisor, depending upon the state's licensure law regarding direct supervision. All fieldwork should be completed within 18 months of the date of successful completion of the academic program. Overall, participating in a Level II fieldwork frequently involves a commitment commensurate to a full-time job.

Level II Fieldwork: Guidelines for the OT

The purpose of Level II fieldwork is to:

Promote clinical reasoning and reflective practice, to transmit the values and beliefs that enable the application of ethics related to the profession, to communicate and model professionalism as a developmental process and a career responsibility, and to develop and expand a repertoire of OT assessments and treatment interventions related to human performance. (ACOTE, 1995a, p. 10)

Students are required to complete the equivalent of 6 months or 940 total hours of Level II fieldwork on a full-time basis with various persons throughout the life span, including those with psychosocial and physical problems impacting their performance and ability to function. The fieldwork should occur in settings with "service delivery models reflective of current practice" (ACOTE, 1995a, p. 11). Within the 6-month period, there should be opportunities for practice of entry-level roles which are supervised by an "OTR, with a minimum of 1 year of experience" (ACOTE, 1995a, p. 11). If equivalent time is used, it should be "appropriate to the setting selected, student needs, and continuity of client services, (e.g., consecutive half days)" (ACOTE, 1995a, p. 11). The student's schedule should align with that of the on-site supervisor, depending upon the state's licensing law regarding direct supervision. All fieldwork should be completed within 24 months of the date of successful completion of the academic program. Overall, participating in a Level II fieldwork frequently involves a commitment commensurate to a full-time job.

CERTIFICATION

Students must successfully complete both the academic and fieldwork components of the curriculum to meet eligibility requirements to sit for the Certification Examination for Occupational Therapists and Occupational Therapy Assistants, administered semi-annually by the National Board of Certification in Occupational Therapy.

EVALUATION OF STUDENT PERFORMANCE ON LEVEL II FIELDWORK

Formally, the AOTA (1983, 1987) has developed standardized fieldwork evaluation forms for the OTA and OT. The Fieldwork Evaluation (FWE) is the instrument adopted by the AOTA to evaluate and formally rate OT student performance in all fieldwork education centers. It is strongly recommended that you consult your academic program fieldwork coordinators and faculty/instructors to find out how you can become familiar with these forms prior to your fieldwork experience.

The FWE for the OTA consists of two sections. The first section consists of 24 behavioral statements depicting competent performance in four areas reflecting the domains of practice: evaluation, treatment, communication, and professional behavior. Each competency is evaluated based upon the percent of time that the desired behavior is demonstrated. Generally, the form instructs the rater to justify any scoring at the high (96% to 100% of the time) or low (0% to 20% of the time) ends of the scale. Space is reserved for the rater's comments and justifications of high/low scores. The second section is reserved for additional comments which might include information about caseload, strengths, weaknesses, and your potential in the area of practice related to the fieldwork experience. The AOTA outlines the standards as: "The highest possible total score is 120, appropriate for students exceptional in every way. The score achieved by a student who attains *normal* or *expected* competence in every item is 94" (AOTA, 1983, p. 16).

The FWE for the OT also consists of two sections. The first section has 51 behavioral statements depicting competent performance in five areas which reflect the scope of practice: assessment, planning, treatment, problem solving, and administration/professionalism. Each competency is evaluated on the basis of performance, judgment, and attitude. The rating scale ranges from excellent (5) to poor (1). The rating "good" or "3" on the rating scale is considered entry-level performance. The second section is a written summary of performance indicating particular strengths, areas for growth, and any other information useful in documenting professional growth and learning experience(s).

The purposes of student performance appraisals encompass a variety of objectives. Their primary purpose is to help determine a student's current level of functioning, including what you are doing well and areas needing improvement. Also, it is important to use this time as a sounding board to clarify whether your perceptions of performance match those of your supervisor. Through this process, change or improvement can be facilitated by the development of a plan that identifies possible barriers to performance and outlines specific learning needs as well as ways to address them.

The FWE is designed to assess students' performance upon completion of their fieldwork experience. The *Guidelines for Occupational Therapy Fieldwork* (COE, 1992b) encourage supervisors to evaluate and keep students informed of their performance status on an ongoing basis. The FWE can also be used at the midpoint of the experience, or as needed, as a means to check and document satisfactory/unsatisfactory student progress.

The FWE process should be carried out with consideration given to all legal and ethical implications. These implications include the right to non-prejudicial evaluation, the right to privacy of information, and the right to appeal. Overall, a passing score on the FWE certifies that the student is competent and signifies a readiness for entry-level practice. The FWE may become part of your official academic record. Most academic programs regard fieldwork as a pass/fail grade. However, students should be aware of their specific academic program's policies relating to criteria for grading.

HOPES AND FEARS: KNOWING YOURSELF

In anticipation of your move from the classroom to the clinic, it is useful to reflect on your hopes, fears, and expectations. Being able to examine and articulate your concerns and aims for fieldwork are good starting points for talking with your supervisor about realistic expectations and learning goals for the experience. Worksheet 23-1 can be used to clarify and identify your hopes and fears related to fieldwork.

Worksheet 23-1

What are you afraid will be expected of you on your fieldwork?

_____

_____

_____

What do you wish or expect from the fieldwork experience?

_____

_____

_____

In considering expectations for the fieldwork experience, students and supervisors may share common hopes and fears (Curtis, 1985). Similar concerns of students and supervisors are:

- That each will expect the other to be perfect
- That each will expect the other to remember facts and theoretical information
- That time demands of the setting will limit or compromise the supervisory relationship and process (i.e., students may feel like a burden; therapists may feel unavailable)

Some of the typical hopes and expectations that students and supervisors share are:

- That students will feel challenged and enter the experience enthusiastically
- That there will be trust, mutual respect, and acknowledgment commensurate with each other's experience, knowledge, and skills
- That students will have an active role as adult learners in their progress in the fieldwork process (Curtis, 1985)

With the insight that you and your supervisor actually may have similar feelings about the fieldwork experience, demonstrating a positive attitude and openness to discussing them can facilitate effective communication. This can be accomplished by showing initiative and willingness to apply skills used in the classroom in the clinical setting. For example, listening skills developed during your academic program in learning new information are translated into a variety of attending skills in the clinic. Attending skills can include observation, reflecting verbally and/or nonverbally that you have understood what has been communicated to you, and being aware of how your own personal values and biases can influence your perceptions (Myers & Swinehart, 1995).

Sharing your experiences and learning style (see Chapter 6) can build a foundation for establishing trust with your supervisor. Communicating and clarifying your learning needs and goals reinforce your adult learner role and responsibilities. Embedded in this process of how we communicate are factors such as age, cultural and family background, values, and level of education. Our backgrounds also affect our appreciation, understanding, and expression of cultural diversity. In striving to become a culturally sensitive and competent practitioner, it is important to reflect upon and recognize individual differences as part of the learning experience.

Included in this process of self-disclosure is the responsibility to identify and discuss your own special needs, if applicable. As Kornblau (1995) states, "The Americans With Disabilities Act (ADA) and other laws have changed the rules by requiring fieldwork sites and academic programs to make accommodations for students with disabilities" (p. 139). It is recommended that students openly dialog as outlined by Kornblau (1995) in her article, "Fieldwork Education and Students With Disabilities: Enter the Americans With Disabilities Act." This method can facilitate "a smooth transition to ADA compliance" (p. 139) in preparation for and during the fieldwork experience (see Chapter 11).

ANALYSIS OF THERAPEUTIC SELF

One of the most important applications of self-knowledge occurs in the interactive nature of OT. This phenomenon has been called the therapeutic use of self (Frank, 1958). To be effective, the therapist must also have a clear realization of his or her own abilities and limitations (Worksheet 23-2) (see Chapter 19).

This framework for self-evaluation can also be used to identify your application of

---

Worksheet 23-2

Think about a recent interaction with someone who was relying on you for help. Rate your use of each of the following therapeutic qualities during that interaction.

Scale: 1-Never used, 2-Sometimes used, 3-Frequently used, 4-Consistently used

_____ Display of affect (please describe)

_____ Attending and listening

_____ Cognitive style (determine: detail or whole-picture oriented)

_____ Confidence

_____ Empathy

_____ Confrontation/limit setting

_____ Humor

_____ Probing

_____ Touch

_____ Verbal communication

_____ Nonverbal communication

_____ Balance of power (identify: need for control vs. empowering others)

_____ Recognizing your own emotions/reactions (please describe)

Adapted from Neistadt, M., Cohn, E. S., & Pinet, D. (1993). Assignment for clinical reasoning seminar. Medford, MA: Tufts University—Boston School of Occupational Therapy.

---

these therapeutic qualities during client interactions. Therapeutic use of self is an inherent part of the profession's increasing focus on client-centered service delivery. This process emphasizes the importance of engaging collaboratively with the client. It is vital that you realize your potential and move beyond "helping people" to become an active participant in the treatment process. Through the therapeutic relationship, your aim is to do treatment with the client as opposed to doing treatment to (or for) them (AOTA, 1995).

PROFESSIONAL DEVELOPMENT

It is clear that a critical element in student success is the ability to demonstrate professional behaviors. Within the profession, some of these characteristics have been defined as self-awareness, contributions to the learning of others, empathy, and cooperation. Additional characteristics of professional development include application of knowledge, dependability, initiative, communication with staff and clients, professional appearance/presentation, organization, and professional growth (Worksheet 23-3) (Barnes & Evenson, 1995; Fidler & Gerney, 1994; Kasar, 1994).

Self-evaluation such as this can help you become more aware of your strengths and areas for growth as you progress through your Level I and Level II fieldwork experiences. It may be beneficial to repeat Worksheet 23-3 periodically as you progress through your academic and fieldwork education programs as a method to empower yourself or to monitor your professional development. Developing these professional qualities will enable

Worksheet 23-3

Review the following list of professional behaviors. Rate your current ability to perform these items based upon past work, volunteer work, classroom performance, and/or Level I fieldwork experience(s).

Scale: 0-Do not demonstrate even when situation/opportunity arises, 1-Demonstrate behavior 0% to 25% of the time, 2-Demonstrate behavior 26% to 50% of the time, 3-Demonstrate behavior 51% to 75% of the time, 4-Demonstrate behavior 76% to 95% of the time, 5-Demonstrate behavior 96% to 100% of the time, NA-Not applicable to the situation/setting

_____Able to make observations and interpret cues effectively

_____Able to identify theory/frame of reference guiding reasoning

_____Able to use professional terminology verbally and in writing

_____Reliable

_____Prompt

_____Responsible

_____Respectful of others

_____Generate relevant questions

_____Discuss related course assignments

_____Flexible/responsive: maturely adjust to changes/demands of situation

_____Contribute in class, meetings, supervision

_____Able to constructively share concerns, feelings regarding experiences with supervisor, instructor

_____Polite, able to judge timing of when to add input

_____Interact with client-centered focus

_____Able to establish rapport

_____Nonjudgmental

_____Culturally sensitive

_____Consider impact of interactions: verbal and nonverbal

_____Present with professional demeanor: confident body posture and eye contact

_____Suitably dressed for environment and related tasks/activities

_____Demonstrate knowledge of AOTA's Standards of Practice and Code of Ethics

_____Modify behavior according to demands of situation

_____Manage time and materials safely and efficiently

_____Are prepared with proper forms (i.e., health/immunization) and/or documentation/assignments due

_____Seek feedback

_____Incorporate feedback into future behavior (modify behavior)

_____Identify areas in which additional information/learning is needed

_____Seek resources to address growth needs

+(Add points to achieve Total Score)

_____Total Score

Interpreting Your Total Score

Where you are on the path to Professional Development:

113-140: This reflects a very advanced degree of professional development. A word of caution: you may have a tendency to be overconfident. Seek feedback from others and/or increase challenges to help you gauge the accuracy of your self-rating.

85-112: You are well on your way to becoming competent in your ability to demonstrate professional behaviors.

57-84: You are off to a good start. This assessment should help you in identifying and targeting behaviors and needed opportunities for growth.

56 and under: Your journey has just begun. At this level, you should seek resources and learning experiences to help you take a more active role in your professional development.

Adapted from Barnes, M., & Evenson, M. (1995, April). From bookbag to briefcase: Engaging everyone in the acculturation process via level I fieldwork. *Paper presented at the American Occupational Therapy Association National Conference; Commission on Education, Denver, CO.*

---

you to become an effective practitioner in the future as you negotiate through an ever-changing health care environment.

Another method of tracking your growth and professional development is by keeping a journal or log during your fieldwork experience. It can serve many functions, becoming "a means for self-evaluation and an opportunity to increase one's understanding of self and others, perceive changing attitudes as well as blocks to learning and growth " (Fidler, 1966, p. 6). In addition, it can provide you with a chronological description of your observations, interactions, feelings, reactions, and accomplishments.

SUPERVISION

Supervision is described as a mutual undertaking between supervisor and supervisee (Cohn, 1992). It is an evolving process, intended to promote growth and development while evaluating performance and maintaining standards of the profession. Supervision is a dynamic process of managing your learning in relation to the expectations outlined in the FWEs (AOTA, 1983, 1987).

OT supervisors' roles, responsibilities, and styles vary. However, roles consistent to all supervisors include: establishing expectations, perhaps in conjunction with the student; explicitly communicating standards of performance; and providing feedback, monitoring, and evaluation of performance. Supervision is structured to provide quality care for clients while simultaneously facilitating learning for the OT student. Working toward mastery of entry-level skills required for competence is a collaborative process between the supervisor and the supervisee.

In engaging in the supervisory process, both the supervisor and student are responsible for seeking a balance in this relationship. The supervisor may function as "a resource person, as an advisor, a facilitator, a coach, a sounding board, and a teacher" (Curtis, 1985, p. 10). Although they can serve as a major source of support for you while learning, it is unrealistic for students to expect supervisors to tell them the answers or to direct all of their activities.

In addition, it is important to acknowledge that the most valued characteristics in a role model are different than those of a friend. If there is confusion regarding these roles on either the part of the student or the supervisor, it can disrupt the balance in the relationship. A more social relationship, although easing the stress of a new situation, may lead to autonomy/dependency issues. This will most likely interfere with the giving and receiving of feedback when the supervisor assumes his or her role as evaluator of student performance.

For Level II fieldwork, the COE recommends that time be scheduled at least once a week for formal supervision meetings. However, there may be numerous opportunities for interaction on a more frequent basis, both formally and informally. The supervisor and student are responsible for sharing in the process of ongoing evaluation of student progress and modifying the learning experience within the existing environment accordingly.

Reflecting on certain clinical situations can help you generate relevant questions and identify your agenda for supervision. Journaling may facilitate your highlighting areas in which you need additional help or information. It can be useful in preparing for supervision as well as a way to organize and look at what you are experiencing. Some fieldwork settings have assignments involving the use of journaling to examine specific topics related to clinical practice, group process, or the fieldwork experience. Use of this method should be discussed and clarified with your immediate supervisor.

Students can also actively participate in the supervisory process by preparing an agenda of questions/issues to discuss, generating problem lists and potential solutions for review, submitting documentation/assignments for review in a timely manner, and identifying specific learning needs. These strategies may facilitate more efficient and productive use of supervision times.

It is expected that the nature of supervision will change, evolving over the course of your fieldwork. As you develop your skills and a better understanding of what is required, your supervisor may become less directive and adopt a coaching style. During these initial phases of supervision, the student is expected to actively participate by sharing ideas, opinions, and feelings, and by following through with designated plans. Generally, at the midpoint of your fieldwork, as you take on more responsibility and demonstrate increased confidence, the supervisor may assume more of a supportive role. At this time, you should be actively engaging in problem identification, problem solving, and goal setting. Decision making becomes a shared responsibility with the supervisor providing assurance and resources to facilitate learning. In the final stages of fieldwork, the learner assumes responsibility for decision-making and carrying out work activities which are monitored by the supervisor (Ebb, McCoy, & Pugh, 1993).

Formally, the student's performance on Level II fieldwork is evaluated by the supervisor(s) using the FWE. This should occur at least once before the final evaluation is done at the end of the fieldwork. Often this interim evaluation is done at the midpoint of the experience. At this point, it is used as a counseling tool to identify what has been accomplished and what remains to be achieved in order to successfully complete the fieldwork. Although your FWE serves as a guide regarding the student role, there is variability from site to site in how these expectations are operationalized. In addition, it is recommended that students perform self-evaluations at the midpoint and final evaluation periods to compare their assessment of their skills with that of the supervisor's. This process can validate the accuracy of your perceptions around your performance. Hopefully, this can also serve as a way to open a dialog to clarify any misperceptions if there are differences in ratings.

Another way to effectively participate in the supervisory relationship is to be sure that you are familiar with and clearly understand the expectations of the setting. Expectations of the student specific to the setting are usually outlined in behavioral objectives designed by the site. These serve to clarify criteria specific to the setting for meeting each of the items on the FWE. In addition, the fieldwork setting may have general guidelines or timelines identifying what they anticipate students should achieve by target points in the fieldwork experience.

Occasionally, problems arise in the supervisory relationship. If this occurs, students should make every attempt to communicate with their immediate supervisor. If this is not successful, students should follow the identified channels of communication for further assistance (i.e., clinical coordinator for Level II fieldwork). Frequently, the academic fieldwork coordinator at your program can be a source of support. If necessary, the academic fieldwork coordinator may act as a third party to mediate between student and supervisor. Students should recognize and respect the importance and proper use of these lines of communication in the event of personal or professional problems that might interfere with successful completion of the fieldwork experience. Formal resources also exist within AOTA through the use of the regional fieldwork consultants and the education department's fieldwork education program manager.

Some fieldwork settings have adopted the use of a collaborative model of supervision, one supervisor to two or more student learners. Intrinsic to this model is a value of cooperation and teamwork among the learners as peers. This approach facilitates the students working together as a cohesive pair for mutually responsible feedback and problem solving, typically carried out prior to consulting the supervisor for direction and guidance. Various sites implementing this model of supervision provide students with an orientation to the policies and procedures of its use specific to the setting.

A third approach is a shared supervisor model. In this configuration, one student has two (or more) supervisors. When using this model, it is vital that the student take responsibility to clarify and communicate expectations and feedback when interacting with his or her supervisors. Carrying a communication book or log between supervisors can be helpful. You may also experience a supervision model that represents a hybrid or combination of any of the above mentioned models.

DOMAINS OF LEARNING AND PRACTICE

An inherent aspect of doing involves use of the cognitive, affective, and psychomotor domains of learning. Another way of thinking about these domains is that learning relates to our "head, heart, and hands" (Curtis, 1985).

Cognitive aspects address our judgment and intellectual understanding. At the most basic level, this involves knowing facts, understanding, and being able to apply this knowledge in a variety of situations. Higher levels of thinking are analysis and synthesis, leading to the ability to evaluate information and make judgments regarding the need for action.

The affective domain includes our feelings, attitudes, and values. Basically, this involves receiving and responding to emotional stimuli. Higher level functions relate to emotional control, and having a growing repertoire of responses, as well as control of one's behavior.

The psychomotor realm involves the physical skills you perform in carrying out tasks.

Like learning to ride a bicycle, you must be able to perceive and respond to the demands of the activity, such as knowing how to balance and how to brake or stop. In the beginning stages, this may seem awkward to some and require a lot of energy and attention until you habituate your response which becomes more automatic. Frequently during fieldwork, students use their supervisor as a model, observing and imitating as a method to learn new skills. In the latter stages of fieldwork, it is expected that a student will advance to a level where he or she can improvise and adapt according to the demands of the situation. This process will take time and practice. A new skier begins with snowplowing and it would be unrealistic to expect to be able to negotiate a black diamond (expert) slope.

As you learn to differentiate between therapeutic and social caring, it is important to be familiar with and aware of your own range of emotions. Everyone has some emotions that are more difficult to deal with than others (Worksheet 23-4).

Worksheet 23-4

Review the following list of emotional states. Circle up to five feelings that you may have trouble managing.

Accepted	Competitive	Hurt	Repulsed
Affectionate	Confused	Inferior	Respect
Afraid	Defensive	Intimate	Sad
Angry	Disappointed	Jealous	Satisfied
Anxious	Free	Joyful	Shy
Attracted	Frustrated	Lonely	Superior
Belonging	Guilty	Loving	Suspicious
Bored	Hopeful	Rejected	Trusting

From Egan, G. (1982). Exercises in helping skills (2nd ed.). A training manual to accompany The Skilled Helper. *Belmont, CA: Wadsworth Inc, p. 39.*

Examine the emotions identified above. Think about when you have had difficulty with these feelings. Describe the types of situations and the trouble you have had with managing your feelings (verbally or in writing).

Now, analyze your story contents to identify possible patterns or beliefs you may hold. Look for beliefs that may not be rational and are possibly adding stress to your experience. These include irrational thoughts or beliefs that fall into the following three categories and examples.

Shoulds

1. Other people should know what I need without my having to tell them.
2. People should always be nice (to each other and to me).
3. I should help everyone who needs assistance or asks me for help.

Absolutist Thinking

1. Any mistake is terrible./Anything less than perfect is no good.
2. Every problem has a "right" solution.
3. It's not my fault./It's always my fault.

Catastrophizing

1. Being criticized is awful—I can't stand it./They must not like me.
2. It would be a catastrophe./I would be a total failure if I don't do this exactly right/make a mistake.
3. I can't stand this situation.

Curtis, 1985.

Now that you've identified your patterns, examine them to screen for any of the following beliefs or thoughts that can further contribute to your stress and possibly get you stuck in a negative cycle. These may include:

- Even though this strategy has failed often in the past, it will work this time (gambler's fallacy).
- It's not fair.
- Other people can do it, so I can too (drinker's fallacy).
- Strong people don't ask for help.
- Perfection is usually possible.
- You can never be too rich or too thin.
- Only bad people have problems (Ellis, 1975).

One way to get unstuck or to break/counter these negative cycles of thinking is to try to challenge any of the illogical thoughts (or portions of them) by using rational thinking. Some examples of how to engage in rational thinking are to enlist the following thought patterns or to ask yourself the following questions:

- Is there another way to look at the situation?
- Is this getting me into trouble with people (i.e., pushing others away, causing them to avoid me)?
- This thought is pointless and interferes with my goals. It doesn't help me to work better, feel better, or get help.
- What are my options?
- I can feel better about this—I need to relax and gain some perspective (Ellis, 1975).

Examining and learning to understand your feelings and ways of thinking can help you in multiple ways. Ideally, it can help you to have realistic expectations of yourself and others, develop your therapeutic use of self, identify your learning needs and level of professional development, effectively engage and participate in the supervisory process, and cope with student role stress.

COPING WITH STUDENT ROLE TRANSITIONS

Stress is a part of everyday living. It has both positive and negative effects. Tension, frustration, and anxiety are other common words used to describe stress. When experiencing role stress, you may feel tension related to or resulting from the role that you are learning or occupying. As an OT student, you experience additional stresses because of the transitional and changing nature of your role(s) as you juggle your academic and fieldwork demands. Unrelieved stress, tension, and anxiety can lead to a psychological condition commonly referred to as "burnout." It can impair a person's physical and mental health, as well as ability to perform work/school tasks (Haack, 1987, 1988).

Academically, research shows that the majority of students surveyed identified their top stressors to consist of exams, extent of classwork, limited free time, extended hours of study, and grades (Everly, Poff, Lamport, Hamant, & Alvey, 1994). Professional education requires that students learn to combine new attitudes, new ways of responding to situations, standards of a professional image/appearance, new values and norms, with a "vast amount of new knowledge and specialized skills...all within a relatively short time" (Butler, 1972, p. 401). Part of the challenge of adjusting to a new situation is taking in a variety of new information. In instances where you feel overstimulated, the "orientation response" as described by Toffler (as cited in Butler, 1972, p. 4) may be triggered, which can result in an adaptive reaction. This in turn can drain the body's energy supply and affect your body chemistry. In addition, "'information overload' can interfere with the ability to think...individuals seem to fall into maladaptive behavior, first displaying confusion, then tension, and finally withdrawal" (as cited in Butler, 1972, p. 404). You may notice that you are feeling more easily fatigued and are having difficulty with paying attention or remembering information as you initially become accustomed to your new situation.

Soon after becoming acclimated to one of your fieldwork placements, you move on to a new one. This represents another role set (Butler, 1972) consisting of different variables such as the site, policies and procedures, staff, clients, and various diagnoses/conditions. Additionally, other life/career transitions such as full-time employee to student role, relationship/marriage/family changes or losses, financial status, living situation, and transportation needs may also have an impact your fieldwork experience.

An exploratory study examining the coping strategies and perceptions (Mitchell & Kampfe, 1990) of students on Level II fieldwork showed that the students "used the Problem-Focused and Seeks Social Support strategies more than the Blamed Self, Wishful Thinking, and Avoidance strategies" (p. 543). It is important to note that the productive coping strategies involved taking action as opposed to the others which consist of negative and/or irrational thought patterns. Overall, "most of the students perceived the fieldwork experience as important, controllable, and stressful, but not disruptive to their lives" (p. 543). In your academic and fieldwork education, it is important that you pace yourself to avoid mounting role stress and potential burnout.

DEALING WITH WITHDRAWAL OR TERMINATION FROM FIELDWORK

Problems may arise at any time during your fieldwork. High risk times are early on, at midterm, and in the later stages when you need to be performing at the capacity of an entry-level practitioner. Early on, some students experience difficulty moving from an orientation/observer role to a more active, "doing" role in providing OT services. At midterm, there should be a general sense of your overall performance in the setting, with specific feedback given on areas to be addressed in the remainder of the fieldwork. In the latter stages of fieldwork, some students are unable to meet the level of expectation which would make their performance equivalent to that of an entry-level practitioner.

Students should be familiar with their academic program's policies regarding withdrawal and/or termination from fieldwork. In most instances, these policies become formalized through legally binding contractual agreements between the academic program and the fieldwork site. Communication about student performance and degree of risk for potential failure is crucial between student and supervisor, supervisor and academic fieldwork coordinator, and academic fieldwork coordinator and student. If logistics permit, the academic fieldwork coordinator may make a site visit to participate in the problem-solving and decision-making processes regarding an individual student's situation. If this is not possible, these same discussions should occur via phone contact.

At the time that the student is identified to be at risk for failure, several options may exist. Some of these may include: contracting terms for remaining at the site (frequently done on a week-by-week or 2-week contract basis), developing a remedial plan for the student to fulfill, extending the length of the fieldwork, the student opting to withdraw from the fieldwork placement, or terminating the fieldwork. In many cases, contractual agreements may outline terms where, to ensure client welfare, the site may take immediate corrective measures without prior consultation with the academic program. This may involve removing a student from a clinical assignment or requesting that a student leave the treatment area/site. In a situation not immediately involving client welfare and in which a student is not performing related duties satisfactorily (i.e., failing to do documentation), resolution of the situation is generally agreed upon between the site and the academic program representing the student.

In the instance that a student withdraws or the site terminates a fieldwork, students must refer to the policies and procedures of their academic program. Your academic program may have formal and/or informal procedures for reviewing your situation and status in the program. The issues that arose and led to an incomplete fieldwork should be processed. The format may involve a step-by-step debriefing which looks at specific feedback and related examples/scenarios that illustrate areas of difficulty. The focus should be on identifying a problem list and developing a remedial plan aimed at understanding and addressing the student's areas of needed growth and change.

The goal of this process is to examine what was learned by this experience in order to be proactive in planning and preparing for future fieldwork. This type of occurrence may require that a student seek additional support services, frequently available from the school in the form of academic advising, personal counseling, and stress reduction. Although few students face failure, it is a time for reflection. Through continued participation in activities which address areas for growth, students can be provided with increased understanding about the demands of the profession. Also, the student may gain insight which helps him or her assess his or her readiness for successful fieldwork performance and OT practice. Engaging in opportunities that build confidence and skills can help the student to regroup, to more realistically anticipate the future, and to make plans accordingly.

SUMMARY

In preparing to become an OT practitioner, accepting responsibility for your learning and development of professional behaviors can empower you to be effective. The need for self-awareness is strongly emphasized as it impacts your relationships with your clients, colleagues, and supervisor. Furthermore, it is essential that you apply the foundations of OT practice learned in your academic preparation. Reviewing this primer can assist you with this process. Being resourceful, reliable, flexible, mature, polite, ethical, and self-directed will help you as you strive to achieve a high level of professional development. If you are diligent about obtaining knowledge about the system, such as the norms, expectations, demands, resources, and constraints, and are equipped with strong skills in communication and interaction, you have effectively laid the groundwork toward becoming a competent OT practitioner. Today's rapidly evolving health care system challenges practitioners to continuously assess and match the available resources to best meet their clients' needs.

BIBLIOGRAPHY

Accreditation Council for Occupational Therapy Education. (1995a). *Essentials and guidelines for an accredited educational program for the occupational therapist* (Rev. ed.). Bethesda, MD:

American Occupational Therapy Association.

Accreditation Council for Occupational Therapy Education. (1995b). *Essentials and guidelines for an accredited educational program for the occupational therapy assistant* (Rev. ed.). Bethesda, MD: American Occupational Therapy Association.

American Occupational Therapy Association. (1983). *Fieldwork evaluation form for occupational therapy assistant students.* Bethesda, MD: Author.

American Occupational Therapy Association. (1987). *Fieldwork evaluation for the occupational therapist.* Bethesda, MD: Author.

American Occupational Therapy Association. (1994a). Occupational therapy code of ethics. *American Journal of Occupational Therapy, 48,* 1037-1038.

American Occupational Therapy Association. (1994b). Standards of practice for occupational therapy. *American Journal of Occupational Therapy, 48,* 1039-1044.

American Occupational Therapy Association. (1994c). Uniform terminology for occupational therapy. *American Journal of Occupational Therapy, 48,* 1047-1055.

American Occupational Therapy Association. (1995). Concept paper: Service delivery in occupational therapy. *The American Journal of Occupational Therapy, 49,* 1029-1931.

Barnes, M., & Evenson, M. (1995, April). *From bookbag to briefcase: Engaging everyone in the acculturation process via level I fieldwork..* Paper presented at the American Occupational Therapy Association National Conference; Commission on Education, Denver, CO.

Berger-Rainville, E. (1992). *Student fieldwork manual.* Springfield, MA: Springfield College.

Bloom, B. (1959). Taxonomy of educational objectives. In *Handbook I: The cognitive domain.* New York, NY: David, McKay, Inc.

Butler, H. F. (1972). Education for the professions: Student role stress. *American Journal of Occupational Therapy, 26,* 399-405.

Cohn, E. S. (1992). *Student fieldwork manual.* Medford, MA: Tufts University—Boston School of Occupational Therapy.

Cohn, E. S., & Crist, P. A. (1995). Back to the future: New approaches to fieldwork education. *American Journal of Occupational Therapy, 49,* 103-106.

Commission on Education. (1992a). *Guidelines for occupational therapy fieldwork—Level I.* Bethesda, MD: American Occupational Therapy Association.

Commission on Education. (1992b). *Guidelines for occupational therapy fieldwork—Level II.* Bethesda, MD: American Occupational Therapy Association.

Crist, P. A. (1995, April 24). Students, it takes more than clinical skills to succeed. *Advance for Occupational Therapists,* 5.

Curtis, K. A. (1985). *Coaching for student success: Skills for the clinical instructor.* Miami, FL: Educational Services for the Health Professions.

Ebb, W., McCoy, C., & Pugh, S. (1993). *Identifying the developmental needs of the fieldwork student.* Paper presented at the American Occupational Therapy Association National Conference, Seattle, WA.

Egan, G. (1982). *Exercises in helping skills* (2nd ed.). *A training manual to accompany* The Skilled Helper. Belmont, CA: Wadsworth Inc.

Ellis, A. (1975). *A new guide to rational living.* Englewood Cliffs, NJ: Prentice Hall.

Everly, J. S., Poff, D. W., Lamport, N., Hamant, C., & Alvey, G. (1994). Perceived stressors and coping strategies of occupational therapy students. *American Journal of Occupational Therapy, 48,* 1022-1028.

Fidler, G. (1966). Eleanor Clarke Slagle Lecture—Learning as a growth process: A conceptual framework for professional education. *American Journal of Occupational Therapy, 20,* 1-8.

Fidler, G., & Gerney, A. (1994, July). *Development of professional behavior.* Paper presented at Can-Am Conference, Commission on Education, Boston, MA.

Frank, J. D. (1958). The therapeutic use of self. *American Journal of Occupational Therapy, 12,* 215-225.

Haack, M. R. (1987). Alcohol use and burnout among nursing students. *Nursing and Health Care, 8,* 289-292.

Haack, M. R. (1988). Stress and impairment among nursing students. *Research in Nursing and*

Health, 11, 125-134.

Haggard, E. E. (1964). Psychological causes and results of stress. In D. S. Lindsley (Ed.), *Human factors in undersea warfare*. Washington, DC: National Research Council.

Herzberg, G. L. (1994). The successful fieldwork student: Supervisor perceptions. *American Journal of Occupational Therapy, 48*, 817-823.

Hughes, C., & Opacich, K. J. (1990, April). *Academic assessment beyond the cognitive domain*. Paper presented at the American Occupational Therapy Association National Conference, New Orleans, LA.

Kasar, J. (1994, July). *Enhancing professional behaviors: The professional development assessment*. Paper presented at Can-Am Conference, Commission on Education, Boston, MA.

Kornblau, B. L. (1995). Fieldwork education and students with disabilities: Enter the Americans With Disabilities Act. *American Journal of Occupational Therapy, 49*, 139-145.

Miller, J. G. (1964). A theoretical review of individual and group psychological reactions to stress. In G. H. Grosser, H. Wechsler, & M. Greenblatt, M. (Eds.), *Threat of impending disaster* (pp. 11-33). Cambridge, MA: Massachusetts Institute of Technology Press.

Mitchell, M. M., & Kampfe, C. M. (1990). Coping strategies used by occupational therapy students during fieldwork: An exploratory study. *American Journal of Occupational Therapy, 44*, 543-550.

Myers, S. K., & Swinehart, S. (1995). *Creating a positive level I fieldwork experience*. Bethesda, MD: American Occupational Therapy Association.

Neistadt, M., Cohn, E. S., & Pinet, D. (1993). *Assignment for clinical reasoning seminar*. Medford, MA: Tufts University—Boston School of Occupational Therapy.

Nelson, D. L. (1996, April). *Why the profession of occupational therapy will flourish in the 21st century*. Eleanor Clarke Slagle Lecture presented at the American Occupational Therapy Association National Conference, Chicago, IL.

Occupational Therapy Roles Task Force. (1994). Occupational therapy roles. Rockville, MD: American Occupational Therapy Association.

Purtilo, R. (1978). *Health professional/patient interaction*. Philadelphia: W. B. Saunders Co.

Toffler, A. (1971). Part five: The limits of adaptability. In *Future Shock* (pp. 325-365). New York: Bantam Books, Inc.

Towle, C. (1954). *The learner in education for the professions*. Chicago, IL: University of Chicago Press.

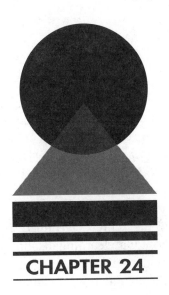

CHAPTER 24

CERTIFICATION AND RÉSUMÉ WRITING

Rosellen S. East, CPRW
Sandra L. Hastings, PhD

CERTIFICATION

Once you've completed all of your coursework, make sure you pause to celebrate your accomplishments. You've worked hard and you're going to graduate. Now there's only one obstacle remaining—certification. The National Board for Certification in Occupational Therapy (NBCOT) is a private, nonprofit agency that manages the certification of all OT personnel. Attainment of this certification ensures prospective employers and clients that you are fully trained and capable of providing high quality service to those you serve. Since most agencies (e.g., government, regulatory, insurance) only hire OTRs and COTAs who are certified by the NBCOT, it's a good idea to obtain this certification. In fact, many state licensing boards consider certification the minimum employment standard.

Certification Exam Procedures

The certification exam is administered in March and September. Once you complete all of the prerequisites, the program director at your college will submit your name to the NBCOT. Mail the postcard you receive from your program director according to the directions. The application for the exam is sent with the candidate's handbook. Carefully follow the instructions for the completion of the application and return the application and the exam fee to NBCOT as instructed.

The Certification Exam

The certification exam is designed to assess a candidate's ability to practice as a newly trained OT personnel. Therefore, the exam measures entry-level skills only. Use *Uniform Terminology for Occupational Therapy* (3rd ed.) (1994) as a terminology reference guide. Call 301-652-2682, or 1-800-SAY-AOTA if you are a student member of AOTA, to order a copy of this publication.

The certification exam uses multiple choice questions. You will attain certification if you are able to meet or exceed the score determined as the minimum passing score. Special needs test takers (e.g., those with learning disabilities) must document their needs before taking the exam. Accommodations will be made in accordance with the Americans With Disabilities Act. Refer to the candidate's handbook for specific instructions.

Preparation for the Exam

In-depth preparation for the exam will greatly improve your chances for success. Some ideas for helping you achieve certification are:

- Studying with a group of friends.
- Attending an exam review conference. Call AOTA or any OT school to find out when a conference is scheduled for your area.
- Review your lecture/class notes.
- Reread sections of your textbooks that you need to review in detail.
- Ask your OT program for suggested study guidelines.

An Additional Note

The NBCOT is creating a new program to renew OT personnel certifications effective March 1997. This additional certification, a tool to promote lifelong learning, will be implemented in two phases. The NBCOT believes implementation of this additional certification will meet customers' demands for the demonstration of lifelong competency. This program will ensure accountability and will ensure the maintenance of high ethical standards for the profession.

RÉSUMÉ WRITING

Once you've finished your OT program and met your certification requirements, you are ready to define your personal and professional goals. Clarification of your goals will determine the skills you want to use, as well as the kind of organization that you want to work for. Taking time to identify your goals will also help you write a résumé that will effectively market your talents to potential employers.

Getting Started—Know Yourself

Before you can write your résumé you must "know yourself" or be able to identify your strengths, work values, interests, transferable skills, and priorities. Many books with self-assessment tools are readily available in bookstores and libraries (e.g., *What Color Is Your Parachute* by Richard Bolles) to help you determine your unique job qualifications. You can also use the Bibliography at the end of this chapter to find a book that might meet your specific needs. Or, you might go the Career Center on your college campus to obtain additional job search assistance.

Since much of the résumé is a chronological listing of your work history and achievements, it's important to identify all relevant experience that might be used to demonstrate your marketability. Although many people may find compiling work history information a tedious process, the information can be used again to create résumés in the future. Often, students state that their greatest challenge is to effectively use their preprofessional experience to obtain their first professional job. Using a self-assessment tool to identify your skills and related experiences will simplify the résumé writing process.

To create a competitive résumé, it's also important to know all of the job duties associated with OT jobs. *The Dictionary of Occupational Titles* (U.S. Department of Labor, 1991) defines the Occupational Therapist 076.121.010 (med. ser.) as:

> Plans, organizes, and conducts occupational therapy program in hospital, institution, or community setting to facilitate development and rehabilitation of mentally, physically, or emotionally handicapped. Plans program involving activities, such as manual arts and crafts; practice in functional, prevocational, vocational, and homemaking skills, and activities of daily living; and participation in sensorimotor, educational, recreational, and social activities designed to help patients or handicapped persons develop or regain physical or mental functioning or adjust to handicaps. Consults with other members of rehabilitation team to select activity program consistent with needs and capabilities of individual and to coordinate occupational therapy with other therapeutic activities. Selects constructive activities suited to individual's physical capacity, intelligence level, and interest to upgrade individual to maximum independence, prepare individual for return to employment, assist in restoration of functions, and aid in adjustment to disability. Teaches individuals skills and techniques required for participation in activities and evaluates individual's progress. Designs and constructs special equipment for individual and suggests adaptation of individual's work-living environment. Requisitions supplies and equipment. Lays out materials for individual's use and cleans and repairs tools at end of sessions. May conduct training programs or participate in training medical and nursing students and other workers in occupational therapy techniques and objectives. May plan, direct, and coordinate occupational therapy techniques and objectives. May plan, direct, and coordinate occupational therapy program and be designated Director, Occupational Therapy (medical ser.).

The Occupational Therapy Assistant 076.364.010 (medical ser.) is defined as:

> Assists OCCUPATIONAL THERAPIST (med. ser.) 076.121.010 in administering occupational therapy programs in hospital, related facility, or community setting for physically, developmentally, mentally retarded, or emotionally handicapped clients. Assists in evaluation of clients daily living skills and capacities to determine extent of abilities and limitations. Assists in planning and implementing educational, vocational, and recreational programs and activities established by registered OCCUPATIONAL THERAPIST (medical ser.), designed to restore, reinforce, and enhance task performances, diminish or correct pathology, and to promote and maintain health and self-sufficiency. Designs and adapts equipment and working-living environment. Fabricates

splints and other assistant devices. Reports information and observations to supervisor. Carries out general activity program for individuals or groups. Assists in instructing patient and family in home programs as well as care and use of adaptive equipment. Prepares work materials, assists in maintenance of equipment, and orders supplies. May be responsible for maintaining observed information in client records and preparing reports. May teach basic living skills to institutionalized, mentally retarded adults.

Use these definitions of OT jobs as a guide as you begin to develop a listing of your skills. In addition, you can complete the OT Résumé Worksheet (Worksheet 24-1) to develop a listing of all your skills and achievements. This listing can be used now, as you begin your career, and can be updated later, as you advance through your career. If you take the time to complete the OT Résumé Worksheet, you will have identified the key skills you'll want to highlight on your résumé which will make writing your résumé easier.

Whenever possible, determine what skills are most important to prospective employers before you write your résumé. You may gather this information by:
- Reviewing a job description prepared by the employer's organization
- Calling the employer to ask pertinent questions
- Having a pre-employment/information interview

You can then customize your résumé by highlighting the job duties most relevant to each employer's needs. If, for example, a community-based employer was most interested in hiring someone to work with elderly clients with sensorimotor impairments, you would provide examples of your experiences that would demonstrate your ability to perform this specific job duty. Although this customization of your résumé may be time consuming, it will give you an advantage over your competition.

Since you've also identified skills that may be transferable to other jobs you might want to keep the OT Résumé Worksheet information for future use. You will find that the time you have invested in this worksheet will facilitate your career seeking activities for many years to come. Updating your résumé will be easier if you create a basic blueprint now.

Choosing the Appropriate Résumé Format

Now that you've defined your skills and related experiences, you can determine what kind of résumé you want to use to sell yourself to prospective employers. Although all OT students have earned the same degree, related job experiences, educational backgrounds, and real life experiences create unique worker profiles. Therefore, the goal is to choose the résumé format that will most effectively market you as a potential employee.

You may choose to write a functional résumé (Figure 24-1 and Worksheet 24-2), a chronological résumé (Figure 24-2 and Worksheet 24-3), or a combination résumé (Figure 24-3 and Worksheet 24-4). The distinctions are listed below.

A Functional Résumé
- Allows you to categorize achievements from different positions, fields, or jobs under a single skill heading

Worksheet 24-1

OT Résumé Worksheet

For each section of the worksheet, list the duties you have performed that relate to those job tasks. List any duties you have performed whether in OT or not. Some of this experience may have been gained from volunteer experience, internships, hobbies, or other activities.

- Stress leadership roles you have taken in campus activities or internships.
- Emphasize the quality of your past achievements.
- Include relevant outside interests.
- Highlight part-time work.
- Be self-assured and stress confidence in the quality of your achievements even if they are limited at this point.

Plans, organizes, and conducts OT program in hospital, institution, or community setting to facilitate development and rehabilitation of mentally, physically, or emotionally handicapped.

_____

_____

Plans program involving activities, such as manual arts and crafts; practice in functional, prevocational, vocational, and homemaking skills, and activities of daily living; and participation in sensorimotor, educational, recreational, and social activities designed to help patients or handicapped persons develop or regain physical or mental functioning or adjust to handicaps.

_____

_____

Consults with other members of rehabilitation team to select activity program consistent with needs and capabilities of individual and to coordinate OT with other therapeutic activities.

_____

_____

Selects constructive activities suited to individual's physical capacity, intelligence level, and interest to upgrade individual to maximum independence, prepare individual for return to employment, assist in restoration of functions, and aid in adjustment to disability.

_____

_____

Teaches individuals skills and techniques required for participation in activities and evaluates individual's progress.

_____

_____

Designs and constructs special equipment for individual and suggests adaptation of individual's work-living environment.

_____

_____

Requisitions supplies and equipment.

_____

_____

Lays out materials for individual's use and cleans and repairs tools at end of sessions.

_____

_____

May conduct training programs or participate in training medical and nursing students and other workers in OT techniques and objectives.

_____

_____

May plan, direct, and coordinate OT techniques and objectives.

_____

_____

May plan, direct, and coordinate OT program and be designated Director, Occupational Therapy (medical ser.).

_____

_____

Other relevant interests or achievements.

_____

_____

- Showcases old accomplishments at the front of the résumé, rather than buried at the end
- Allows the opportunity to highlight skills, experiences, and qualifications gained through internships, volunteer work, college, and other activities not necessarily related to employment experiences
- Eliminates the need to be repetitive if a large majority of your career has been within the same industry or same professions

Your Best Choice If...
- You are a career/job changer
- You lack experience in an occupational area
- You are a recent college graduate
- You are an older worker
- You are an individual returning to the workforce
- Your skills and experiences are more impressive than job titles or employers
- You are returning to a previous line of work

A Chronological Résumé
- Lists work history in reverse chronological order (most recent to past)
- Most commonly used style
- Highlights dates and places of employment
- List job titles, employment, and dates first
- Responsibilities and achievements follow
- Demonstrates strong job-related background

Your Best Choice If...
- Your career includes progressively responsible experience
- You want to advance within your present occupational area
- Your employment has been with well-known employers
- You are seeking employment in a field where a nontraditional style of résumé would be unacceptable
- Your career includes steady work history with key accomplishments in your most recent position

A Combination Résumé

- Begins with a summary of skills and qualifications followed by the customary chronological work history
- Allows the opportunity to highlight significant skills and qualifications, but then provides back-up of these statements with definitive information regarding work history
- Provides the format to highlight industry buzz words most suited to your objectives
- Allows the reader to get a quick glimpse of your talents
- Best used if you have over 15 years experience
- Also known as the "targeted" résumé

Your Best Choice If...
- You have a strong work history and progressively responsible experiences
- You prefer the chronological format but want to highlight qualifications from positions early in your career
- You want to quickly and effectively target your experience to the criteria of the employer

Students with limited job experience may discover that the functional or combination format best highlights their accomplishments and skills. Other students may choose to highlight work experience in a chronological résumé. In addition, each student may choose to match each résumé to the prospective employer's stated needs (i.e., a chronological résumé might be best if an employer is most interested in "years of experience").

SPECIFIC RÉSUMÉ WRITING TIPS

Contact Information

Regardless of the résumé format you choose, the most important information goes first.

Example

Your Name	Adele L. Anderson
Street Address	589 Elm Street
City, State, Zip Code	Provo, UT 84111
Phone	801-624-1289

The information in this section is centered if there is only one address. If, however, it is desirable to list a school address as well as a home address use the following format.

MARIA STEPHENS

412 South 11th Place	853 Sunflower Drive
Arlington, VA 22201	Dallas, TX 76712
(703) 528-0012	(817) 767-8402

OBJECTIVE

Motivated individual seeking entry-level position in urban environment which utilizes my organizational and communications abilities. Skilled in extracting, synthesizing, and conveying information through observation and analysis. Excellent interpersonal skills.

EDUCATION

University of Virginia, B.A. Foreign Affairs, May 1994. Dean's List.
Business-related coursework included 14 hours Math, 6 hours Economics.

Valedictorian, Waynesboro High School, VA, June 1990.

SPECIAL EVENTS PLANNING EXPERIENCE

International Projects Assistant, Division of Continuing Education, University of Virginia, August 1993-May 1994.
Witnessed day-to-day operation of diverse organization, responsible for planning all continuing education programs. Helped create and organize academic seminars for government officials, professionals, and alumni. Wrote biographies, organized and critiqued correspondence, edited brochures, developed conference ideas, conducted research, and analyzed survey results.

Assistant Fundraiser, Alpha Omicron Pi Sorority, March 1993-March 1994.
Success crucial to buy and furnish house. Helped organize all projects including direct-mail network of parents and alumni and community-wide Battle of the Bands. Gained experience with publicity, sales, and coordination of people and facilities for $2500 earning event.

Swim Team Coach, SMAC Summer League, Waynesboro, VA, Summers 1989-1993.
Organized practices and events for group of nearly 100. Required motivational, analytical, and teamwork abilities to develop team and support staff to highest potential. Demanded flexibility and difficult decision making. Advanced from 4th place in 1989 to League Champions in 1993.

WORK EXPERIENCE

Lifeguard, various pools in Waynesboro, VA, and at the University of Virginia, August 1988-August 1993.
Strengthened communication skills by allowing interaction with people of all ages and socio-economic backgrounds. Utilized ability to think and react quickly and to be diplomatic under stress.

Swim Instructor, YMCA and city pool, Waynesboro, VA, August 1988-August 1993.
Led beginners aged 3 to adult. Highlighted strong interpersonal abilities and ability to remain positive and calm. Received numerous commendations from superiors and patrons.

SKILLS AND INTERESTS

WordPerfect, MSWord, Excel. Some French and Italian.

Figure 24-1. Sample of a functional résumé.

Worksheet 24-2

Worksheet for Functional Résumé

Name _____

Address _____

City, State _____

Phone _____

Summary or Objective _____

_____

Education _____

Degree_____ Major_____ Date _____
Optional

Institution_____ City, State_____

Other Related Training _____

_____   _____

Course   School or Company

_____   _____

Course   School or Company

List of Skills _____

* _____

* _____

* _____

* _____

* _____

Work Experience: Job #1 or Fieldwork #1 _____

Name of Company_____

City, State_____ Dates Worked _____

Job Title_____

Work Experience: Job #2 or Fieldwork #2 _____

Name of Company _____

City, State_____ Dates Worked _____

Job Title_____

_____

```
Work Experience: Job #3 or Fieldwork #3 _____

Name of Company _____

City, State_____ Dates Worked _____

Job Title_____ _____


Extras _____

_____

_____

```

Use your OT Résumé Worksheet to list accomplishments.

Example

Your Name   **Sam Jones**

School Street Address   Home Street Address   Box 3298   17 Hebron Road
University   City, State, Zip Code Trinity College   Elmira, NY 14901
City, State, Zip Code   Telephone Number   Hartford, CT 06109 607-649-5587
Telephone   860-565-3391
Email Address   SJones@aol.com

Objective

An objective tells the reader what job you want. It is also referred to as a Job Objective, Career Objective, or Career Goal. Make sure your objective is specific enough to give the potential employer a clear understanding of the position that interests you. Avoid writing an objective that is either too general or too short.

Example: Too General

"Seeking a professional position with an employer offering potential for advancement." This objective does not really tell the reader where you want to go or what you want from them. It does not really say anything.

Example: Too Short

"Seeking a position in Occupational Therapy." This objective does not say enough about the kind of job that interests you. Keep in mind that the reader probably knows you want a job as an OT.

Example: Appropriate OT Objective

"Seeking entry-level therapist position in field of traumatic brain injury with focus on community re-entry."

As an OT student seeking a position only as an OTR or COTA, the use of an objective most likely is appropriate because your career objective is specific. However, if you want to create a résumé that can be used to apply for a variety of positions you would use a summary instead.

GEORGE TYSON, OTR
1921 Woodlawn Avenue
Flint, MI 48503
(810) 488-5868

CAREER SUMMARY
- Occupational Therapist with over 5 years experience
- Strong clinical background
- Considerable written, oral, and interpersonal skills
- Proven leader and team player

EXPERIENCE
1990-Present

HENRY T. FORD REHABILITATION CENTER, Dearborn, MI
Occupational Therapist
- Planned, managed, and coordinated individual and group treatment in a community program
- Evaluated and treated patient population with traumatic brain injury, spinal cord injuries, and orthopedic conditions
- Interacted with treatment teams to plan and implement programs
- Supervised staff including three COTAs
- Formulated a comprehensive training program for COTA student interns
- Wrote reports, articles, and other communications

MELLING COMMUNITY HOSPITAL, Cincinnati, OH
1989-1990
OT Fieldwork Level II
- Assisted in treatment planning and implementation
- Ran life skills and self-esteem groups
- Maintained progress notes and discharge summaries
- Performed sensory integration techniques
- Planned and instructed gross motor group activities

WEST VILLAGE BEHAVIORAL HEALTH CENTER, Gary, IN
1988-1989
OT Fieldwork Level I
- Assisted patients with daily living skills
- Used reality orientation, psychodrama, and cognitive rehabilitation techniques
- Charted progress and discharge summaries
- Provided feedback to treatment teams

EDUCATION

PURDUE UNIVERSITY, West Lafayette, IN
B.S.—Occupational Therapy, May 1990
Summa Cum Laude

PROFESSIONAL AFFILIATIONS

American Occupational Therapy Association
National Board for Certification in Occupational Therapy

Figure 24-2. Sample of a chronological résumé.

Worksheet 24-3

Worksheet for Chronological Résumé

Name _____

Address _____

City, State _____

Phone _____

Summary or Objective _____

_____

Work Experience: Job #1 or Fieldwork #1 _____

Name of Company _____

City, State_____ Dates Worked_____

Job Title _____

General Job Description _____

_____

_____

Accomplishments _____

_____

_____

_____

Work Experience: Job #2 or Fieldwork #2 _____

Name of Company _____

City, State_____ Dates Worked_____

Job Title _____

General Job Description _____

_____

_____

Accomplishments _____

_____

_____

_____

Work Experience: Job #3 or Fieldwork #3 _____

Name of Company _____

City, State_____ Dates Worked _____

Job Title _____

General Job Description _____
_____
_____
_____

Accomplishments _____
_____
_____
_____
_____

Education _____

Degree_____Major_____ Date _____
                                            Optional

Institution_____ City, State_____

Other Related Training _____

_____   _____
Course   School or Company

_____   _____
Course   School or Company

Special Skills or Activities (Optional) _____
_____
_____

Use your OT Résumé Worksheet to list accomplishments.

Summary

In place of the objective, you may prefer to write a career summary that highlights your accomplishments. This summary immediately identifies what skills you have that will be useful to a potential employer. It tells the reader what unique qualities you will bring to the job. It is also referred to as Skills, Strengths, Special Skills, and Career Focus. A summary tells the reader where you have been, and what you can do for him or her.

Example

- Developed arts and crafts program at U.S. Veterans Hospital
- Redesigned existing programs to facilitate growth and learning
- Conducted training program for new hires

Overall, the use of an objective or career summary allows you to customize your résumé for each position. This section of the résumé is most critical. If your objective or summary is interesting, it's likely the potential employer will read the rest of your résumé. Make sure this section markets your abilities well by using action words.

NYDIA GARCIA-ROBLES
115 Elm Street
New Haven, CT 06511
413-555-7613

SUMMARY

- Proven skills in working with youth groups
- Effective program planning skills
- Fluent in Spanish
- Manage time effectively

EDUCATION

BS, Occupational Therapy, Expected May 1997
Quinnipiac College, Hamden, CT
AS, Human Services, May 1990
Dade County Community College, Deerfield, FL

RELATED EXPERIENCE

Teen Counselor
- Supervised children during various athletic events (tennis, water sports, basketball, track and field)
- Assisted with daily living skills (dressing, bathing, toileting)
- Supervised large and small groups on a 24-hour basis

Tutor
- Interacted with teens gaining skills in English speaking
- Developed action plans for continuing skills practice
- Integrated Hispanic cultural heritage in lessons

Internship
- Assisted in program development for teens with dyslexia and developmental disorders
- Kept progress records
- Coordinated workshops for special needs youths
- Scheduled daily activities and field trips

WORK HISTORY

4/96 - 6/96   *Occupational Therapy Intern*—Martindale Center Inc. Thomaston, CT
1/96 - 3/96   *Occupational Therapy Intern*—Group Care Rehab Center Torrington, CT
5/94 - 8/94   *Camp Counselor*—Warm Springs Teen Center Atlanta, GA
5/92 - Present   *English Tutor*—Farnham Neighborhood House New Haven, CT

Figure 24-3. Sample of a combination résumé.

Worksheet 24-4

Worksheet for Combination Résumé

Name _____

Address _____

City, State _____

Phone _____

Summary or Objective _____

_____

Education _____

Degree_____Major_____ Date _____
                                                   Optional

Institution_____ City, State_____

Other Related Training _____

_____   _____

Course   School or Company

_____   _____

Course   School or Company

Selected Accomplishments _____

_____

_____

_____

_____

_____

Work Experience: Job #1 or Fieldwork #1 _____

Name of Company_____

City, State_____ Dates Worked_____

Job Title_____

Work Experience: Job #2 or Fieldwork #2 _____

Name of Company_____

City, State_____ Dates Worked_____

Job Title_____

Work Experience: Job #3 or Fieldwork #3 _____

Name of Company_____

City, State_____ Dates Worked_____

Job Title_____

Extras _____

_____

_____

_____

Refer to any of the résumé preparation manuals included in the Bibliography at the end of this chapter for an action word list. If you choose to use a summary you can state your objective in the cover letter.

Work Experience

This section of your résumé highlights relevant job information. It is also referred to as Professional Experience, Career History, and Work History. The type of résumé you write will determine how the information should be written. Review the work experience sections of the sample résumés before you write this section.

Example

1985-1994   Seaview Rehabilitation Center, Lawrence, CA
Occupational Therapy Student
- Ensured constructive daily activities for vocational rehabilitation patients
- Designed arts and crafts programs appropriate to physical capacity of clients
- Taught patients skills necessary for participation in program to facilitate return to work setting

Education

In this section of your résumé you will list the degrees you have earned with the highest degree listed first. This section is generally either the second section or the last section of the résumé. It is also referred to as Academic Credentials, Educational Background, and Relevant Coursework. Check the résumé samples for guidelines.

Example

A. S. Occupational Therapy, May 1995
Greenwood Technical College, Greenwood, SC

Other Activities

This section is an optional section that should be included only if you have a skill or interest that might strengthen your application. It is also referred to as Skills and Interests. Specific examples include: academic awards or honors, software expertise, computer skills, community activities, language proficiencies, military experience/honors, patents or published writings, organizational affiliations, or licenses or certifications. Hobbies should only be listed if they are relevant to your career. Do not include personal information such as marital status, health, number of children, and birthdate.

Example

Use WordPerfect, MSWord, Excel; speak Spanish

References

It is not necessary to include this section. Employers assume that you will provide references when requested.

EDITING SUGGESTIONS

Creating your résumé is an experience in writing and as such requires editing and proofreading. The challenge is to incorporate your marketing strategy in a document that is perfectly written.

- Rely on your college mentors or counselors for feedback on your résumé.
- Be sure to ask for help in proofreading your résumé.
- Ask your friends in other programs, family, and fellow OT students to proofread your résumé.

As with all written forms of communication, consistency in format is critical. For example, you can choose one of several formats for phone numbers: (904) 288-6777 or 904/288-6777 or 904-288-6777. The important thing is to be consistent throughout in the format you choose. Being consistent applies to other areas such as spelling out the name of a state (Maine) or using the two-letter postal abbreviation (ME).

Check reference books for the rules regarding use of punctuation and grammar, such as capital letters, hyphenation, periods, spelling, and parallel construction. Use short, concise sentences to create your résumé. Choose action words and active voice whenever possible.

The Bibliography in this chapter includes handbooks that can help you write your résumé. Do not guess about proper usage! Remember the résumé and cover letter package sell you and your skills. Even one spelling error can say to the prospective employer that you are a risky candidate. Your potential employer decides whether or not to grant you an interview based on the résumé package you present.

Again, we cannot overemphasize the need for editing and then proofreading your résumé and cover letter until it is error free. The résumé package represents you. Even if you hire a professional résumé writer to produce your résumé, you will want to edit and proofread the document to be sure it is error free. You also need to be sure the résumé is an accurate representation of you and your skills for the prospective employer.

THE COVER LETTER

The cover letter is a letter to your prospective employer which literally "covers" the résumé. As such, it is the first thing that the reader, your prospective employer sees. Consider the cover letter another opportunity to market yourself with pizzazz (Table 24-

1). Think of a cover letter as a great opportunity to share your unique qualities with a prospective employer to pique curiosity and obtain a personal interview. Use the cover letter to:

- Sell yourself to the prospective employer
- Show your ability to organize thoughts and get to the point
- Include your objective, if you did not include an objective in your résumé
- Give yourself the competitive edge over other applicants for the same job
- Call attention to your skills and abilities
- Explain unusual circumstances such as gaps in employment or why you are changing fields

A template of a good cover letter is included in this chapter (Figures 24-4 and 24-5). Many of the books in the Bibliography give sample cover letters that you can use as a guide in constructing this critical part of your résumé package.

COMMONLY ASKED QUESTIONS IN RÉSUMÉ PREPARATION

I can't seem to fit my résumé on one page. Do you have any ideas or pointers on making a one-page résumé?

First of all, it may not be necessary to have a one-page résumé, for example, if you have an extensive background with a lot of relevant experience you may choose to use a multi-page résumé. If, however, you decide you want to use a one-page résumé, you may have to change the format to get everything on one page. For example, using a functional résumé, which simply lists your experience, may save some space and get the information needed to the reader more effectively. You might also use a smaller font and decrease your margins to consolidate your information. Minor adjustments can make a big difference.

I don't have much related work experience and my scholastic achievements are not outstanding. I have always been a hard worker but am not a good test taker. What can I do to make my résumé effective?

You need to market yourself to your prospective employer. Your résumé should reflect your strong points. Look for transferable skills (skills that can be applied in any field) that you used in part-time jobs. Stress achievements, rather than scholastic records. In reality, most employers will be more impressed by accomplishments than by high scholastic marks.

How do I make my chronological résumé stand out from the rest? In other words, how do I explain my skills in a way that doesn't sound generic and like everyone else's?

You can personalize your résumé through the use of a career summary. Individuals may have similar work histories, but each individual has distinct skill strengths. Use your accomplishments to create interest in your résumé. You can then include your objective in the cover letter.

How do I decide whether to create a functional or chronological résumé?

Use the OT Résumé Worksheet (see Worksheet 24-1) included in this chapter to identify your skill strengths. Then, contact the potential employer to determine what specific skills are needed for the job that interests you. Review the three types of résumés and when it's most appropriate to use them. Based on all of this information, choose the

Table 24-1
Suggestions for Common Cover Letter Problems

Don't	Instead
Mail your résumé without a cover letter.	Write a letter to sell the skills listed in the résumé.
Address cover letter "To Whom It May Concern" or "Dear Sir" or "Dear Madam."	Address cover letter to a specific individual. Check with your local library or call the company to get the name and title of the individual to whom the letter most logically should be addressed, such as the personnel director.
Include salary requirements in cover letter unless specifically requested by employer.	Salary discussion may be more appropriate at the job interview.
Try to list all your skills in the cover letter.	Be clear, brief, and businesslike. Say you are enclosing your résumé and do so.

résumé format that best fits your immediate needs.

What do you do if your job title does not accurately reflect your duties?

Present your job duties in a straightforward manner. Specify your duties accurately by listing the skills you used on your jobs. If you think it is necessary, you can explain the discrepancy in your cover letter.

Where do I go to get help and materials to write my résumé?

There are many resources available to help you write your résumé. Even the smallest local libraries have a section devoted to job seekers with a myriad of publications devoted to résumé writing. Bookstores also offer résumé writers all the current resources available; Career Centers on college campuses offer résumé materials and assistance. For the computer literate, there are resources on the Internet. Remember that a good résumé is the result of many hours of preparation. Use multiple resources to identify the skills and work experiences that will best market your potential.

Should I list a career objective and/or summary of qualifications?

Base your decision to use an objective or a summary on your personal credentials. Review the section in this chapter that outlines the benefits of both options. Current thinking is that the summary is generally more effective than the objective because it calls attention to specific skills at the beginning of the résumé. If, however, you have limited experience then the objective may be the best option.

What hobbies should I include on my résumé?

Most of the literature today suggests that you include only hobbies or outside interests that are directly related to the job you are seeking. For example, if you are a running enthusiast seeking a job in OT you might not include running on the résumé. If, however, you are applying for a sales position with a company that sells running shoes you would include your accomplishments and/or interests as a runner.

Leave 3 to 5 blank lines from top of page depending on length of letter **Your Address**	Street Address City, State, Zip Code Area Code and Home Phone Number Area Code and Work Phone Number (Optional)
Leave 1 blank line **Date of Cover Letter** Leave 3 to 5 blank lines depending on length of letter	Today's Date
Name and Address of **Prospective Employer** Personalized, to a name **not** To Whom It May Concern	Name of Addressee Title Company Street Address City, State, Zip Code
Leave 1 blank line **Salutation** Leave 1 blank line **Introduction**	Dear Mr. Phipps: Include who you are and why you are sending letter. If you have not included an objective in your résumé you may include it here.
Leave 1 blank line **Qualifications** This section may be broken into more than one paragraph.	Sell yourself, use this paragraph to make it clear you should be considered for this position. You may include reasons for gaps in employment or change in career here.
Leave 1 blank line **Action**	Include action to be taken such as date and time for an interview.
Leave 1 blank line **Closing** Leave 3 to 4 blank lines for your handwritten signature **Type your name** Leave 1 blank line **Enclosure(s), if any**	Sincerely, Your Name Enclosure

Figure 24-4. Template for cover letter.

BIBLIOGRAPHY

Asher, D. (1992). *From college to career: Entry-level résumés for any major.* Berkeley, CA: Ten Speed Press.

Beatty, R. N. (1989). *The perfect cover letter.* New York: Wiley.

Bolles, R. N. (1991). *What color is your parachute?* Berkeley, CA: Ten Speed Press.

Corbin, B., & Wright, S. (1993). *The edge résumé & job search strategy.* Carmel, IN: Beckett-Highland Publishing.

Fein, R. (1994). *Cover letters, cover letters, cover letters.* Hawthorne, NJ: Career Press.

132 West Main Street
Waltham, MA 02135
215-555-4439

April 25, 1997

Lucille Murphy
C.D.A.
Community Health Network
8 Terrace Drive
Newton, MA 02161

Dear Ms. Murphy:

I am submitting my résumé in response to the advertisement for occupational therapy personnel listed in the April 22 *OT Week*. As a recent college graduate with excellent communication skills, treatment planning experience, and a high degree of professionalism, I may be the candidate you seek.

I graduated from the University of Virginia in May 1996 and I am seeking to relocate to the Washington, DC metro area. While a student, I gained experience in treatment planning through a 1-year internship at the Johns Hopkins University Hospital and as planning chairperson for a student organization fundraiser. As a fieldwork intern, I worked in a stroke recovery program helping organize and implement educational seminars. These experiences enhanced my ability to organize large amounts of material and information, handle multiple tasks, and work under pressure. I am also proficient in WordPerfect and Macintosh applications and type 50 words per minute. Finally, I am mature, flexible, and dedicated as demonstrated by my 7 years of success as a swim instructor and coach. I feel that my character and experiences as described above qualify me to meet the demands of this position.

I would like very much to be part of your team and would welcome the opportunity to prove myself in an interview. I will contact your office next week to inquire about setting up a meeting. Thank you for your consideration.

Sincerely,

Joan Richmond
Joan Richmond, OTR/L

Figure 24-5. Sample cover letter.

Freeman, L. H., & Bacon, T. (Eds.). (1995). *Style guide*. Bountiful, UT: Shipley Associates.
Fry, R. W. (1988). *Your first résumé: The comprehensive preparation for high school and college students*. Hawthorne, NJ: Career Press.
Hirsh, S., & Kummerow, J. (1989). *Lifetypes*. New York: Warner Books
Krannich, R. L., & Krannich, C. (1992). *Dynamite cover letters*. Woodbridge, VA: Impact.

Lewis, A. A. (1985). *Better résumés for college graduates.* Woodbury, NY: Barron's Educational Services.

Miller, A. F. , & Mattson, R. T. (1989). *The truth about you.* Berkeley, CA: Ten Speed Press.

Noble, D. F. (1994). *Gallery of best résumés.* Indianapolis, IN: JIST Works Inc.

Noble, D. F. (1996). *Gallery of best résumés for two-year degree graduates.* Indianapolis, IN: JIST Works Inc.

Parker, Y. (1987). *The resume catalog: 200 damn good examples.* Berkeley, CA: Ten Speed Press.

Sabin, W. A. (1995). *The Gregg reference manual.* New York: McGraw-Hill.

Schuman, N., & Lewis, A. (1993). *From college to career: Winning résumés for college graduates.* Happauge, NY: Barron's Educational Services.

Tieger, P. D., & Barron-Tieger, B. (1995). *Do what you are.* Boston: Little, Brown and Company.

U.S. Department of Labor. (1991). *Dictionary of occupational titles (DOT)* (4th ed.). Washington, DC: DOL Employment & Training Administration.

Weinstein, B. (1993). *Resumes don't get jobs: The realities and myths of job hunting.* New York: McGraw-Hill.

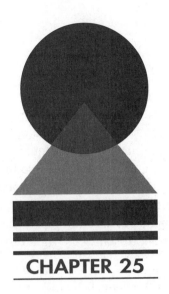

CHAPTER 25

INTERVIEWING AND NETWORKING FOR YOUR FIRST JOB

Linda Waak, RPT

INTRODUCTION

Now that you have completed your OT program, your fieldwork, your licensure requirements, and your résumé, it's time to prepare for your first job. OT jobs are currently plentiful, but finding the right one for you can be a challenge. This chapter will assist you in preparing for a job interview, which is the first step in your search for an ideal job.

PREPARING FOR THE INTERVIEW

The interview stands as a critical step between your earlier contacts with the organization and an offer. Networking can be a valuable tool to help you land your ideal job. It has been estimated that about 80% of all new jobs are found through informal networking channels. Once you have found a few organizations that are interesting to you, begin a search to find personal contacts within them.

Find out whether any of your friends, relatives, or acquaintances know anyone connected with the organization. Do not forget people from your past that might be good connections. Personal contacts can provide you with insight about how the organization runs. Often times these individuals can offer you information that they have heard through the grapevine. In other words, "organizational gossip" can be a valuable resource. These personal contacts can offer you assistance in getting your foot in the door and an opportunity to interview with an organization you are interested in.

If you have been invited to interview, you can assume that your cover letter, résumé, and/or phone calls have created an interest in your qualifications and background. This face-to-face meeting will give you a chance to reinforce the employer's positive impression of you and also provide you an opportunity to learn more about the organization. The interview is a mutual exchange of information in which both you and the interviewer are selling and evaluating. As the applicant, a good basic mindset would be "I have a product that is good (myself), and I want to sell to the right buyer (best organization)."

INTERVIEW OBJECTIVES

The primary objectives for the interviewer are to:

- Determine the relevance of your experience and training in terms of the demand of a specific job, and assess whether or not you meet the criteria established for the position.
- Ascertain how well you as a person would fit into the organization by appraising your personality, motivation, and character.
- Evaluate your mental ability to see whether or not you will make a contribution to the organization and provide it a good return on investment.

This objective is of particular importance in selecting people for higher level jobs. Most organizations prefer to hire individuals with potential for advancement so that they can promote from within the organization.

The primary objectives of the applicant are to:

- Determine how comfortable you feel in that specific organization's environment.
- Evaluate the match between your personal and professional needs and goals, the organization's personality, and the personalities and managerial styles of your potential co-workers and superiors.

COMPONENTS OF AN INTERVIEW

It is important to understand the main components of an interview so that you are not caught off guard or left unprepared. Most thorough interviews take 1 to 2 hours to complete. Make sure you have scheduled ample time for the interview so you do not feel rushed or pressured to finish.

The interview usually begins with some small talk to establish initial rapport and comfort. Upon meeting, greet the interviewer with a firm handshake and address him or her by name. You should know who you will be interviewing with ahead of time. Remember, we form our initial impressions about people within the first 30 seconds of meeting them. We will discuss how to make a good first impression later in this chapter. Often the interview will begin with a tour of the OT department and facility. This is an opportunity for the interviewer to provide you with information about the organization and specific job requirements. This is also an opportunity for you to begin addressing specific questions you might have for the interviewer, as well as carefully observe the working environment of the organization.

The interview usually continues in a quiet place where there are no interruptions. The interviewer will seek further information by asking questions about your skills, qualifications, and traits. The interviewer might also present hypothetical scenarios to assess your maturity and ability to problem solve. Questions should be asked in an open-ended manner allowing you to elaborate on your education, work experience, student clinical experiences, and personal traits that will be an asset to the organization. You as the applicant will have center stage throughout the interview. It is the job of the interviewer to encourage you to do most of the talking. Probing questions will be used to encourage you to complete an idea or thought in greater depth. An interview is considered successful if the applicant has talked 80% to 85% of the time (Table 25-1).

The interview might also entail a brief meeting with a human resource representative to discuss your application and obtain permission to check personal references. At this time, the organization's benefit package will be presented. Larger organizations will typically have a human resource representative available to assist with this portion of the interview. In smaller organizations, the interviewer is responsible for presenting this material.

As part of the interview you may have the opportunity to meet with key personnel such as the medical director, supervisors, and senior OT clinicians. This is your opportunity to gain further knowledge about the personality of the organization and the cohesiveness of the team you will potentially be working with. If you are not given this opportunity you may wish to request a meeting and/or ask to observe a treatment session with a therapist. Doing so will allow you to evaluate the dynamics of the treatment area as well as gain understanding about the various patients the organization serves.

What Are the Important Questions an Applicant Could Ask?

Asking the right questions at the right time will strengthen your image with the interviewer and provide you with information to evaluate the organization. Table 25-2 is a list

---

Table 25-1
What Does the Interviewer Expect From You?

- You are expected to arrive on time for the interview.
- You should present yourself with a neat and polished professional image.
- You are expected to remain composed throughout the interview. The interviewer will want to know if you can handle yourself in a situation that may present stress or pressure.
- You are expected to be prepared to answer questions about job skill, qualifications, and personal character in a clear and concise manner.
- You will be expected to ask questions about the organization and the specific job for which you are applying. Asking these questions demonstrates your interest in the job.
- Do your homework and research the organization so you have valuable knowledge on which to base your questions. The fact that you are well informed and are asking well thought-out questions will impress the interviewer.
- You should express your ideas in an organized and clear way.
- You should remember that the interviewer expects your salary expectations to be reasonable in terms of your experience and the job market. Do your homework and know what competitors are offering for your same level of experience.

Table 25-2
Questions for the Interviewer

1. How many staff members are presently in your department?
2. What is the ratio of COTAs to OTRs?
3. Can you describe the level of experience of your staff?
4. How would you describe your staff?
5. How would you describe a typical day as a staff therapist?
6. How many patients would I be responsible for treating each day?
7. How long do I spend with each patient?
8. What are the common diagnoses of the patients your staff treat?
9. What would be my work hours? Are the work hours flexible?
10. Is there weekend work involved? If so, how often?
11. Do you have a productivity standard for your staff? If so, would you explain the productivity standard?
12. How would you describe the rapport of your OT department with the physicians and various departments with which you work?
13. What documentation is required in your department?
14. What is the organizational structure of your department? Who would I directly report to? How long has this individual been in his or her current position?
15. What is the retention rate of your therapists?
16. What would you describe as the strengths and weaknesses of your department?
17. Do you develop yearly objectives for your department and are your therapists involved with this process?
18. What professional learning experiences are available for your staff?
19. Do you have a student program? What OTR/COTA programs do you affiliate with?
20. What changes has your department and organization made to be successful in the reforming health care system?
21. Do you have a copy of a job description and performance appraisal for me to review?
22. What realistic advancement opportunities are available in your organization for staff therapists?
23. Does a structured career ladder exist for your staff? Can you explain this ladder to me?
24. Do you feel your workplace is conducive for the development of new graduates?

of important questions that you as the applicant could ask, if they have not been addressed.

What Important Questions Will the Interviewer Ask You?

A major purpose of the interview is for the interviewer to gain information about your qualifications, traits, and character. Questions that the employer would target focus on emotional maturity and control, assertiveness, self-discipline, self-confidence, initiative, analytical capacity, critical thinking, adaptability, attitude, interpersonal skills, values and integrity, and problem-solving abilities. The information obtained must enable the interviewer to make an intelligent decision regarding the suitability of you for the job. Table 25-3 is a list of questions that the interviewer might ask. Before you go to an interview,

Table 25-3
Potential Questions the Interviewer May Ask You

Job Objective Questions

These particular questions will give the interviewer an idea about the specific objectives you are looking for, or wishing to avoid, in a job or career.

1. What are some of the things in a job that are important to you, and why?
2. What are some of the things you would like to avoid in a job, and why?
3. What made you choose the OT profession?
4. What qualifications do you have that will make you a successful clinician?
5. What do you know about our organization?
6. What is your overall career objective?
7. What kind of position would you expect to progress to in 5 years? In 10 years?
8. As a new graduate, what areas would you like to continue to develop?

People Skills Questions

These questions will help the employer to get a feel of how you interact with people, co-workers, and supervisors.

1. What was your clinical instructor's or supervisor's greatest strengths?
2. Describe your favorite supervisor or clinical instructor. What was it that made that person special?
3. What kind of people do you like working with?
4. What kind of people do you find it most difficult to work with?
5. How have you successfully worked or dealt with this type of person in the past?

Academia Questions

These questions may provide clues to your abilities and motivation as a professional.

1. What was your best and most difficult subject during college?
2. How were your grades? Were they average? Above average? Below average?
3. What activities did you participate in during high school? College?
4. How conscientious a student were you? How many hours a day did you study?
5. Did you receive any special awards or achievements during high school? College?
6. Have you given any thought to attending graduate school?
7. Did you help to finance your college education?

Motivation Questions

These questions will give the interviewer more information on your level of motivation and abilities to be successful.

1. Why are you interviewing with us?
2. Why did you apply for this position?
3. What about this organization makes you want to work here?
4. How will this job help you reach your long-term goals?
5. Where else are you applying?
6. What reservations, if any, do you have about working here?

Teamwork/Social Sensitivity Questions

These questions will assist the interviewer on assessing your comfort level and success when working in a team situation.

1. Have you ever worked within a team?
2. What are the advantages and disadvantages of working on a team?

3. Tell me about an occasion when you pulled a team together. What was your particular role on the team?

4. In working with new people, how do you go about getting an understanding with them?

5. Define cooperation.

6. What difficulties do you have in tolerating people with backgrounds and interests different from yours?

Communication Skills Questions

These questions will provide the interviewer with insight into your abilities to exercise effective communication skills.

1. How important was communication and interaction with others on your clinical affiliation?

2. Describe a time when you had a confrontation with someone. How did you handle it?

3. What do you think are essential communication skills to possess as a health care professional?

4. What communication skills do you feel you could improve?

Self-Confidence/Self-Esteem Questions

These questions will help distinguish how well you regard yourself.

1. How would you describe yourself?

2. What would you consider your greatest strength as a person?

3. What do you feel you could most improve upon?

4. What are some of the things that motivate you?

5. What personal qualities do you think are necessary to be successful in this job?

6. Do you consider yourself successful? Why?

7. What have you done that you are proud of?

Self-Discipline and Initiative Questions

These questions will help the interviewer establish an idea of your level of self-initiative.

1. How do you define a successful career?

2. Recall a major project you worked on in school. How did you organize and plan for it?

3. What professional goals have you set for yourself?

4. What are you doing to reach them?

5. Do you always reach your goals?

6. Tell me about a time when you failed to reach your goals.

7. What can you do for us that someone else cannot?

Problem-Solving and Decision-Making Questions

These questions can help determine your abilities and maturity in problem solving and making difficult decisions.

1. Tell me about a time when a quick decision had to be made. What did you do?

2. What are examples of problems you find difficult to solve?

3. What decisions do you find difficult to make?

4. Where do you turn for help?

Grace Under Pressure Questions

These questions will provide insight into how you react in stressful and crisis situations.

1. What was the most difficult situation you have ever faced? How did you react?

2. What do you do when you have a great deal of work to accomplish in a short time span? How have you reacted?

3. Tell me about an occasion when your performance did not live up to your expectations.

4. Can you recall a time when you went back to a failed project to give it another shot? Why did you do it and what happened?

Worksheet 25-1

Now that you have an idea of what questions you should ask the interviewer and what questions might be asked of you, it is time to practice and mentally prepare for the interview.

1. Take a couple of days to review the questions that the interviewer might ask you. How would you respond to these questions? Create a mental response for several questions in each trait category.

2. Set up a mock interview with another classmate. One student will be the interviewer, the other the applicant. The interviewer will ask one question from each of the trait categories. The applicant should have a detailed response for each question asked. Tape record the session and listen to it. How did you come across? Was the interview successful? Why or why not?

3. Provide feedback to the student who is playing the role as the applicant. How did he or she come across? Was he or she prepared? Were his or her responses detailed, yet clear and concise? Vocal tone appropriate? (Lowered pitched voice?) How was the volume of his or her voice? (Too loud? Too soft?) How was his or her nonverbal communication? Good eye contact? Body posture? Gestures? Facial expressions? Did it sound overrehearsed?

4. Reverse roles and repeat steps 2 and 3.

5. Review the questions listed that you as the applicant could ask about the OT department and organization. What other important questions do you want to ask? Add these questions to your list now.

review the list and how you would answer the questions. Even better, have a friend or family member ask you the questions and give you feedback on your answers. These questions are grouped into categories that provide insight into a specific quality or trait. Use Worksheet 25-1 to practice and mentally prepare for your interview.

WHAT DO EQUAL EMPLOYMENT OPPORTUNITY LAWS MEAN TO YOU?

It is important for you to understand that federal legislation has made it unlawful for employers to ask certain question that are discriminatory against an applicant prior to hiring that person. This legislation has been titled equal employment opportunity (EEO). It is designed to provide equal opportunity to be hired, retained, trained, and promoted for all persons regardless of sex, race, ethnic origin, religion, physical condition, or age.

Equal employment opportunity laws state that the employer should also refrain from asking your views on the following areas: politics, military history (unless the job specifically requires it), sexual preference, future personal plans such as children or marriage, arrest records, emotional or psychological issues, labor unions, credit ratings, disabilities, and workers' compensation claims. Any questions related to these issues may be unlawful if the answers might eliminate you from consideration for a job that you are actually qualified.

In a majority of cases it is the manner in which a question is phrased that makes it illegal. Questions can often be phrased a different way to eliminate the discriminatory overtone (Table 25-4).

> ### Table 25-4
> ### Avoiding Discriminatory Overtones
>
> | Interviewer Should Not Ask | Bona Fide Job Questions |
> |---|---|
> | Do you have any physical or mental impairments? | Are you able to handle the work tasks the job you're applying for involves? |
> | Are you married? | Do you have any personal responsibilities that may affect your schedule? |
> | Do you plan to have children? | This job requires occasional work on Saturdays and Sundays. How do you feel about that? |
> | Are you pregnant? | |
> | How old are your children? | Are you a U.S. citizen or a resident alien with the right to work in the United States? |
> | Do you live alone? | Will you be able to perform the tasks the job requires? |
> | Where are you from? | |
> | Where were you born? | What professional organizations do you belong to that may assist you in the job that you are applying for? |
> | I love your accent. What ethnic background do you have? | |
> | How is your health? | |
> | Have you ever filed a workers' compensation claim? | |
> | Have you ever been treated for a mental or emotional problem? | |
> | Are you taking any prescribed drugs? | |
> | What organizations do you belong to? | |

What will you do if an interviewer asks you a question that you believe is discriminatory? How will you handle this difficult situation? Table 25-5 lists some possibilities and techniques you can use. Use Worksheet 25-2 to practice your responses.

THE IMPORTANCE OF PERSONAL REFERENCES

Personal references are used as another way for the potential employer to verify that they have selected a good applicant. References are usually checked after an employer has selected, interviewed, and screened the applicant for a particular job. Often times, employment is contingent upon receiving acceptable reference checks.

It is therefore important that you spend some time deciding whom you should give as a reference prior to the interview. Since you may have little or no work experience upon

Table 25-5
Handling Inappropriate Questions

Technique	Applicant's Response
Sidestep the question by not responding to it. Example: What arrangement have you made for the care of your children?	My personal responsibilities will not interfere with my job.
Downplay the question by answering as briefly as possible and move on to a related topic. Example: Will your husband object to your working on weekends?	What kind of weekend work does the job entail?
Challenge the relevance of the question as a requirement for the job. Example: Do you plan to have children?	Is motherhood an essential requirement for this job?

Worksheet 25-2

1. Ask a friend to play the role of an interviewer that is asking discriminatory questions. Use each of the techniques above to respond to these questions.
2. Ask your friend for feedback on how you came across while responding to the discriminatory questions. Did you maintain good eye contact? Were you tactful? Were you appropriate with your response?
3. How comfortable did you feel using these techniques? Which technique was most comfortable for you and why?

completion of your academic degree, it is appropriate to ask a teacher or others who are familiar with your academic performance to serve as a reference. Other individuals who would be appropriate references would be clinical instructors from your affiliations, supervisors from volunteer work, or a professional person who is well respected in the community and who has known you for several years. Former bosses or anyone who can give an objective evaluation of your personal habits and characteristics would also be appropriate.

These individuals should be contacted ahead of time to seek permission to use their name as a reference. Make sure to update them on the type of position you are seeking and your qualifications. Give them the names of the employers who might be contacting them (Worksheet 25-3).

It is unnecessary to advertise references on your résumé. Doing so protects the privacy of the individual and eliminates them from being contacted unnecessarily. Typically, employers will not check references unless you are considered a top applicant for the position. Usually the employer will contact the reference by telephone and ask the individual questions about your personal traits and qualifications. Sometimes a written letter of recommendation is requested so it may be kept as part of the permanent personnel file. You may wish to request a written letter of recommendation from those willing to assist you and bring them to the interview.

Worksheet 25-3

1. Think about who you would like to ask to provide a personal reference for you. You should have at least three people.
2. Call each of them to request permission.
3. Send each of them your résumé so that they will be familiar with your recent accomplishments.
4. Ask them if they would write a personal letter of recommendation and mail it to you.
5. Complete a reference sheet with the persons' names, titles, addresses, and current phone numbers to give to the interviewer.

The employer must obtain prior permission from the applicant to check references. Usually there is a statement for authorization to check references located on the employment application. This authorization is usually confirmed during the interview process.

It is important that once you have received a job that you acknowledge those individuals serving as personal references with a note of thanks or phone call. You should make sure to update them about your new position.

THE INTERVIEW

Now that all the preparation has been completed for the interview you are ready to present your best self and land the right job.

What can you bring to the interview? It is appropriate to bring a notebook to take notes during the interview. Take only brief notes during the interview and fill in the details after you leave. Often applicants will bring a list of specific questions that they would like to address. This is acceptable as long as you are discrete in using this list, not appearing overrehearsed or too mechanical. Other important information to have available at the interview would be an extra copy of your résumé, a copy of your temporary or permanent license to practice, a copy of your diploma from an accredited program, personal reference sheet if requested, and written letters of recommendation if requested.

Dress for Success

The way you dress communicates a great deal about your self-concept and the person you are. Your image is crucial during a job interview and what you wear sends powerful signals to the interviewer. Remember this will be the first meeting with a potential new employer and first impressions are usually lasting impressions. When dressing for a job interview you usually know very little about the person you will be meeting. This is why it is important to wear something that appeals to the general public. Many books and articles have been written on the subject of appropriate dress for the professional. Here are some basic suggestions from the experts.

- Select a conservative approach, classic style and simple lines. For women, the best outfit would be a business suit, conservative dress, or classic pant suit. For men, a business suit and tie are most acceptable.
- Avoid extremes. Do not be swept away by the latest fashion.
- Wear styles and colors that you look best in and feel most comfortable with.

- Neutral colors are always safe—grey, navy, browns, and black. Several surveys have been done in regard to colors and the perceptions that people have of various colors. Neutral colors allow you to concentrate on the individual and not their clothes. Black is considered a power color for both men and women. Pastels are regarded as feminine and weaker. Women perceive cream/off-white color on other women as powerful.
- You can add your own touches of individuality with jewelry, scarves, accessories, or choice of tie.
- Remember hair, fingernails, and make-up also leave impressions. Hair should never hang in your face and keep make-up conservative.
- Take the time and make the effort to find out what looks best on you. Solicit advice from friends and professionals.

Effective Interviewing Techniques

- When you greet the individual, whether it be a male or female, shake his or her hand firmly and address the individual by name.
- Breathe deeply and relax. You have adequately prepared for the interview.
- Do not chew gum or eat candy.
- Have a positive attitude. Keep in mind the mindset of really wanting a job, and demonstrating this attitude frequently separates the winning applicants from the losers.
- Show excitement and enthusiasm during the interview process. This will put you in a separate league than the average applicant.
- Strive for a natural dialog with the interviewer as quickly as possible, but allow him or her to control the interview.
- As you answer questions, remember to be clear and concise, do not ramble.
- Be sure that you understand the question. If a question is not clear, rather than guess, ask for clarity.
- Be consistent in your answers.
- Do not alter your response because a question is asked a different way.
- Always turn a negative question into a positive by replying using positive terms. For example, use words such as "challenge" or "opportunity." Avoid words such as "problem."
- Avoid saying anything negative about any person or organization that you have been involved with.
- The job interview is not a time to be shy or modest. Toot your own horn.
- Watch for opportunities to ask the kinds of questions that show you've done some homework on the organization.
- Be cooperative and courteous throughout the interview.
- Remember to be conscious of your nonverbal communication. This is your silent language. Maintain good eye contact. An erect posture demonstrates confidence. Do not fidget with your hands. Be aware of your gestures and facial expressions.

How to Handle the "Money Question"

The money question always seems to be a difficult question to handle. As the applicant, you should always allow the interviewer to broach this subject first. Often the interviewer will ask, "What salary range are you looking for?" Some of the best ways to address this question are the following:

- "I am looking for a good career opportunity and a position where I am able to grow professionally."
- "I will accept an offer that is competitive with other organizations for my same level of experience."

You should avoid naming numbers at the first greeting. As a general rule, if salary is not addressed by the interviewer at an interview, do not mention it. You do not want to appear as if salary is the primary motivator for accepting a position. The interviewer will follow up with you by phone and negotiate salary requirements once he or she has decided that you are a top applicant.

Closing the Interview

How you close the interview is as important as how you open the interview. First and last impressions are always the most powerful. In order to guarantee success, close the interview with the following thoughts.

- Express enthusiasm about the organization and your desire to be part of it.
- Communicate your interest in the specific position.
- State that you are confident that you will be an asset to the organization and possess the ability to be successful.
- Ask when you can expect to receive follow up from the interview.
- Thank the interviewer for his or her time.

INTERVIEW FOLLOW-UP

After the interview, you should take the time to follow up with a note of thanks. The note should reiterate your interest in the position and your strengths as a top applicant. This gesture will leave a good impression with the potential employer and place your name back in his or her mind.

Follow up with any person that has offered to be a personal reference to inform them that they may be getting contacted by the employer. Mentally review the interview to evaluate what went well and what could have been better. Assess what you would do differently in the next interview.

BIBLIOGRAPHY

Bolles, R. N. (1991). *What color is your parachute?* Berkeley, CA: Ten Speed Press.

Brown, C. (1989). *Dynamic communication skills for women.* Shawnee Mission, KS: National Press Publications.

Carline, S. (1995) *How to interview and hire the right people.* Boulder, CO: Career Track Publications.

Carr-Ruffino, N. (1993). *The promotable woman advancing through leadership skills* (2nd ed.). Belmont, CA: Wadsworth Publishing Company.

Fear, R. A., & Chiron, R. J. (1990). *The evaluation interview* (4th ed.). McGraw-Hill, Inc.

Jackson, C. (1987). *Color me beautiful.* NY: Ballantine Book.

Medley, A. H. (1984). *Sweaty palms: The neglected art of being interviewed.* Berkeley, CA: Ten Speed Press.

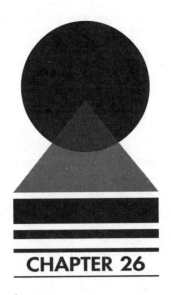

CHAPTER 26

GRADUATE SCHOOL AND CONTINUING EDUCATION

Karen Sladyk, MS, OTR/L

INTRODUCTION

You're just about to finish your OT program. It's been a long, exhausting trip. It seems you have been going to school forever, and that may be true. You are looking forward to free time and no homework when, all of a sudden, you're thinking about continuing education and maybe another degree. This chapter is about continuing your professional growth.

CONTINUING EDUCATION VS. TRADITIONAL FORMAL EDUCATION

There are many experts in education who will argue that one type of education is better than another type. You will likely get much advice about which type is better even if you do not seek the advice. The ultimate opinion is of course yours. The bottom line is that you continue to educate yourself and stay current in your field. Before you form an opinion about formal education vs. continuing education, you should make sure you understand all the options available to you.

Continuing Education

Continuing education has seen an explosion of ideas in OT. Pick up any of the weekly OT newspapers and you will find pages of educational opportunities. Not only are conferences listed but AOTA has developed self-study programs, on-line computer education, and a national OT conference that attracts 5,000 people at one time. There is no want for topics. Just about everything is available. Examining 1 week's worth of OT newspapers found the following continuing education opportunities:

- AOTA Annual Conference
- On-line computer conference and on-line practice support
- Several state associations' conferences
- Self-study packages
- *American Journal of Occupational Therapy (AJOT)*, SIS newsletters, *OT Practice*
- New books recently published

AOTA offers an annual conference, as well as a yearly special interest conference. These conferences allow you to get a variety of experiences packed into 5 days. There is something very exciting about sitting in an auditorium with 5,000 other COTAs and OTRs to hear a motivating keynote speaker. Most OT state associations offer yearly conferences with mixed topics. These conferences are usually inexpensive and allow you to meet COTAs and OTRs from your area. Networking at these conferences provides you with a wealth of future resources.

Many OT schools offer free or inexpensive conferences related to educational issues such as fieldwork. These conferences allow attendees to enjoy the latest information about education at a greatly reduced price. In addition, OTs can share experiences and educational models that are effective in the clinic. Sometimes OT schools offer certificates of advanced training. When you take a cluster of four master level classes you earn the certificate. Those interested in continuing on to an advanced degree can count the certificate classes toward a master's degree.

On-line classes or self-study programs allow COTAs and OTRs to study a topic at their own pace without leaving their home or workplace. These self-contained conferences award certificates of completion and some can be accepted for master's degree credits. With these types of continuing education opportunities, rural COTAs and OTRs can participate without leaving home. The self-study programs can be done in a small group, allowing for questions and feedback, as well as networking. Other on-line services are available from AOTA including resources for help on special problems.

Many individual and specialty groups also offer conferences. You will find these listed in the weekly OT newspapers. Fees for these conferences vary greatly and the topics are usually specific with some advanced skills required. The best way to stay up-to-date on these specialty topics is to scan the conference listings regularly.

Many continuing education opportunities are mailed directly to your home. *AJOT* provides you with monthly, up-to-date research in OT. Readers are sometimes intimated by the level of writing but the editor and reviewers work hard to make the articles clear. The more you read the journal, the more you will understand. *AJOT* makes an excellent continuing education opportunity because it is delivered to you, is self-paced, and is available at no cost with your membership. *OT Practice* magazine provides a more informal continuing education opportunity by focusing on current practice in a practical format. Like *AJOT*, it comes right to your home and is included with your AOTA membership.

Traditional Formal Education

Traditional formal education means returning to college or a university to seek a higher degree than the one you currently possess. The benefits of another degree might include self-esteem, promotion, pay raise, and mastery of a subject. Generally, the workplace or the general public recognizes your scholarship more easily with a formal degree. Some workplaces offer promotion or pay raises with another degree, while others do not. Many workplaces even encourage college study by offering special discounts, time off, or tuition reimbursement programs. If you think you are likely to return to college after you start working, be sure to check into tuition assistance programs with the personnel department when you interview.

College degrees are offered in four levels: associate, bachelor's, master's, and doctorate. Traditionally, the first three levels of degrees are focused in either the arts or sciences. This means that you can have an associate in arts (AA) or an associate in sciences (AS). The same is true of the bachelor's (BA or BS) and the master's (MA or MS) degrees. Some schools offer specialty degrees which follow state laws and accrediting rules. Examples of these specialty degrees include the master's in OT (MOT) or a master's in social work (MSW). Traditionally, the doctoral level is a PhD, a research-focused doctoral degree. Other doctoral level degrees are now available such as an EdD (education), ScD (science), JD (law), and a new program emerging in OT called a Clinical Doctorate. Each type of degree has different requirements and each school can design the degree as necessary within the laws of the state. Generally, each degree requires the following as the minimum:

- Associate: 60 credit hours
- Bachelor's: 120 credit hours
- Master's: 36 credit hours above a bachelor's degree
- Doctorate: Varies greatly depending on degree

As an OT student, your degree is likely to be over the minimum credit requirements. This is because there is a lot to learn in OT and fieldwork is a required component.

So how do you know which degree is for you? Once you decide you want to go back to school, you have to do some research. Two helpful places to use are your school's placement center and your local library. Just explain to the people who work in either place that you are thinking about going back to school and do not know where to start. Librarians are particularly good resources because many enjoy solving these types of puzzles. Either place is likely to direct you to career information and local school catalogs. Scan the school catalogs for something that interests you and then write to the school for more information.

You will have to decide if you want a degree in OT or if you want a degree in a related area. The decision is totally up to your needs and goals. Only you can evaluate what area of study you want to pursue. Consider your interests and long-term plans. Discuss your thoughts with people who have done what you are thinking about. Use Worksheet 26-1 to stimulate your thinking.

You may be lucky enough to be able to pack up and move to another area to go to school full-time. More than likely, your viable choices will be limited by several factors. These include:

- Driveable from your home
- Within your budget and the tuition reimbursement rules of work
- Willing to take part-time students
- Some flexibility to fit into your schedule, including your family's schedule

Often local city newspapers will publish a "back to school" section in the paper in August. This section might have a list of all the colleges and universities in your state.

Worksheet 26-1

OT Degree or Related Area

Question	Yes	No
Have I developed my goals in earning another degree?		
Do I plan to continue to work at my current job?		
Is OT something I want to study more?		
Is there another area that will enhance my skills in OT?		
What areas do I have interest in?		
Do I want to be promoted to a higher skill level position?		
Do I want to teach OT?		

The AOTA can provide you with a list of accredited and developing OT degree programs. Request a catalog and application from each school that interests you. Some schools require you to pay for the catalog because they have so many requests. This is usually true of ivy league schools such as Yale University in New Haven, Connecticut. Once you get the catalogs, look for programs of interest. Also check with peers and co-workers about the different programs and the reputation. Consider the tuition costs and what you can afford.

The choices of possible degrees are endless but you may be restricted by a geographical area. If so, the best way to find a degree that interests you is to review the local college catalogs you find in your library. Some of the more common areas of study are included in Table 26-1. When you have decided which program is for you, complete the application and apply.

Some schools at the master's and doctorate level require scholastic tests such as the Graduate Record Exam (GRE). Several different exams are available but the GRE is the most common. The GRE is similar to the SAT you took in high school. Although taking the GRE is no walk in the park, it will not be nearly as bad as you remember the SAT. The key is being prepared and reviewing before the test. Do not take the GRE cold, without preparation. You can take the GRE as many times as you want but all your scores are reported until the score becomes 5 years old and is dropped from the record.

GRE review classes are available but they can be expensive. If you own a computer, you can get a review class on disk. Computer programs are nice because they score practice tests for you. Prices vary greatly on GRE computer programs. The least costly approach to GRE reviews can be found at your local bookstore. GRE review books generally cost less than $25 and provide you with the wealth of knowledge you need for the exam. If possible, buy at least one book 3 months or more ahead of the exam. When it comes time to study for the exam, review Chapter 7 in this primer on how to memorize what needs to be memorized.

DEGREES OF SPECIAL INTEREST FOR OT

If you have decided to further your education in OT, the first step is calling AOTA and requesting a list of approved OT degree programs. If you keep prior *AJOT*s in your home,

Table 26-1
Areas of Study

OT	Related Areas
• COTA to OTR programs	• Adult learning
• MOT with focus in developmental disabilities, mental health, physical rehabilitation, pediatric, management, education, research, or occupational science	• Community health
	• Counseling
• Doctoral programs specific to OT	• Education
	• Management
	• Marriage and family
	• Neuroscience
	• Psychology
	• Public health
	• Rehabilitation
	• Social work

you can likely find the list in a former issue. This will save time on your part. Once you have narrowed down the list, request catalogs from each school. Do not be discouraged if only one meets your criteria. By deciding OT, you have already narrowed the field down to the program you want.

GETTING A BACHELOR'S DEGREE AFTER YOUR ASSOCIATE DEGREE

Many times COTAs transfer the credits they earned at the associate degree level into a bachelor's degree. This may be in OT or in a related area mentioned above. COTAs usually become frustrated when they discover that many of the COTA classes do not easily transfer. This is not unusual to any student who transfers. Many classes at the technical level are not considered to be at the same level as a bachelor's degree. Just like your associate degree, getting a bachelor's degree can be hard work. If it wasn't, everyone would have a degree. Stay focused and make a plan. Do not get frustrated but examine your options fully.

Start with your school and read your catalog. Does your COTA school have an agreement with another school to transfer credits more easily? Does the state that you live in have a college without walls that gives credit for life experience? (Check Higher Education Department in blue pages of phone book.) Does the school you are going to give life experience, portfolio assessment, college-level examination program exams, or allow you to test out of some classes? See as many academic advisors on each campus as possible. Ask each person to put what they agreed to in writing.

COTA TO OTR PROGRAMS

There are times when a COTA decides to become an OTR and there are special programs that are designed just for this option. Keep in mind that the profession supports both COTAs and OTRs and there is never any assumption that COTAs must work to become OTRs. When a COTA does wish to become an OTR, AOTA will provide a list of special programs. At the time of this printing there were seven accredited COTA to OTR programs with several developing for the future. Unfortunately for many people, most of the accredited programs are east of the Mississippi River. Most of the COTA to OTR programs have classes in the evenings or on weekends. This allows the COTA to continue to work full-time until it comes time to do fieldwork.

If there are no COTA to OTR programs available to you, it is still possible to become an OTR through a traditional OTR program. If the OTR program is a bachelor's degree, consider making an appointment with either the admissions director or the department chairperson. Bring with you a copy of all your transcripts. Explain your background and ask for an evaluation of your transcripts. Ask that a tentative plan of study be developed so you can make an educated decision. Keep in mind that you will have to do 2 years of liberal arts and sciences core classes as part of your degree. Almost every college or university requires this. Remember college was not designed to provide job training. The purpose of college is to graduate an educated person with solid thinking skills, capable of leading the world into the future.

Sometimes it is easier to become an OTR through an entry-level master's degree than a traditional bachelor's degree. If you have a lot of different classes from different schools it is sometimes easier to finish a bachelor's in general studies (BGS) and then apply to OTR school. In this way, you are more likely to avoid the inflexible 2 years liberal arts and sciences core required by traditional bachelor's degrees. Consider college without walls (see above) or a more flexible liberal arts college for your bachelor's degree. Plan ahead and make sure you take all the prerequisites needed for OT school as part of your BGS. Do not think that a BGS is an easy thing. Getting any college degree should be a challenge to your thinking or it is not worth the time. A BGS simply allows you more flexibility in class design.

OTR EARNING AN ADVANCED MASTER'S DEGREE

The practicing OTR will have to decide if an advanced master's in OT is his or her preference or a master's in a related area. Most OTRs earning master's degrees in the past had little choice. A master's in OT was fairly rare. This has changed and many schools offer advanced degrees to OTRs. Many advanced degrees allow students to specialize in an area of interest such as developmental disabilities, pediatrics, or management. Some degrees focus on education or research. If you are interested in an advanced degree in OT, call AOTA and request a list of advanced degree programs. As mentioned above, you can also find a list of programs in *AJOT*. Request a catalog and application from the program. If the program looks of interest, call the school and ask to speak to a student in the program. The student should be able to address your questions on pace, requirements, teachers, and content of classes. You may be able to sit in on a class or attend an open house.

DOCTORAL DEGREES

At this time you may be thinking, "Is she crazy?" I know the doctoral idea is not appealing to a lot of you, but there are a few who have been hiding this thought in the back of their mind. Doctoral level work is most certainly a challenge, but a challenge that many OTRs have succeeded at. If you hold as your goal a faculty appointment, doctoral level education is highly desirable. It is possible to get and maintain a faculty position without a doctorate but having one makes promotion and tenure a lot easier.

Just like the master's degrees mentioned above, doctorates can be in OT or a related area. At the time of this writing, there were only five up and running doctorates in OT.

All are located in or near major U.S. cities. This may limit the choices of OTRs not living near an OT program. For those interested in other related areas, it is possible to combined your love of OT with a new study area. For example, most doctoral programs will allow you to transfer in up to two classes. Most will allow independent studies. So if you are an OTR studying adult learning, you may be able to transfer a class in clinical reasoning and a class on fieldwork into your program. An independent study can compare and contrast clinical reasoning with theories on critical thinking in adulthood. Lastly, you can use OT as a component of your dissertation. Check with the doctoral program you are interested in for the rules and regulations.

If you think a doctorate is in your future, consider looking at combination programs that give you a master's degree on your way to your doctorate. Also, carefully weigh out the benefits of a PhD, ScD, EdD, or Clinical Doctorate. Each has its own benefits. Although all require great disciplined study, the PhD has a long history of being well established and is often privately acknowledged as the preferred degree. Lastly, understand the program requirements before you start. Will you be required to do a full-time residency? Can you take classes part-time? How is the research component of the degree managed? The more you know before you start, the easier it will be to finish.

SUMMARY

This chapter addressed the very important issue of continuing to learn after graduation. It is your professional responsibility to stay current in the practice of OT. Furthering your education can take two different roads. First, formal education such as returning to a college or university for another degree can develop or refine skills. Second, less formal continuing education allows the learner to be specific in his or her learning needs. Educational experts disagree as to which type is best. The learner must evaluate his or her own needs when developing a plan for further education.

BIBLIOGRAPHY

Gardner, J. N., & Jewler, A. J. (1989). *College is only the beginning.* Belmont, CA: Wadsworth.

Gardner, J. N., & Jewler, A. J. (1995). *Your college experience: Strategies for success.* Belmont, CA: Wadsworth.

Peters, R. L. (1992). *Getting what you came for: The smart student's guide to earning a master's or a PhD.* New York: The Noonday Press.

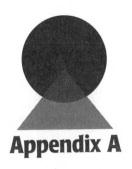

Appendix A

RESOURCE GUIDES AND MONOGRAPHS RELATED TO EMPOWERING STUDENTS WITH DISABILITIES

Association on Higher Education and Disability. An international, multicultural organization of professionals commited to full participation in higher education for persons with disabilities. Institutional membership cost: $187.50. Contact: 614-488-4972 (phone), 614-488-1174 (fax).

Health resource directory (1993-1994). Health Resource Center. One free copy. Contact: 800-331-3761.

Guiding the learning disabled student: A directory of programs and services at NACAC member institutions. (1991). Cost: $10.00. Contact: 703-836-2222.

The national directory of four year colleges, two year colleges and post high school training for young people with learning disabilities. (1994). Partners in Publishing. Cost: $32.95. Contact: 918-584-5906.

FROM THE ASSOCIATION ON HIGHER EDUCATION AND DISABILITY (AHEAD)

Farrell, M. (1993). *Support services for students with learning disabilities in higher education: A compendium of readings.* Cost: $40.00.

Gimblett, R. (1992). *Peer mentoring: A support model for students with disabilities.* Cost: $23.00.

Support service for deaf/hard of hearing students in postsecondary education. (1989). Cost: $25.00.

Unlocking the doors: Making the transition to postsecondary education. (1987). Cost: $12.50.

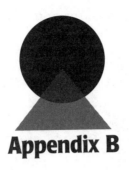

Appendix B

RESOURCES FOR THERAPEUTIC ACTIVITIES

Students often complain that they run out of ideas for activities. With experience this changes. The following is a partial list of resources for therapeutic activities. The list includes activities for both groups and individual sessions across the age span and diagnostic categories. Resources that are primarily (90% to 100%) therapeutic activities are marked with an ** before the reference. Check your local public library for sources of activity books related to community groups such as scouting, education, leisure, social clubs, homemaking, and crafts. Although the community books will not discuss the therapeutic aspect of a particular activity, a creative COTA or OTR can use activity analysis to make the project meaningful.

Allen, C. K., Earhart, C. A., & Blue, T. (1992). *Occupational therapy treatment goals for the physically and cognitively disabled.* Bethesda, MD: American Occupational Therapy Association.

Case-Smith, J., & Pehoski, C. (1992). *Development of hand skills in the child.* Bethesda, MD: American Occupational Therapy Association.

**Drake, M. (1992). *Crafts in therapy and rehabilitation.* Thorofare, NJ: SLACK Inc.

**Fink, B. E. (1977). *Sensory motor integration: An activity curricula.* Lowell, MI: Author.

Hemphill, B. J., Peterson, C. Q., & Werner, P. C. (1991). *Rehabilitation in mental health: Goals and objectives for independent living.* Thorofare, NJ: SLACK Inc.

**Korb, K. L., Azok, S. D., & Leutenberg, E. A. (1991). *Life management skills I.* Beachwood, OH: Wellness Reproduction, Inc.

**Korb, K. L., Azok, S. D., & Leutenberg, E. A. (1991). *Life management skills II.* Beachwood, OH: Wellness Reproduction, Inc.

**Korb, K. L., Azok, S. D., & Leutenberg, E. A. (1995). *Life management skills III.* Beachwood, OH: Wellness Reproduction, Inc.

**Korb-Khalsa, K. L., & Leutenberg, E. A. (1996). *Life management skills IV.* Beachwood, OH: Wellness Reproduction, Inc.

Leslie, D. K. (1989). *Mature stuff: Physical activity for the older adult.* Reston, VA: American Alliance for Health, Physical Education, Recreation, and Dance.

**Lobdell, K., Johnson, C., Nesbitt, J., & Clare, M. (1996). *Therapeutic crafts: A practical approach.* Thorofare, NJ: SLACK Inc.

Reed, K. L. (1991). *Quick reference to occupational therapy.* Gaithersburg, MD: Aspen Publications.

**Rider, B. B., & Gramblin, J. T. (1981). *The activity card file.* Kalamazoo, MI: Author.

Ross, M. (1987). *Group process.* Thorofare, NJ: SLACK Inc.

**Simon, S. B., Howe, L. W., & Kirschenbaum, H. (1978). *Value clarification.* Hadley, MA: Values Associates.

**Simmons, P. L., & Mullins, L. (1981). *Acute psychiatric care.* Thorofare, NJ: SLACK Inc.

Zoltan, B. (1996). *Vision, perception, and cogntion: A manual for evaluation and treatment of the neurologically impaired adult* (3rd ed.). Thorofare, NJ: SLACK Inc.

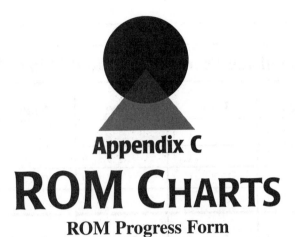

ROM CHARTS

ROM Progress Form

Patient Name:

Therapist:

	Date:				
S	Flexion				
H	Extension				
O	Abduction				
U **L** **D**	Internal Rotation				
E **R**	External Rotation				

F **O** **R**	**E** **L**	Extension/ Flexion			
E **A**	**B** **O**	Supination			
R **M**	**W**	Pronation			

	Flexion				
W	Extension				
R **I**	Ulnar Deviation				
S **T**	Radial Deviation				

Key: ↑=increase, ↓=decrease.

Reprinted with permission from Gaylord Hospital, Wallingford, CT.

Patient Name:

Therapist:

Occupational Therapy Hand ROM Flow Sheet

Date	Index	Long	Ring	Small	Thumb
MP	( )	( )	( )	( )	( )
PIP	( )	( )	( )	( )	( )
DIP	( )	( )	( )	( )	( )
TAM	( )	( )	( )	( )	( )
Date	**Index**	**Long**	**Ring**	**Small**	**Thumb**
MP	( )	( )	( )	( )	( )
PIP	( )	( )	( )	( )	( )
DIP	( )	( )	( )	( )	( )
TAM	( )	( )	( )	( )	( )
Date	**Index**	**Long**	**Ring**	**Small**	**Thumb**
MP	( )	( )	( )	( )	( )
PIP	( )	( )	( )	( )	( )
DIP	( )	( )	( )	( )	( )
TAM	( )	( )	( )	( )	( )
Date	**Index**	**Long**	**Ring**	**Small**	**Thumb**
MP	( )	( )	( )	( )	( )
PIP	( )	( )	( )	( )	( )
DIP	( )	( )	( )	( )	( )
TAM	( )	( )	( )	( )	( )

Key: ↑=increase, ↓=decrease.

Reprinted with permission from Gaylord Hospital, Wallingford, CT.

Patient_____ Unit____ Age____ Chart Number_____

Dx _____

Onset_____ Admitted_____ Therapist_____

Comments:_____

Functional Joint ROM/Muscle Strength Evaluation

Left								Action	Average Range	Muscle	Right					
Date			**Date**								**Date**			**Date**		
PROM	AROM	MMT	PROM	AROM	MMT						PROM	AROM	MMT	PROM	AROM	MMT
						SCAPULA		Elevation	0 1/4 1/2 3/4 full	Upper trapezius						
								Depression	0 1/4 1/2 3/4 full	Lower trapezius						
								Protraction	0 1/4 1/2 3/4 full	Serratus anterior						
								Retraction	0 1/4 1/2 3/4 full	Middles trapezius, Rhomboids						
						SHOULDER		Flexion	0 to 90°	Anterior deltoid, Cor. brach.						
								Extension	0 to 60°	Latissimus dorsi						
								Abduction	0 to 180°	Middle deltoid, Supraspin.						
								Adduction	0 to 75°							
								Horizontal Adduction	0 to 135°	Pect. major—clavicular/Pect. major—sternal						
								Horizontal Abduction	0 to 45°	Posterior deltoid						
								Int. Rotation	0 to 70°	Subscap., Teres major						
								Ext. Rotation	0 to 90°	Teres minor, Infraspin.						
						ELBOW		Flexion	0 to 150°	Biceps brachii/ Brachialis/ Brachioradialis						
								Extension	150° to 0	Triceps						
						FORE-ARM		Pronation	0 to 80°	Pron. teres. quad.						
								Supination	0 to 80°	Supinator						
						WRIST		Flexion	0 to 80°	Flex. carpi uln./ Flex. carpi rad./ Palm. longus						
								Extension	0 to 70°	Ext. carpi uln./ Ext. carpi rad. long./ Ext. carpi rad. brev.						
								Ulnar Deviation	0 to 30°							
								Radial Deviation	0 to 20°							

Key:

N (5)=complete ROM, gravity with full resistance.

G+=complete ROM, gravity with full resistance but cannot maintain motion (i.e., "breaks").

G (4)=complete ROM, gravity with moderate resistance.

G-=complete ROM, gravity with minimal resistance.

F+=slight resistance at end of ROM.

F (3)=complete ROM, gravity with no resistance.

F=more than 1/4 A/ROM against gravity with no resistance, but not a full A/ROM.

P+=less than 1/4 A/ROM against gravity with no resistance.

P (2)=complete ROM with gravity eliminated.

P-=less than 1/4 A/ROM with gravity eliminated, but not full A/ROM.

T+=evidence of slight A/ROM with gravity eliminated.

T (1)=evidence of slight contractility, no joint return.

O (0)=no evidence of contractility.

Left				Right	
PROM	**AROM**			**PROM**	**AROM**
		<u>Thumb</u>			
		Palmar Abduction	0 to 50		
		Radial Abduction	0 to 50		
		MP Flexion-Extension	0 to 50		
		IP Flexion-Extension	0 to 90		
		Opposition	cm or inches		
		<u>Index Finger</u>			
		MP Flexion	0 to 90		
		MP Hyperextension	0 to 45		
		PIP Flexion-Extension	0 to 110		
		DIP Flexion-Extension	0 to 80		
		Abduction-Adduction	0 to 25		
		<u>Middle Finger</u>			
		MP Flexion	0 to 90		
		MP Hyperextension	0 to 45		
		PIP Flexion-Extension	0 to 110		
		DIP Flexion-Extension	0 to 80		
		<u>Ringer Finger</u>			
		MP Flexion	0 to 90		
		MP Hyperextension	0 to 45		
		PIP Flexion-Extension	0 to 110		
		DIP Flexion-Extension	0 to 80		
		Abduction-Adduction	0 to 25		
		<u>Little Finger</u>			
		MP Flexion	0 to 90		
		MP Hyperextension	0 to 45		
		PIP Flexion-Extension	0 to 110		
		DIP Flexion-Extension	0 to 80		
		Abduction-Adduction	0 to 25		

Comments:

Reprinted with permission from Gaylord Hospital, Wallingford, CT.

THE GAYLORD HOSPITAL
PHYSICAL THERAPY DEPARTMENT
MUSCULOSKELETAL EVALUATION
p. 4 of 5

DATE: _____ INITIAL/DISCH.

		(normal ROM)	R.O.M.		STRENGTH/SYNERGY		TONE	
			L	R	L	R	L	R
CERVICAL	ROTATION	(60-0-60)						
	FLEXION	(0-45)						
	EXTENSION	(0-45)						
	LAT FLEX	(0-45)						
SCAPULA	ELEVATION							
	DEPRESSION							
	ABDUCTION							
	ADDUCTION							
SHOULDER	ABDUCTION	(0-180)						
	H ABDUCTION	(0-45)						
	H ADDUCTION	(0-135)						
	FLEXION	(0-180)						
	EXTENSION	(0-60)						
	INT ROTATION	(0-80)						
	EXT ROTATION	(0-90)						
ELBOW	FLEXION	(0-150)						
	EXTENSION	(0)						
FOREARM	SUPINATION	(0-80)						
	PRONATION	(0-80)						
WRIST	FLEXION	(0-80)						
	EXTENSION	(0-70)						

CODE DEFINITIONS
(numerator = test result)
(denominator = normal)

STRENGTH
0/5 = zero
1/5 = trace
2/5 = poor
3/5 = fair
4/5 = good
5/5 = normal

G = GONIOMETER
A = APPROXIMATE   P = PAINFUL

SYNERGY
* = 1/3 range
** = 2/3 range
*** = full range

TONE
0/1 = flaccid, hypotonic
1/1 = normal tone
2/1 = minimal resistance to passive lengthening
3/1 = moderate resistance to passive lengthening
4/1 = maximal resistance to passive lengthening
5/1 = rigid, no motion

FORM #710.015   ORG. 4/89   THERAPIST: _____

Reprinted with permission from Gaylord Hospital, Wallingford, CT.

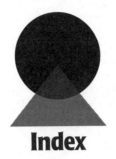

Index

For your information

This book and many others on numerous different topics are available from SLACK Incorporated. For further information or a copy of our latest catalog, contact us at:

Professional Book Division
SLACK Incorporated
6900 Grove Road
Thorofare, NJ 08086 USA
Telephone: 1-609-848-1000
1-800-257-8290
Fax: 1-609-853-5991
E-mail: orders@slackinc.com
WWW: http://www.slackinc.com

We accept most major credit cards and checks or money orders in US dollars drawn on a US bank. Most orders are shipped within 72 hours.

Contact us for information on recent releases, forthcoming titles, and bestsellers. If you have a comment about this title or see a need for a new book, direct your correspondence to the Editorial Director at the above address.

*If you are an instructor, we can be reached at the address listed above or on the Internet at **educomps@slackinc.com** for specific needs.*

Thank you for your interest and we hope you found this work beneficial.